Rectal Cancer

Current Clinical Oncology

Maurie Markman, MD, Series Editor

For other titles published in this series, go to
www.springer.com/series/7631

Rectal Cancer

International Perspectives on Multimodality Management

Edited by

Brian G. Czito

Department of Radiation Oncology, Duke University Medical Center, Durham, NC, USA

Christopher G. Willett

Department of Radiation Oncology, Duke University Medical Center, Durham, NC, USA

Humana Press

Editors
Brian G. Czito
Department of Radiation Oncology
Duke University Medical Center
Durham, NC
USA
czito001@mc.duke.edu

Christopher G. Willett
Department of Radiation Oncology
Duke University Medical Center
Durham, NC
USA
wille009@mc.duke.edu

ISBN: 978-1-61779-695-1 ISBN: 978-1-60761-567-5 (eBook)
DOI: 10.1007/978-1-60761-567-5
Springer New York Dordrecht Heidelberg London

Printed on acid-free paper

Humana Press, a part of Springer Science+Business Media (www.springer.com)

Preface

Rectal Cancer: International Perspectives on Multimodality Management is a timely analysis of the diagnosis, staging, pathology, and therapy of cancer of the rectum. This book is intended as a useful resource for physicians, scientists, medical students, and allied health personnel in the disciplines of radiology, gastroenterology, surgical oncology, medical oncology, radiation oncology, and pathology. Renowned contributors from different medical disciplines have written their chapters in a thoughtful, provocative, and visual fashion. Importantly, these chapters highlight the controversies in the diagnostic, staging, and therapeutic management of patients with rectal cancer while providing practical management recommendations.

This book is divided into 18 chapters. Early chapters address the diagnosis and staging of rectal cancer, highlighting the critical role of contemporary imaging in guiding treatment. The remaining chapters focus on the multimodality management of rectal cancer from the vantage points of surgery, pathology, chemotherapy, and radiation therapy. The major developments in surgery are reviewed first, including contemporary roles of local excision, total mesorectal excision, lateral pelvic lymph node dissection, organ preservation approaches, as well as the management of advanced, recurrent, and metastatic disease. Following is a chapter describing the pathologic evaluation of rectal cancer specimens, with emphasis on proper methodology and its clinical relevance to overall disease management. The final chapters review the contemporary roles of chemotherapy (including with radiation therapy, adjuvant and neoadjuvant settings without radiation therapy, as well as in metastatic disease) as well as radiation therapy (including adjuvant and neoadjuvant approaches, short vs. long course treatments, brachytherapy and contact therapy, nonoperative approaches utilizing definitive chemoradiotherapy, and technical innovations).

We would like to thank the authors for their outstanding contributions which will aid us in the understanding of this malignancy as well as the care of our patients. We would also express thanks to the patients whose willingness has allowed continued therapeutic advances to be made in this disease over the past three decades. We hope you enjoy reviewing this work as much as we have.

Durham, NC

Brian G. Czito
Christopher G. Willett

Contributors

CHRISTOPHE BORG, MD, PhD • Medical Oncology Department, Besançon University Hospital, Besançon, France

JEAN-FRANÇOIS BOSSET, MD • Radiotherapy-Oncology Department, Besançon University Hospital, Besançon, France

MATHIEU BOSSET, MD • Radiotherapy-Oncology Department, Besançon University Hospital, Besançon, France

GINA BROWN, MD • Royal Marsden Hospital, Sutton, Surrey, UK

KRZYSZTOF BUJKO, MD • Department of Radiotherapy, Maria Sklodowska-Curie Memorial Cancer Centre and Institute of Oncology, Warsaw, Poland

MAGDALENA BUJKO, MD • Department of Radiotherapy, Maria Sklodowska-Curie Memorial Cancer Centre and Institute of Oncology, Warsaw, Poland

IAN CHUA, MD • Department of Medicine, Royal Marsden Hospital, Sutton, Surrey, UK

HUEYLAN CHERN, MD • Department of Surgery, Memorial Sloan-Kettering Cancer Center, New York, NY, USA

BRYAN M. CLARY, MD • Department of Surgery, Division of General Surgery, Duke University Medical Center, Durham, NC, USA

GILLES CREHANGE, MD • Radiotherapy Department, Georges François Leclerc Center, Dijon, France

DAVID CUNNINGHAM, MD, FRCP • Department of Medicine, Royal Marsden Hospital, Sutton, Surrey, UK

BRIAN G. CZITO, MD • Department of Radiation Oncology, Duke University Medical Center, Durham, NC, USA

THOMAS A. D'AMICO, MD • Department of Surgery, Division of General Surgery, Duke University Medical Center, Durham, NC, USA

SLOBODAN DEVIC, PhD • Department of Medical Physics, McGill University, Montreal, QC, Canada

SHWETAL DIGHE, MS (Mum), DNB, MRCS • Mayday University Hospital, Croydon, UK

LORETTA ERHUNMWUNSEE, MD • Department of Surgery, Division of General Surgery, Duke University Medical Center, Durham, NC, USA

KATHRYN M. FIELD, MBBS Hons, MD • Royal Melbourne Hospital, Victoria, Australia

JOAQUIM GAMA-RODRIGUES, MD, PhD • Department of Gastroenterology, University of Sao Paulo, Sao Paulo, Brazil

JEAN-PIERRE GÉRARD, MD • Department of Radiation Oncology, Centre Antoine Lacassagne, Nice, France

JOSE GUILLEM, MD, MPH • Department of Surgery, Memorial Sloan-Kettering Cancer Center, New York, NY, USA

ANGELITA HABR-GAMA, MD, PhD • Department of Gastroenterology, University of Sao Paulo, Sao Paulo, Brazil

LAUREN KOSINSKI, MD • Section of Colorectal Surgery, Department of Surgery, Medical College of Wisconsin, Milwaukee, WI, USA

MIRANDA KUSTERS, MSc • Department of Surgery, Leiden University Medical Center, Leiden, The Netherlands

KIRK LUDWIG, MD • MCW/Froedtert Cancer Center and Department of Surgery, Medical College of Wisconsin, Milwaukee, WI, USA

PHILIPPE MAINGON, MD, PhD • Radiotherapy Department, Georges François Leclerc Center, Dijon, France

YOSHIHIRO MORIYA, MD • Department of Colorectal Surgery, National Cancer Center Hospital, Tokyo, Japan

ROBERT MYERSON, MD, PhD • Department of Radiation Oncology, Washington University of Medicine, St, Louis, MO, USA

A. SUN MYINT, FRCP, FRCR • Clatterbridge Centre for Oncology, NHS Foundation Trust, Wirral, UK

HEIDI NELSON, MD • Division of Colon and Rectal Surgery, Mayo Clinic College of Medicine, Rochester, MN, USA

JASON PARK, MD, MEd • Department of Surgery, Memorial Sloan-Kettering Cancer Center, New York, NY, USA

RODRIGO PEREZ, MD • Department of Gastroenterology, University of Sao Paulo, Sao Paulo, Brazil

ERVIN PODGORSAK, PhD • Department of Medical Physics, McGill University, Montreal, QC, Canada

IGOR PROSCURSHIM, MD • Department of Gastroenterology, University of Sao Paulo, Sao Paulo, Brazil

PHILIP QUIRKE, PhD • Department of Pathology and Tumour Biology, Leeds Institute of Molecular Medicine, University of Leeds, Leeds, UK

SRINEVAS K. REDDY, MD • Department of Surgery, Division of General Surgery, Duke University Medical Center, Durham, NC, USA

TIMOTHY RIDOLFI, MD • Department of Surgery, Medical College of Wisconsin, Milwaukee, WI, USA

CLAUS RÖDEL, MD • Department of Radiation Therapy and Oncology, University of Frankfurt, Germany

HARM J.T. RUTTEN, PhD • Department of Surgery, Catherina Hospital, Eindhoven, The Netherlands

ROLF SAUER, MD • Department of Radiation Therapy, University of Erlangen, Germany

STÉPHANIE SERVAGI-VERNAT, MD • Radiotherapy-Oncology Department, Besançon University Hospital, Besançon, France

FIONA TAYLOR, MBBS, MRCS • Mayday University Hospital, Croydon, UK

CORNELIS J.H. VAN DE VELDE, MD, PhD • Department of Surgery, Leiden University Medical Center, Leiden, The Netherlands

TÉ VUONG, MD, FRCPC • Department of Radiation Oncology, McGill University, Montreal, QC, Canada

NICHOLAS P. WEST, MB, ChB • Department of Pathology and Tumour Biology, Leeds Institute of Molecular Medicine, University of Leeds, Leeds, UK

CHRISTOPHER G. WILLETT, MD • Department of Radiation Oncology, Duke University Medical Center, Durham, NC, USA

W. DOUGLAS WONG, MD • Department of Surgery, Memorial Sloan-Kettering Cancer Center, New York, NY, USA

RACHEL WONG, MD • Department of Medicine, Royal Marsden Hospital, Sutton, Surrey, UK

Y. NANCY YOU, MD, MHSc • Division of Colorectal Surgery, Department of Surgery, Mayo Clinic, Rochester, MN, USA

JOHN R. ZALCBERG, MD, PhD • Division of Hematology and Medical Oncology and Department of Medicine, Peter MacCallum Cancer Centre, University of Melbourne, Melbourne, Australia

1 Clinical Staging: Endoscopic Techniques

Hueylan Chern and W. Douglas Wong

INTRODUCTION

The treatment of rectal cancer has advanced tremendously in the last decade, leading to a decrease in local recurrence and an increase in sphincter-sparing rates. The importance of preoperative staging in improving rectal cancer treatment cannot be overemphasized. Accurate preoperative staging guides important management decisions, such as identification of patients who will benefit from neoadjuvant therapy as well as those amenable to local excision or sphincter-sparing surgery rather than abdominoperineal resection.

In randomized controlled trials, preoperative chemoradiation therapy for T3, T4, or N1 rectal cancers has been shown to result in lower toxicity and improved local control compared with postoperative chemoradiotherapy *(2)*. Local excision may be considered for some T1 rectal cancers. However, local excision for T2 or more advanced lesions (including those with positive. lymph nodes) is not generally recommended *(3)*. Thus, it is of utmost importance that initial staging of rectal cancer be accurate and complete, in order to determine individual T stage as well as nodal status.

Contemporary modalities used for preoperative staging of rectal cancer include digital rectal exam (DRE), computed tomography (CT), magnetic resonance imaging (MRI), and endorectal ultrasound (ERUS). The ideal staging modality should be relatively easy to perform, accurate, and cost-effective. This chapter focuses on ERUS, which is the authors' initial staging method of choice.

For "Rectal Cancer: International Perspectives on Multimodality Management", Brian G. Czito, MD and Christopher G. Willett, MD, editors (Humana Press)

From: *Current Clinical Oncology: Rectal Cancer*,
Edited by: B.G. Czito and C.G. Willett, DOI: 10.1007/978-1-60761-567-5_1,

STAGING OF RECTAL CANCER

Many classification systems have been used for the staging of rectal cancer. In the United States, the standard and most commonly used system is the tumor, node, metastasis (TNM) staging system *(4)* (Table 1). Addition of the prefix "u" to a TNM classification indicates that staging has been performed by ultrasound *(5)*. At Memorial Sloan Kettering Cancer Center (MSKCC), a modified ultrasound staging system has been proposed to assist in clinical decision-making (Table 2). In this modified, treatment-oriented ultra-

Table 1
TNM staging system for rectal cancer

Primary tumor (T)	
Tis	Carcinoma in situ
T1	Tumor invades the submucosa
T2	Tumor invades the muscularis propria
T3	Tumor invades the perirectal fat
T4	Tumor directly invades adjacent organs and structures, and/or perforates visceral peritoneum
Regional lymph nodes (N)	
Nx	Tumor cannot be assessed
N0	No regional metastases
N1	Metastases in one to three nodes
N2	Metastases in four or more regional nodes
Distant metastases (M)	
Mx	Distant metastases cannot be assessed
M0	No distant metastases
M1	Distant metastases
Staging	
Stage 0	Tis N0 M0
Stage I	T1-2 N0 M0
Stage IIA	T3 N0 M0
Stage IIB	T4 N0 M0
Stage IIIA	T1-2 N1 M0
Stage IIIB	T3-4 N1 M0
Stage IIIC	Any T N2 M0
Stage IV	Any T Any N M1

Table 2
MSKCC modified ERUS staging system

Stage		*Description*
uTw	uT0/T1	Amenable to local excision
uTy	uT2/superficial uT3	Recommend radical surgery, may require neoadjuvant therapy, pathologic features and nodal status helpful in determining need for neoadjuvant therapy
uTz	Deep uT3/any uT4	Recommend neoadjuvant therapy followed by radical resection
uN1	Probable or definite	Recommend neoadjuvant therapy
uN1	Equivocal	Base treatment on tumor stage and pathologic features

sound staging system, uT0/T1 lesions are classified as potentially amenable to local excision and uT2/superficial uT3N0 tumors as potentially suitable for radical resection without neoadjuvant therapy. Based on extramural depth of the tumor, uT3 lesions are further classified as superficial or deep; deep uT3/uT4 tumors should receive neoadjuvant therapy prior to radical resection.

STAGING ACCURACY OF DIGITAL RECTAL EXAM (DRE)

The staging accuracy of DRE is not optimal and limited only to cancers that are palpable on clinical exam. Starck et al. reported that about half of the patients in their study could be evaluated with digital rectal exam *(6)*. The accuracy of this modality in patients suitable for evaluation by DRE is 68%. Others have reported varying DRE staging accuracies, ranging from 57.9 to 82.8% *(5)*. While DRE by itself is not a good staging modality, it does provide the clinician with valuable information: distance of tumor from the anorectal sphincter complex and tumor location, morphology, and mobility. It also allows the clinician to appreciate the tumor and its relationship to surrounding anatomic structures, such as the vagina or the prostate. In female patients, combining DRE with a vaginal examination enables the assessment of the rectovaginal septum and its possible involvement by the tumor. An accurate evaluation of anorectal sphincter involvement and the distance of tumor from the anorectal sphincter complex are especially important when assessing the possibility of a sphincter-saving procedure. Therefore, DRE remains an important step in the initial evaluation of rectal cancer.

STAGING ACCURACY OF CT, MRI, ERUS

Other staging modalities include CT, ERUS, and MRI. Each has its own advantages and limitations. A meta-analysis by Kwok et al. best summarizes the comparative accuracy of these imaging tools *(1)*. The reported accuracy for T-staging is 84, 80, 74, and 81% for ERUS, CT, MRI, and MRI with endorectal coil, respectively. The possibility of overstaging is 11, 13, 13, and 12% for ERUS, CT, MRI, and MRI with endorectal coil, respectively; the possibility of understaging is 5, 7, 13, and 6% for ERUS, CT, MRI, and MRI with endorectal coil, respectively. In summary, ERUS appears to demonstrate the greatest reported accuracy for assessing T-stage, at approximately 84%.

The accuracy of staging nodal status is 74, 66, 74, and 82% for ERUS, CT, MRI, and MRI with endorectal coil, respectively, *(1)* indicating that MRI with endorectal coil may be the most accurate in predicting nodal status. However, this modality has some limitations, which will be discussed below.

STAGING WITH CT

CT is a useful staging tool given its ability to evaluate primary lesions in the pelvis as well as distant tumor spread. However, one major limitation of CT is its inability to differentiate the individual layers of the rectal wall to accurately assess T-stage. Kim et al. reported that CT has a T-staging accuracy of 82% in the setting of locally advanced T3 and T4 rectal cancers; however, the accuracy drops to 15% for T2 rectal cancers *(7)*. Therefore, while CT accurately assesses the tumor penetrance of the rectal wall, it cannot be used with accuracy to assign T-stage. Staging rectal cancers with CT alone is clearly inadequate, especially in the setting of early tumors.

STAGING WITH MRI

As advances were made in MRI technology, the accuracy of staging rectal cancers with MRI improved significantly as well. While the initial reports on rectal cancer staging using body coil MRI reported accuracy as low as 59%, accuracy as high as 86% has been reported for MRI with phased-array coils *(8, 9)*. The addition of endorectal coils to MRI allows visualization of the individual rectal wall layers, similar to what is visualized on ERUS. Studies have shown comparative staging accuracy between ERUS and MRI with endorectal coils *(10)*. However, MRI with endorectal coils has its drawbacks such as patient discomfort, limited field of view when it is used as a solo modality, and significantly higher cost. Therefore, it is unavailable at most centers.

Even though phased-array MRI is limited in evaluating the T-stage of an early rectal cancer, it is very accurate in determining the likelihood of an involved circumferential resection margin, which is a powerful predictor of local recurrence *(11)*. In addition, phased-array MRI has demonstrated accuracy in evaluating advanced and recurrent tumors that invade other pelvic structures *(8)*. Hence, MRI remains an important tool for assisting surgeons in the treatment of advanced and recurrent rectal cancer.

STAGING WITH ERUS

One of the great advantages of ERUS is that it enables the operator to distinguish the individual layers of the rectal wall. For this reason, it is considered the most accurate imaging tool for the staging of early rectal cancers or benign adenomas. This helps the surgeon determine which patients are suitable candidates for local excision and which patients should be treated with neoadjuvant chemoradiation followed by more extensive resection. ERUS is an especially useful and attractive method of initial evaluation for patients and clinicians alike. Requiring minimal preparation by the patient, ERUS can be performed without sedation during an office visit. The exam is generally well tolerated, and the results are immediately available for use in discussing treatment options.

A limitation of ERUS is its suboptimal evaluation of more proximal, obstructing, or stenotic lesions. It also provides a limited field of view, depending on the acoustic penetrance of the ultrasound waves. Although another drawback of ERUS is that it is operator-dependent, in experienced hands it is extremely accurate. Orrom et al. reported that with increasing operator experience and standardization in interpreting ERUS, its staging accuracy increased from 59.3 to 95% *(12)*.

ERUS TECHNIQUE

During a patient's initial visit to our outpatient clinic, an evaluation form highlighting many important elements necessary to a complete staging of rectal cancer (Table 3) is routinely filled in.

The authors use a dedicated room in the clinic for ERUS. Two different types of ultrasound probes are used: the Brüel & Kjær 1850 and the Brüel & Kjær 2052. Both can be utilized for performing endoanal ultrasound as well as ERUS. The primary difference between the probes is in the setup of the transducer. While the operator must physically move the 1850 probe as the transducer moves along the entire length of the tumor, the 2052 probe remains still, while the transducer rotates through the length of the probe itself.

Prior to ERUS, a balloon is fitted over the probe. When using the 1850 probe, the balloon is usually inflated with 30–40 cc of water. When using the 2052 probe, a balloon is fitted

Table 3
MSKCC outpatient clinic evaluation form

ANAL CANCER / RECTAL CANCER

Date: _________ **Tape:** _________

DIGITAL EXAM: Normal Mobile Slightly Tethered Tethered Fixed Not Palpable

PALPABLE LN: N/A Yes No Other **CLINICAL STAGE:** Benign T1 T2 T3 T4 ____

PROCTOSCOPY: Negative Done Not Done

LOCATION: Left Right Anterior Posterior Lateral Circumferential

CIRCUMFERENCE: _________ (10 – 100) % **DIAMETER:** _________ **cm.**

MORPHOLOGY: N/A Exophytic Ulcerated Other

DISTANCE FROM ANAL VERGE: **Distal** _________ **cm.** **Proximal** _________ **cm.** from Anal Verge

EXAMINED TO: _________ (1 – 20) **cm.** from Anal Verge **Balloon Volume:** _________ **ml.**

ERUS:
WIDTH _________ **mm.**
DEPTH _________ **mm.** @ LEVEL _________ **cm.**
RADIAL _________ **mm.**

SAVED IMAGES:
1. ___________
2. ___________
3. ___________

NODES:
Node 1 Location: Left Right Anterior Posterior Lateral
Node 1 Size: _________ **mm.**
Node 1 Level: _________ **cm.** from Anal Verge
Node 1 Significance: Probable Definite Equivocal

Node 2 Location: Left Right Anterior Posterior Lateral
Node 2 Size: _________ **mm.**
Node 2 Level: _________ **cm.** from Anal Verge
Node 2 Significance: Probable Definite Equivocal

Node 3 Location: Left Right Anterior Posterior Lateral
Node 3 Size: _________ **mm.**
Node 3 Level: _________ **cm.** from Anal Verge
Node 3 Significance: Probable Definite Equivocal

ERUS CLINICAL:
uT Stage: Unsatis Normal Benign uTx uT1 uT2 uT3 uT4
uN Stage: uN0 uN1 uNx
uTw: uT0/ uT1 **uTy:** uT2/superficial uT3 **uTz:** deep uT3/any uT4

EAUS CLINICAL:
Internal Sphincter
Involvement: Yes No
Location: Left Right Anterior Posterior Lateral Circumferential
External Sphincter
Involvement: Yes No
Location: Left Right Anterior Posterior Lateral Circumferential

BX done: yes no
FFS done: yes no
3D done: yes no

Educational form highlighting important elements of clinical staging of rectal cancer

over the entire probe and inflated with approximately 100 cc of fluid; this probe can also be used without a balloon by inserting 100 cc of fluid directly into the rectum. The volume of water depends on the size of the lesion, the diameter of the lumen, and the patient's level of comfort. To minimize the possible creation of artifact, it is important to avoid introducing air into the balloon. Endoanal ultrasound can also be performed with the 1850 probe by fitting a plastic cap over the transducer. It can also be performed with the 2052 probe without a balloon or cap. Three-dimensional ERUS imaging can be undertaken with either probe, utilizing appropriate software support.

Patients are instructed to self-administer two enemas on the morning of their examination. The enema facilitates evacuation of air, stool, and mucous. A DRE is first performed with the patient in the left lateral decubitus position, providing information on tumor location, mobility, distance from the anal verge, and its relation to the anorectal ring. A proctoscope measuring 20 mm in diameter, which accommodates both the 1850 and the 2052 ERUS probes, is utilized next for further evaluation of the lesion's morphology, distance from the anal verge, circumferential involvement, etc. Insertion of the proctoscope also results in evacuation of residual stool, mucus, or enema effluent, further reducing the risk of image artifact.

Once the proctoscope is advanced above the lesion, the ERUS probe is advanced with the proctoscope in place, ensuring complete evaluation of the lesion. This is carried out in a proximal-to-distal manner. It is crucial that the entire lesion be assessed, as depth of invasion may vary. A complete exam may require several passes. It is important to keep the probe centrally in the lumen to avoid artifact and maintain constant echo texture. Nodal status is usually evaluated first, followed by the depth of invasion. Tumor size, radial extension, location, and the size and echo texture of lymph nodes are measured.

In the case of stenotic lesions that prevent the passage of the proctoscope, using the probe alone may enable passage beyond the tumor. Blind insertion of the probe, however, can result in distorted visualization of the lesion and/or omission of its proximal extent.

Following evaluation of the rectal wall and mesorectum, endoanal ultrasound (EAUS) can be done in the setting of more distal rectal cancers, especially tumors that extend down to the anal canal. EAUS is helpful when a sphincter-sparing procedure is contemplated, facilitating assessment of the tumor's relation to the puborectalis and sphincter complex. If these structures are uninvolved by tumor, sphincter preservation can be considered.

NORMAL ERUS ANATOMY

A system developed by Hildebrandt and Feifel divides the rectal wall into five ultrasonographic layers *(13)*. The inner white layer represents the interface between balloon and mucosa. The inner dark layer represents the mucosa and muscularis mucosa. The middle white layer represents the submucosa. The outer dark layer represents the muscularis propria. The outermost white layer represents the interface with the perirectal fat (Fig. 1).

The upper anal canal is identified by the presence of the puborectalis muscle. As a striated muscle, the puborectalis appears as a hyperechoic layer that swings around the rectum posteriorly (Fig. 2). The middle anal canal is identified by a circular layer of internal sphincter muscle which appears as a hypoechoic band, and a circular layer of external sphincter muscle which appears as a hyperechoic band (Fig. 3). The lower anal canal is identified by the presence of a circular, hyperechoic external sphincter muscle, without the presence of the internal sphincter muscle (Fig. 4).

INTERPRETING ERUS

The orientation of an ultrasound image is similar to that of a CT scan. The superior aspect is the patient's anterior, the inferior aspect the patient's posterior, the right aspect the patient's left, and the left aspect the patient's right. However, it is important to note that the patient is examined

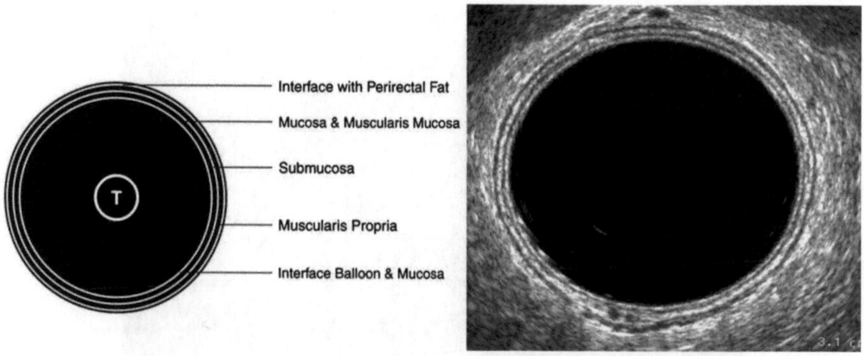

Fig. 1. Endorectal ultrasound: five-layer model.

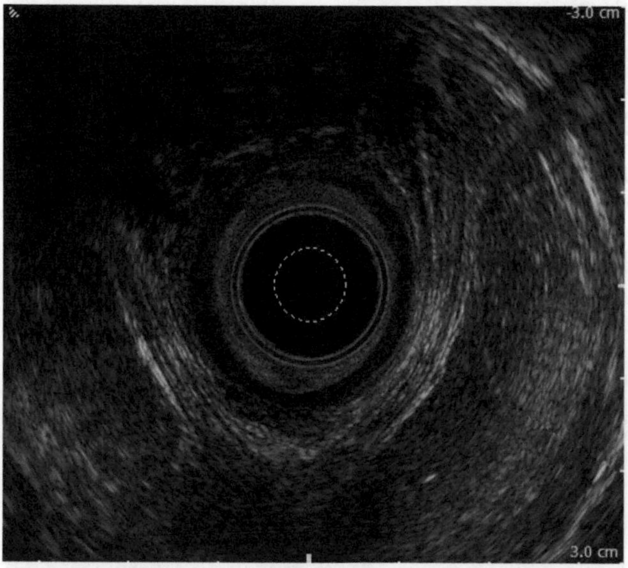

Fig. 2. Proximal anal canal. Note the puborectalis muscle forming a posterior sling.

in the left lateral decubitus position. Therefore, rotating the images 90° clockwise can assist with orientation and ensure that the ultrasound probe is kept in the center of the lumen.

uT0 Disease

uT0 lesions, such as villous adenomas, are noninvasive, benign, and confined to the rectal mucosa. On ERUS imaging, the middle white layer (submucosa) remains intact without any break or irregularity (Fig. 5). ERUS has demonstrated accuracy ranging from 87 to 96% in distinguishing these benign lesions from invasive tumors *(14, 15)*. uT0 lesions can be treated with local excision. Although tissue biopsy is necessary, ERUS should be performed prior to excision to completely evaluate the lesion, as biopsy "sampling error" may result in missing of

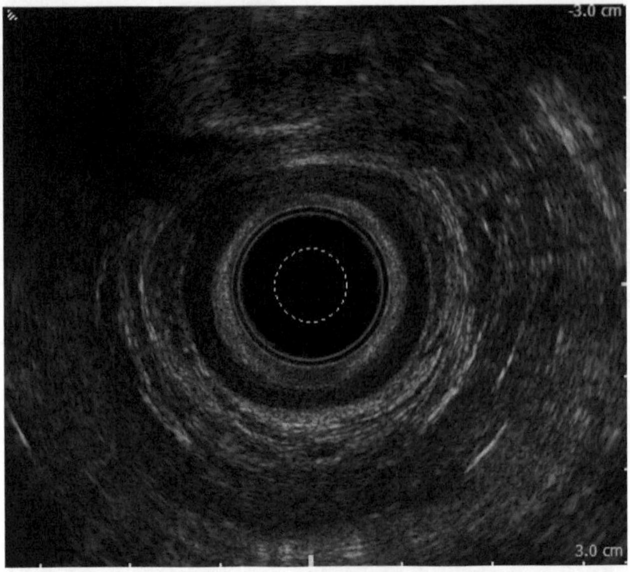

Fig. 3. Middle anal canal. Note the hypoechoic internal sphincter and the hyperechoic external sphincter forming a complete circle.

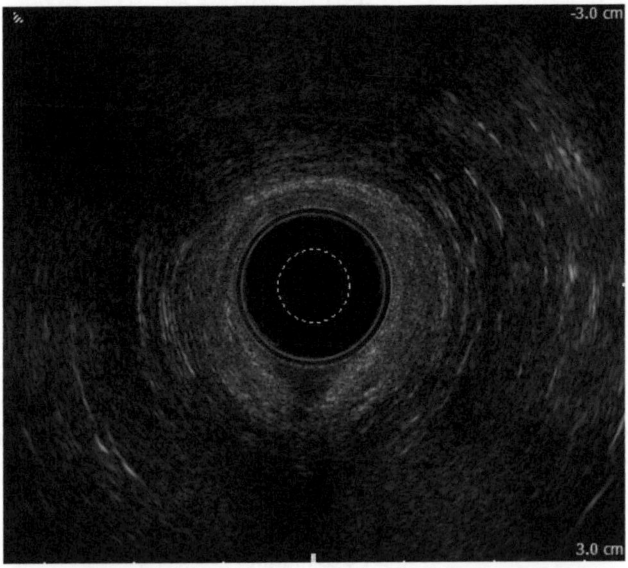

Fig. 4. Distal anal canal. Note the presence of only external anal sphincter.

focal areas of invasion or may fail to reveal a more invasive component *(16, 17)*. If a focal area of invasion is identified within a villous adenoma, it would be inappropriate to perform a submucosal dissection/local excision. Therefore, preoperative evaluation of a biopsy-proven rectal adenoma should include ERUS to rule out any foci of invasion.

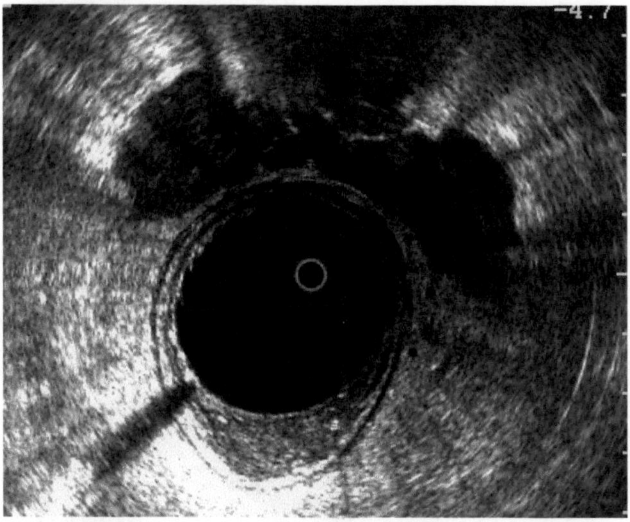

Fig. 5. T0 adenoma. Note the intact submucosa/middle white layer.

uT1 Disease

uT1 cancers invade and penetrate the mucosa but do not extend beyond the submucosa. The ERUS finding shows an irregular middle white layer that may appear thickened or stippled but without any distinct break (Fig. 6). The clinician must carefully evaluate for lymph nodes in these patients, however, as a 10–18% rate of nodal metastasis has been reported in the setting of T1 rectal cancer *(5)*. Some patients with uT1N0 lesions are candidates for local excision, particularly elderly individuals or those with significant comorbidities. However, at MSKCC we generally recommend radical resection for good-risk patients with uT1 rectal cancer because of the increased local recurrence rate following local excision vs. radical resection. The accuracy of ERUS staging of uT1 cancer ranges from 47 to 96% *(1, 14)*. Landman et al. have shown that in the setting of T1 adenocarcinoma, the accuracy of ERUS nodal staging is lower due to occult metastases, which are often micrometastatic (<1 mm) and cannot be visualized *(18)*. This limitation contributes to the higher local recurrence rates observed after local excision of rectal cancer. Bentrem et al. reported a local recurrence rate of 15% for T1 adenocarcinoma following transanal excision, which is five times higher than the rate of local recurrence following radical surgery *(19)*. For this reason, local excision of uT1 rectal cancer should be performed with caution, with an understanding of the limitations of ERUS in preoperative nodal staging and the higher risk of local recurrence.

uT2 Disease

uT2 cancers invade through the mucosa and submucosa and into, but not through, the muscularis propria. The ERUS finding is a distinct disruption in the middle white layer (submucosa) (Fig. 7). uT2 lesions are subdivided into early lesions, which demonstrate minimal expansion of the outer hypoechoic layer (muscularis propria) and deep lesions, which show more dramatic expansion of the outer hypoechoic layer, often characterized by a serrated or "scalloped" appearance (Fig. 8). Because of this scalloping, there is a tendency to

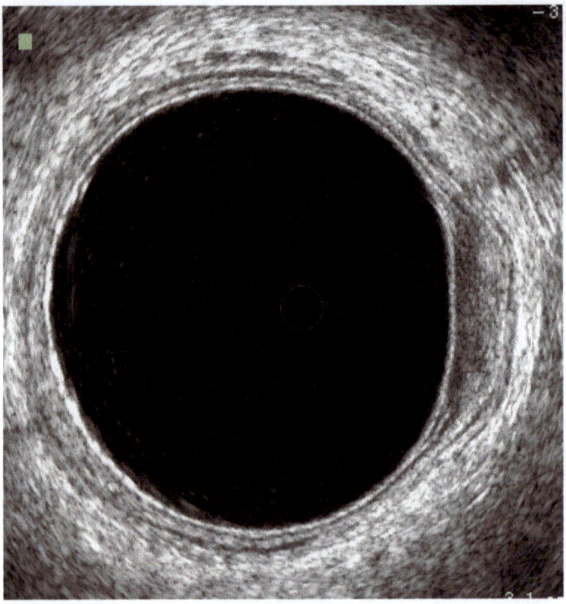

Fig. 6. T1 rectal cancer. Note the irregular but intact submucosa/middle white layer.

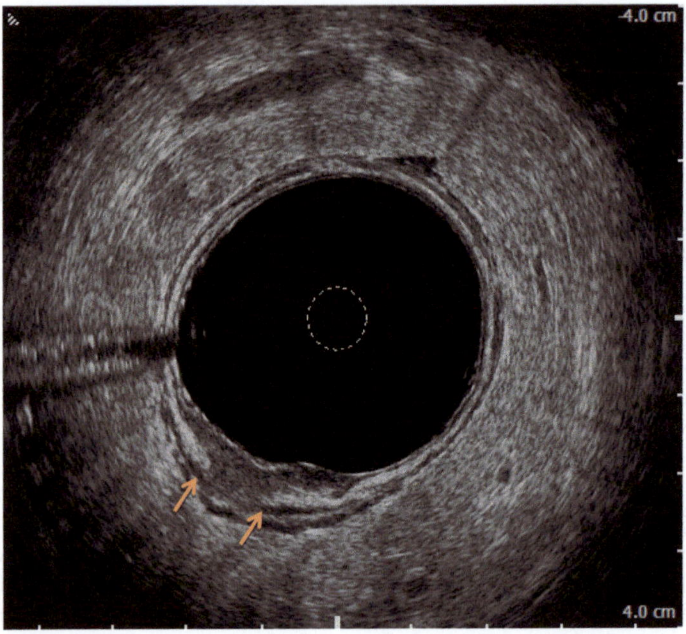

Fig. 7. T2 rectal cancer. Note the distinct break of the submucosa/middle white layer (*arrows*).

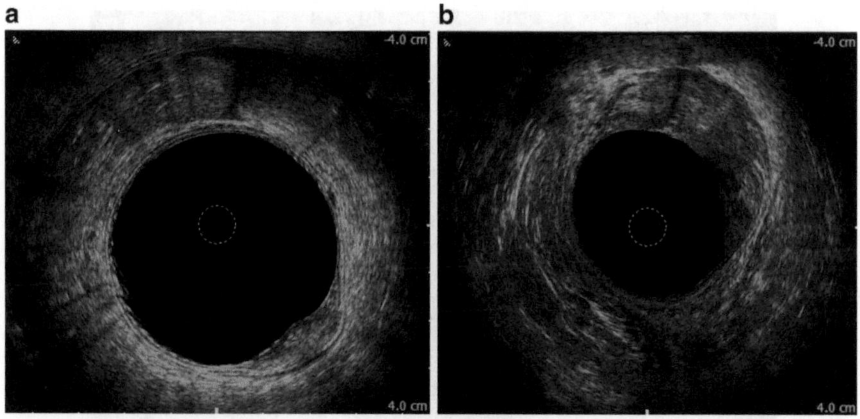

Fig. 8. Early vs. deep T2 rectal cancer. (**a**) Early T2 tumor with minimal expansion of the muscularis propria/outer dark layer. (**b**) Deep T2 tumor with dramatic expansion of the muscularis propria/outer dark layer.

upstage deep uT2 lesions as uT3. However, a lesion should be staged as uT2 if the interface between the muscularis propria and perirectal fat remains intact. The reported accuracy of ERUS staging of uT2 lesions is 68% *(14)*.

A 17–47% rate of nodal metastasis has been reported for T2 lesions *(5)*. uT2N0 lesions are usually treated with radical resection without neoadjuvant therapy. In the setting of a very distal uT2N0 tumor, however, neoadjuvant radiation therapy may be recommended when a sphincter-sparing procedure is planned. Any uT2N1 lesion should be treated with neoadjuvant therapy prior to radical resection.

uT3 Disease

uT3 cancers invade through the full thickness of the bowel wall into the perirectal fat. The characteristic ERUS finding is disruption of the outer white layer with a "thumbprint-like" extension into the perirectal fat (Fig. 9). The reported accuracy of ERUS in staging uT3 lesions ranges from 70 to 81% *(14, 20)*. Measurement of radial extension into the perirectal fat further categorizes uT3 lesions as superficial or deep. Superficial uT3 lesions show radial extension <2 mm, while deep uT3 lesions show radial extension ≥2 mm (Fig. 10). uT3 lesions have been reported to portend a 66% chance of nodal metastasis *(5)*. In the case of select, superficial uT3N0 lesions with favorable histology and tumor location, consideration can be given to forgoing neoadjuvant therapy prior to resection. However, deep uT3N0 and uT3N1 lesions should be treated with neoadjuvant chemoradiotherapy prior to surgical resection.

uT4 Disease

uT4 cancers invade adjacent structures such as the prostate or vagina (Fig. 11). Here, ERUS imaging shows deep radial extension of the tumor, with loss of the normal hyperechoic plane between rectum and prostate in men or rectum and vagina in women.

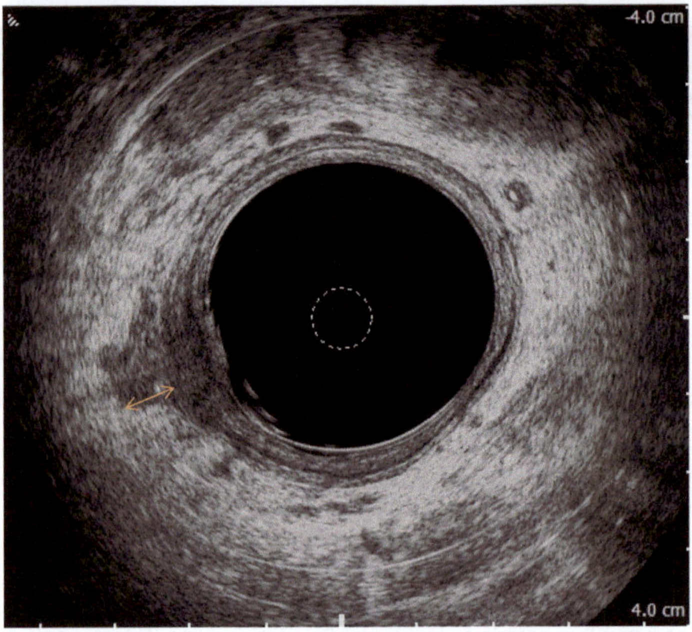

Fig. 9. T3 rectal cancer. Note the radial extension (double arrow) into the perirectal fat/the outer white layer.

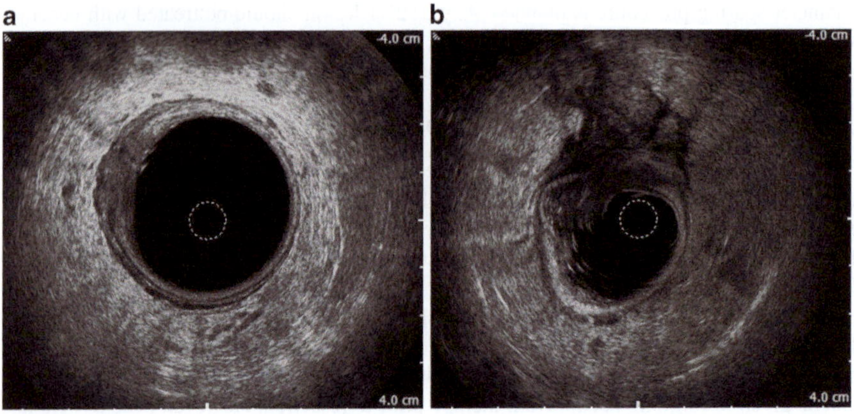

Fig. 10. Early vs. deep T3 rectal cancer. (**a**) Early T3 tumor with superficial radial extension. (**b**) Deep T3 tumor with deep radial extension.

The accuracy of ERUS in this setting is only 50% *(14)*. Pelvic MRI may complement ERUS in the staging of uT4 lesions by demonstrating invasion into other pelvic organs and facilitating assessment of the circumferential resection margin.

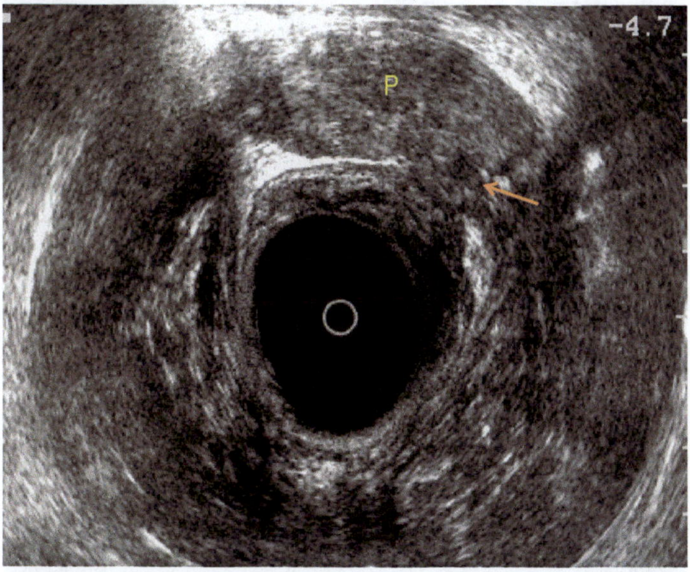

Fig. 11. T4 rectal cancer. Tumor invading into the prostate anteriorly (*arrow*). *P*=prostate.

Nodal Metastasis

In their meta-analysis, Kwok et al. report that the accuracy of lymph node staging by ERUS is 74% *(1)*. Normal, non-enlarged lymph nodes are usually not appreciated on ultrasound. In general, based on echo texture, there are two types of lymph nodes: hyperechoic or hypoechoic. Tio and Tyget first described the hypoechoic texture of metastatic lymph nodes in upper gastrointestinal studies *(21)*. Hildebrandt and Beynon subsequently described hypoechoic lymph nodes in rectal cancer *(22)*. Hyperechoic lymph nodes are usually inflammatory and benign, whereas hypoechoic nodes are frequently metastatic (Figs. 12 and 13). The echo texture of a metastatic lymph node closely resembles that of the tumor.

There is lack of an accepted size threshold for characterizing a lymph node as metastatic. Even small lymph nodes have the potential to harbor malignancy *(23–25)*. While advancing the endosonic probe along the entire length of tumor during an ERUS, any hypoechoic lymph nodes appreciated in the mesorectum should be recorded as potentially positive. At MSKCC, we observe no specific size cut-off for metastatic nodes; a hypoechoic lymph node of any size is considered potentially metastatic (Fig. 13). However, blood vessels can be mistaken for hypoechoic nodes on cross-section. Careful examination of the area with several passes of the probe will generally reveal the branching pattern typical of blood vessels as well as the continuity of a blood vessel over distance beyond the cross-sectional area.

EVALUATING DISTAL RECTAL CANCER WITH ENDOANAL ULTRASOUND

Our ability to perform sphincter-saving procedures has improved greatly for several reasons: (1) preoperative chemoradiaton has increased the rate of sphincter preservation, (2) a distal margin of 1 cm is now considered oncologically acceptable, and (3) intersphincteric

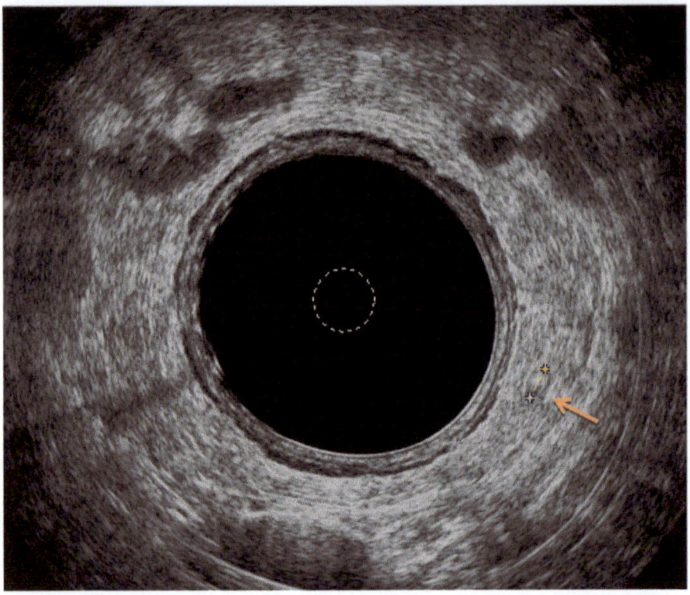

Fig. 12. Hyperechoic lymph node. A hyperechoic lymph node (*arrow*), likely inflammatory in nature.

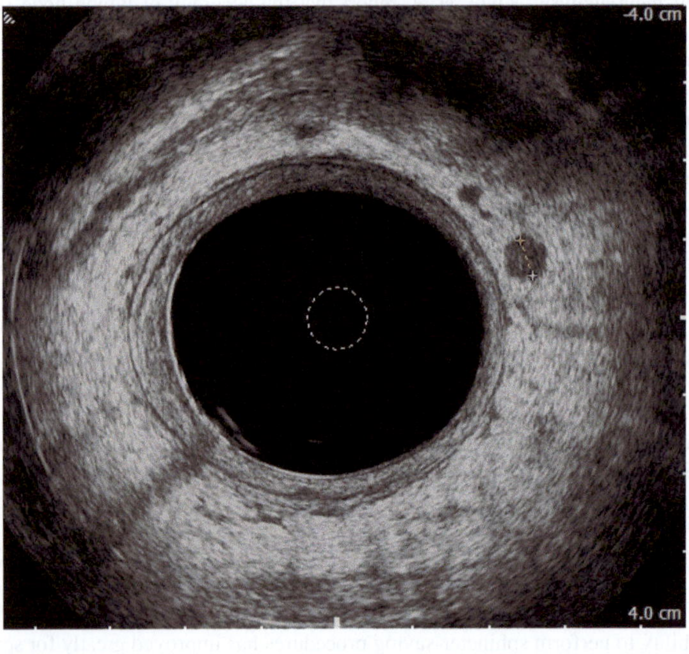

Fig. 13. Hypoechoic lymph node. A hypoechoic lymph node (measurement), likely representing nodal metastasis.

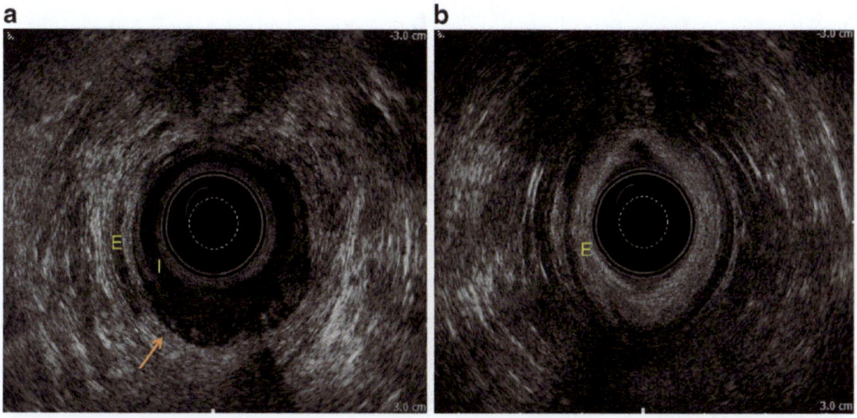

Fig. 14. Distal rectal cancer. (**a**) Tumor involving internal and part of external anal sphincter in the mid- to upper anal canal. I = internal anal sphincter; E = external anal sphincter. Arrow = posteriorly located tumor. (**b**) In the same patient, the distal anal canal is free of involvement by tumor.

resection of distal rectal cancers has been shown to allow sphincter preservation without compromising oncologic outcomes (*2, 26, 27*). However, tumor involvement of the sphincter complex is an absolute contraindication to sphincter-saving surgery. Endoanal ultrasound (EAUS) permits good visualization of the anal canal at different levels, enabling the clinical assessment of sphincter involvement by tumor.

At the level of the upper anal canal, the puborectalis appears as a hyperechoic posterior sling. At the level of the middle anal canal, the internal sphincter is a hypoechoic circular muscle and the external sphincter is a hyperechoic circular muscle. At the distal anal canal, the internal sphincter disappears, leaving a hyperechoic, circular external sphincter muscle. Rectal cancers appear hypoechoic and, when invading the sphincter complex, show extension into the internal and/or external sphincter musculature (Fig. 14). If the sphincter complex is involved, intersphincteric resection in an attempt at sphincter preservation is not advised.

3D ENDORECTAL ULTRASOUND

Three-dimensional endorectal ultrasound (3D ERUS) is endorectal ultrasound with multiplanar display imaging in the coronal, transverse, and sagittal planes. Images are recorded as a crystal passes over the length of tumor. The stored images can be reviewed and analyzed. 3D ERUS is helpful in distinguishing blood vessels from lymph nodes because it shows the anatomic structure of interest in different planes (Fig. 15). The other unique function of 3D ERUS is its ability to calculate the volume of a tumor (Fig. 16). At MSKCC, a protocol investigating 3D ERUS prediction of rectal cancer response to preoperative chemoradiation, by measuring the change in the volume of rectal tumors before and after chemoradiotherapy, is currently underway.

Some studies have shown that 3D ERUS is more accurate than conventional ERUS in staging rectal cancers, while others have shown equivalent accuracy between 3D ERUS, conventional ERUS, and other staging modalities. In a study involving 33 rectal cancer patients assessed by conventional ERUS and 3D ERUS, Kim et al. reported that the accuracy

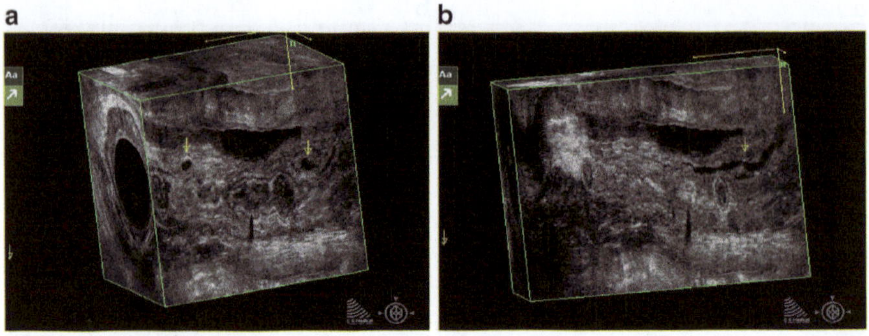

Fig. 15. Differentiation of blood vessel from lymph node with 3D ERUS. (**a**) Two hypoechoice structures, potentially lymph nodes (*arrows*) on cross section. (**b**) Manipulation with 3D endorectal ultrasound demonstrates that one of the hypoechoic structures is a branching blood vessel (*arrow*).

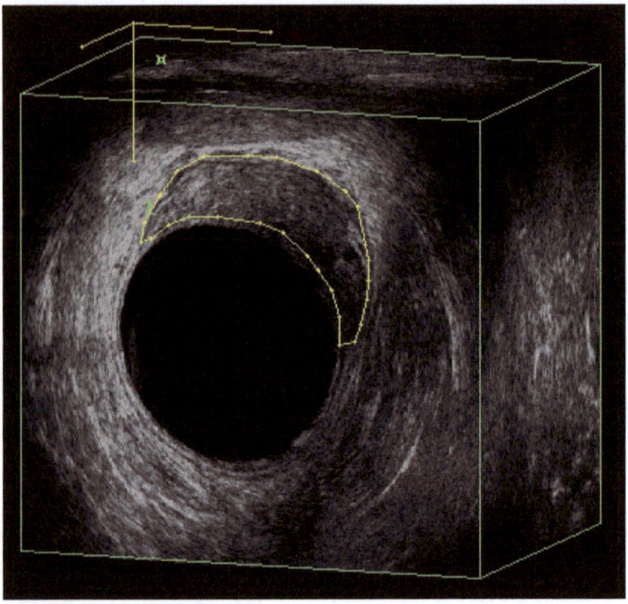

Fig. 16. 3D ERUS measurement.

of conventional and 3D ERUS were similar for both T- and N-staging *(28)*. In a larger study involving 86 patients, Kim et al. compared the accuracy of conventional ERUS, 3D ERUS, and CT in staging rectal cancer *(29)*. The T-staging accuracy was 78% for 3D ERUS, 69% for conventional ERUS, and 57% for CT. The accuracy of lymph node staging was 65% for 3D ERUS, 56% for conventional ERUS, and 53% for CT. These differences were statistically significant. The authors concluded that 3D ERUS is more accurate than either conventional ERUS or CT. Hunerbein et al. compared the accuracy of ERUS, 3D ERUS, and endorectal

MRI in 30 patients, *(30)* reporting comparative accuracies of 84, 88 and 91% for determining T-stage by ERUS, 3D ERUS, and endorectal MRI, respectively. Larger studies are needed to further define the role of 3D ERUS in rectal cancer staging.

ERUS FOLLOWING NEOADJUVANT CHEMORADIATION

ERUS has demonstrated accuracy as an initial staging modality. ERUS distinguishes the individual layers of the rectal wall, thereby facilitating accurate assessment of depth of invasion. However, the ability of ERUS to restage rectal cancer following neoadjuvant chemoradiotherapy is disappointing. In this setting, ERUS is limited by its failure to differentiate residual tumor from radiation-induced edema, inflammation, or fibrosis. Vanagunas et al. reported an accuracy of 48% for ERUS determination of T-stage following chemoradiation therapy, in a study in which 38% were overstaged and 14% understaged *(31)*. They concluded that ERUS should not be routinely used to restage rectal cancer. Unfortunately, the same limitation applies to other modalities such as CT and MRI *(32, 33)*. As mentioned previously, a study is being carried out at MSKCC to investigate the role of 3D ERUS in predicting the response of rectal cancer to preoperative chemoradiation therapy by measuring the change in the volume of rectal tumors before and after chemoradiotherapy.

ERUS IN POSTOPERATIVE FOLLOW-UP

Whether or not intensive surveillance leads to improved rectal cancer survival remains controversial. However, ERUS has been shown to successfully identify asymptomatic, recurrent disease *(34–37)*. Hernandez de Anda et al. reported that approximately 30% of local recurrences following local excision and radical surgery are identified by ERUS only and are missed by DRE and proctoscopic exam *(36)*. Additionally, recurrence identified on ERUS can be confirmed histologically by ultrasound-directed biopsy *(37)*. A baseline ERUS can be performed at 3 months postoperatively, and serial ultrasounds utilized to follow any postoperative scarring or to identify recurrence. At MSKCC, ERUS is not routinely performed following radical surgery. However, a program utilizing ERUS is used to follow patients after local excision. ERUS is initially performed at 3 months after surgery, and again every 4 months for 3 years, followed by every 6 months for another 3 years thereafter.

CONCLUSION

While many staging modalities for rectal cancer exist, ERUS has demonstrated good overall accuracy in tumor and nodal staging. It has the advantage of comparatively low cost, requires no sedation, can be performed in the outpatient setting after simple preparation, and the results can be interpreted and discussed immediately. ERUS should be the initial staging modality of choice for rectal cancer, and every colorectal surgeon should be familiar with this technique.

REFERENCES

1. Kwok H, Bissett IP, Hill GL. Preoperative staging of rectal cancer. *Int J Colorectal Dis*. 2000;15:9–20.
2. Sauer R, Becker H, Hohenberger W, et al. Preoperative versus postoperative chemoradiotherapy for rectal cancer. *N Engl J Med*. 2004;351:1731–1740.

3. Tjandra JJ, Kilkenny JW, Buie WD, et al. Practice parameters for the management of rectal cancer (revised). *Dis Colon Rectum*. 2005;48:411–423.
4. Compton CC, Greene FL. The staging of colorectal cancer: 2004 and beyond. *CA Cancer J Clin*. 2004;54:295–308.
5. Schaffzin DM, Wong WD. Endorectal ultrasound in the preoperative evaluation of rectal cancer. *Clin Colorectal Cancer*. 2004;4:124–132.
6. Starck M, Bohe M, Fork FT, Lindström C, Sjöberg S. Endoluminal ultrasound and low-field magnetic resonance imaging are superior to clinical examination in the preoperative staging of rectal cancer. *Eur J Surg*. 1995;161:841–845.
7. Kim NK, Kim MJ, Yun SH, Sohn SK, Min JS. Comparative study of transrectal ultrasonography, pelvic computerized tomography, and magnetic resonance imaging in preoperative staging of rectal cancer. *Dis Colon Rectum*. 1999;42:770–775.
8. Beets-Tan RGH, Beets GL. Rectal cancer: review with emphasis on MR imaging. *Radiology*. 2004;232:335–346.
9. Gagliardi G, Bayar S̆, Smith R, Salem RR. Preoperative staging of rectal cancer using magnetic resonance imaging with external phase-arrayed coils. *Arch Surg*. 2002;137:447–451.
10. Gualdi GF, Casciani E, Guadalaxara A. d'Orta C, Polettini E, Pappalardo G. Local staging of rectal cancer with transrectal ultrasound and endorectal magnetic resonance imaging: comparison with histologic findings. *Dis Colon Rectum*. 2000;43:338–345.
11. Beets-Tan RG, Beets GL, Vliegen RF, et al. Accuracy of magnetic resonance imaging in prediction of tumour-free resection margin in rectal cancer surgery. *Lancet*. 2001;357:497–504.
12. Orrom WJ, Wong WD, Rothenberger DA, Jensen LL, Goldberg SM. Endorectal ultrasound in the preoperative staging of rectal tumors. A learning experience. *Dis Colon Rectum*. 1990;33:654–659.
13. Hildebrandt U, Feifel G. Preoperative staging of rectal cancer by intrarectal ultrasound. *Dis Colon Rectum*. 1985;28:42–46.
14. Garcia-Aguilar J, Pollack J, Lee S-H, et al. Accuracy of endorectal ultrasonography in preoperative staging of rectal tumors. *Dis Colon Rectum*. 2002;45:10–15.
15. Pikarsky A, Wexner S, Lebensart P, et al. The use of rectal ultrasound for the correct diagnosis and treatment of rectal villous tumors. *Am J Surg*. 2000;179:261–265.
16. Adams WJ, Wong WD. Endorectal ultrasonic detection of malignancy within rectal villous lesions. *Dis Colon Rectum*. 1995;38:1093–1096.
17. Worrell S, Horvath K, Blakemore T, Flum D. Endorectal ultrasound detection of focal carcinoma within rectal adenomas. *Am J Surg*. 2004;187:625–629.
18. Landmann RG, Wong WD, Hoepfl J, et al. Limitations of early rectal cancer nodal staging may explain failure after local excision. *Dis Colon Rectum*. 2007;50:1520–1525.
19. Bentrem. T1 Adenocarcinoma of the rectum: transanal excision or radical surgery? *Ann Surg*. 2005;242:472–479
20. Herzog U, von Flüe M, Tondelli P, Schuppisser JP. How accurate is endorectal ultrasound in the preoperative staging of rectal cancer? *Dis Colon Rectum*. 1993;36:127–134.
21. Tio TL, Tytgat GN. Endoscopic ultrasonography in the assessment of intra- and transmural infiltration of tumours in the oesophagus, stomach and papilla of Vater and in the detection of extraoesophageal lesions. *Endoscopy*. 1984;16:203–210.
22. Beynon J, Mortensen NJ, Foy DM, Channer JL, Rigby H, Virjee J. Preoperative assessment of mesorectal lymph node involvement in rectal cancer. *Br J Surg*. 1989;76:276–279.
23. Katsura Y, Yamada K, Ishizawa T, Yoshinaka H, Shimazu H. Endorectal ultrasonography for the assessment of wall invasion and lymph node metastasis in rectal cancer. *Dis Colon Rectum*. 1992;35:362–368.
24. Akasu T, Sugihara K, Moriya Y, Fujita S. Limitations and pitfalls of transrectal ultrasonography for staging of rectal cancer. *Dis Colon Rectum*. 1997;40:S10-S15.
25. Sunouchi K, Sakaguchi M, Higuchi Y, Namiki K, Muto T. Limitation of endorectal ultrasonography: what does a low lesion more than 5 mm in size correspond to histologically? *Dis Colon Rectum*. 1998;41:761–764.

26. Guillem JG, Chessin DB, Shia J, et al. A prospective pathologic analysis using whole-mount sections of rectal cancer following preoperative combined modality therapy: implications for sphincter preservation. *Ann Surg*. 2007;245:88–93.
27. Chamlou R, Parc Y, Simon T, et al. Long-term results of intersphincteric resection for low rectal cancer. *Ann Surg*. 2007;246:916–921.
28. Kim JC, Cho YK, Kim SY, Park SK, Lee MG. Comparative study of three-dimensional and conventional endorectal ultrasonography used in rectal cancer staging. *Surg Endosc*. 2002;16:1280–1285.
29. Kim JC, Kim HC, Yu CS, et al. Efficacy of 3-dimensional endorectal ultrasonography compared with conventional ultrasonography and computed tomography in preoperative rectal cancer staging. *Am J Surg*. 2006;192:89–97.
30. Hünerbein M, Pegios W, Rau B, Vogl TJ, Felix R, Schlag PM. Prospective comparison of endorectal ultrasound, three-dimensional endorectal ultrasound, and endorectal MRI in the preoperative evaluation of rectal tumors. Preliminary results. *Surg Endosc*. 2000;14:1005–1009.
31. Vanagunas A, Lin DE, Stryker SJ. Accuracy of endoscopic ultrasound for restaging rectal cancer following neoadjuvant chemoradiation therapy. *Am J Gastroenterol*. 2004;99:109–112.
32. Huh JW, Park YA, Jung EJ, Lee KY, Sohn S-K. Accuracy of endorectal ultrasonography and computed tomography for restaging rectal cancer after preoperative chemoradiation. *J Am Coll Surg*. 2008;207:7–12.
33. Maretto I, Pomerri F, Pucciarelli S, et al. The potential of restaging in the prediction of pathologic response after preoperative chemoradiotherapy for rectal cancer. *Ann Surg Oncol*. 2007;14:455–461.
34. Tjandra JJ, Chan MKY. Follow-up after curative resection of colorectal cancer: a meta-analysis. *Dis Colon Rectum*. 2007;50:1783–1799.
35. Löhnert MS, Doniec JM, Henne-Bruns D. Effectiveness of endoluminal sonography in the identification of occult local rectal cancer recurrences. *Dis Colon Rectum*. 2000;43:483–491.
36. de Anda EH, Lee S-H, Finne CO, Rothenberger DA, Madoff RD, Garcia-Aguilar J. Endorectal ultrasound in the follow-up of rectal cancer patients treated by local excision or radical surgery. *Dis Colon Rectum*. 2004;47:818–824.
37. Morken JJ, Baxter NN, Madoff RD, Finne CO. Endorectal ultrasound-directed biopsy: a useful technique to detect local recurrence of rectal cancer. *Int J Colorectal Dis*. 2006;21:258–264.

26. Cuthbert JG, Chessin DB, Shia J, et al. A prospective pathology analysis using whole-mount sections of rectal cancer following preoperative combined modality therapy: implications for sphincter preservation. Ann Surg 2006;243:28–33.
27. [illegible]
28. [illegible]

2 Clinical Staging: CT and MRI

Gina Brown, Shwetal Dighe, and Fiona Taylor

INTRODUCTION

Currently, spiral CT and multidetector CT (MDCT) allow faster acquisition times, and a whole staging scan of the chest, abdomen, and pelvis can be completed in a single breath-hold. This allows structures in the abdomen to be scanned at different vascular phases, following injection of intravenous contrast agents to optimally detect target lesions. Also, with collimation as thin as 1 mm, the image quality of the study has improved remarkably *(1)*. The computer software available to view these detailed scans allows image reconstruction in multiple planes to provide the radiologist with a 3D image, further improving the accuracy of staging scans.

In the United Kingdom, the National Institute for Clinical Excellence (NICE) recommends that for rectal cancer patients who are being considered for surgery, MRI should be performed before the treatment begins, to determine who might benefit from either neoadjuvant therapy or surgery alone.

MRI offers the benefit of objective assessment of all relevant anatomy. It has been shown to be helpful in identifying important surgical and pathological risk factors such as prediction of a tumor-free circumferential resection margin (CRM), lymph node metastases, depth of extramural invasion, involvement of the serosa at or above the peritoneal reflection, and extramural vascular invasion (EMVI) *(2,3)*.

Early studies were performed using an endorectal coil. Although this approach initially showed good results, it was problematic for stenotic lesions *(4,5)*. Both endorectal coil and EUS allow highly accurate differentiation of the layers of the intestinal wall. However, they share the same disadvantages, namely a field of view that is small, allowing adequate evaluation of early tumors alone. Additionally, insertion of an endoluminal coil or probe in advanced or stenotic lesions is not feasible. The development of high resolution phased array surface coil systems, which combine high spatial resolution with a large field of view, has enabled detailed evaluation of the relevant anatomy, without the need for an invasive technique.

From: *Current Clinical Oncology: Rectal Cancer*,
Edited by: B.G. Czito and C.G. Willett, DOI: 10.1007/978-1-60761-567-5_2,

ANATOMY AND SURGICAL IMPLICATIONS

The understanding of colon anatomy in relation to the peritoneum and the retroperitoneum is crucial to staging rectal tumors. The rectum is only covered by a serosal layer, the peritoneum, over its upper third, anterior, and lateral surfaces. The distal two thirds of the rectum has no serosa, but is instead surrounded by fatty mesorectum that is enveloped by a visceral fascial layer that is commonly known as the mesorectal fascia. This distinction is important because if the tumor breaches the peritonealized covering of the colon, it is classified as T4 disease, while tumor extension into the mesorectum and the mesorectal fascia classifies the tumor as T3 unless it invades an adjacent organ. Tumors in the rectum grow radially into the mesorectum and disease spread tends to be confined to the mesorectum. The mesorectal fascia that surrounds the mesorectum forms the anatomical plane for surgical resection in total mesorectal excision (TME) of the rectum. The significant reduction in local recurrence associated with TME rectal cancer surgery is considered to be a consequence of complete removal of the mesorectum containing tumor and local disease spread within a distinct and enclosed surgical "package." This radial margin of excision surgery is called the circumferential radial margin (CRM). Once the tumor extends beyond the mesorectal fascia, it invades the pelvic sidewall and adjacent organs, making curative surgical resection more challenging.

Subsequent nodal drainage from the mesorectum lymph nodes falls into three main groups. The first group is the paracolic lymph nodes that lie in the peritoneum close to the colon. The second group lies along the main vessels supplying blood to the colon. The third group is the para-aortic nodes that cluster around the root of the SMA and IMA and are classified as distant metastases. While rectal lymph nodes are confined within a well-defined mesorectal envelope, colonic lymph nodes spread along the much broader mesentery. As a consequence, staging is easier in the case of rectal cancers, as potentially involved nodes will be visualized within the defined compartments of the mesorectum.

PROGNOSTIC FACTORS

Circumferential Margin

In rectal cancer, the distance between the tumor and the CRM is an important prognostic factor *(6–8)* and has been shown to be associated with a higher risk of pelvic recurrence *(9,10)*. A minimum clearance of 1 mm is needed to achieve R0 resection and reduce the chances of local failure. As the decision for neoadjuvant chemoradiotherapy may be dependent on the risk of circumferential involvement, staging investigations are essential to identify this variable accurately. Prognosis in rectal cancer is directly related to the extent of extramural spread into the mesorectum *(11,12)* and the ability to achieve clearance at the CRM *(7,10,11,13)*. Hall *(13)* demonstrated that CRM involvement was more an indicator of advanced disease than inadequate surgery and postulated that patients with an involved margin may die from distant disease before local recurrence becomes apparent. The quality of surgery also has a significant role in the prediction of a positive CRM, and MRI will only predict a positive resection margin for those patients undergoing TME. Nagtegaal et al *(14)* looked in detail at 180 patients who entered into the Dutch rectal cancer study and found that 24% of patients had incomplete TME specimens, which increased their risk for local and distant recurrence. Since CRM involvement can be due to direct extension of tumor into the mesorectal fascia, the presence of malignant nodes within 1 mm of the CRM or tumor within veins extending to the CRM, preoperative assessment of all of these variables is important.

Nodes

The prognosis of patients with rectal cancer is known to be influenced by the number of involved lymph nodes, *(15)* and this identification is important in guiding preoperative therapeutic approaches (see below).

Extramural Venous Invasion

EMVI is a reported poor prognostic factor in colorectal cancers resulting in reduced overall and disease-free survival *(16)*. EMVI has previously been identified using MRI in rectal cancer and is described as serpiginous extension of tumor within a vascular structure *(2)*. EMVI can also be visualized on CT *(17)* and is characterized by nodularity and expansion of the perirectal vessels.

Peritoneal Involvement

T4 disease or evidence of peritoneal involvement, with or without penetration of adjacent organs, has been shown to be a poor prognostic indicator in colorectal cancer *(18)*. Peritoneal involvement without invasion of adjacent organs can be difficult to predict as the serosa is a particularly thin layer of the bowel wall. Previous studies have not described T staging of tumors in the context of peritoneal anatomy but instead have limited assessment of T4 staging as invasion into adjacent organs shown by loss of fat planes *(19)*. Using different criteria and with knowledge of peritonealized surfaces of the colon, accuracies of 70–85% can be achieved through an understanding of peritonealized versus nonperitonealized colonic surfaces *(20)*. Local tumor perforation (pT4b) through the peritoneal membrane is common and also indicates an unfavorable prognosis, not only due to associated peritonitis, but also because of the risk of dissemination of malignant cells within the abdominal cavity resulting in transcoelomic spread and peritoneal involvement *(18)*. Tumor cells may be present in peritoneal washings in up to 42% of patients *(21)*. Transcoelomic metastases favor certain sites, such as to the lower right small bowel mesentery (superior and inferior ileocolic recesses), the intersigmoid recess and the rectovesical or rectouterine pouch (pouch of Douglas). This has implications for both surveillance of patients at a high risk of recurrence (T4b disease) and the identification of the likely patterns of recurrence.

STAGING

The international TNM staging system *(22)* is the most widely used pathological staging system, based upon the depth of tumor in and beyond the bowel wall, the number of nodal metastases, and the presence of distant metastases (Table 1) *(22)*.

CT STAGING

The main criterion for identification of tumor on CT is the focal thickening of the rectal wall. The usual bowel wall thickness on CT is 3 mm, with 6 mm being considered abnormal *(19)*. Asymmetrical bowel wall thickening with or without an irregular surface is likely to be a tumor. Extension into pericolonic tissues is indicated by the irregularity of the border of the colonic wall and nodular extension of soft tissue density extending into pericolonic fat (Fig. 1).

Table 1
Definitions of TNM components in the sixth edition of the AJCC and UICC system for staging cancer of the colon and rectum, 2002

Category	*Description*
TX	The primary tumor cannot be assessed
T0	No evidence of primary tumor
Tis	Carcinoma in situ (intraepithelial or intramucosal carcinoma)
T1	Tumor invades into the submucosa
T2	Tumor invades into the muscularis propria
T3	Tumor invades through the muscularis propria into the subserosa, or into nonperitonealized pericolic or perirectal tissues
Optional subdivision of T3	
T3a	Minimal invasion: <1 mm beyond the border of the muscularis propria
T3b	Slight invasion: 1–5 mm beyond the border of the muscularis propria
T3c	Moderate invasion: >5–15 mm beyond the border of the muscularis propria
T3d	Extensive invasion: >15 mm beyond the border of the muscularis propria
T4	Tumor directly invades into other organs or structures (T4a) or perforates the visceral peritoneum (T4b)
NX	Regional lymph nodes cannot be assessed
N0	No regional lymph node metastases
N1	Metastatic tumor in 1–3 pericolic or perirectal lymph nodes
N2	Metastatic tumor in 4 or more pericolic or perirectal lymph nodes
MX	The presence of distant metastasis cannot be assessed
M0	No distant metastasis
M1	Distant metastasis present

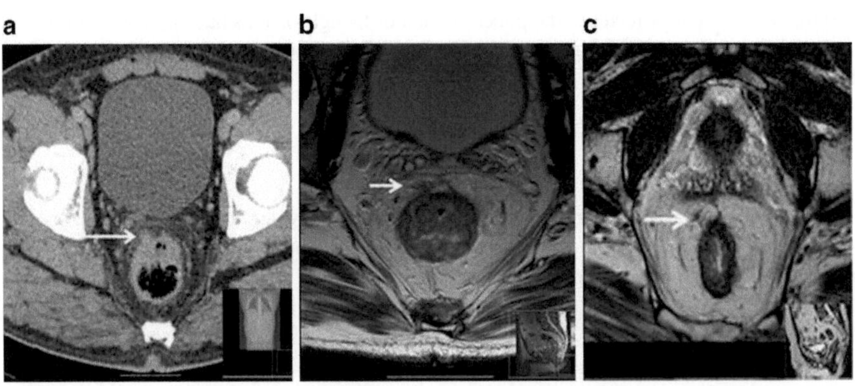

Fig. 1. (**a**) Axial CT images in a 77-year-old male showing an anterior mid-rectal T3c tumor extending towards the mesorectal fascia anteriorly, (**b**) T2-weighted axial rectal MRI in the same patient. The *arrow* shows the tumor extending anteriorly and lying close to the mesorectal fascia, (**c**) T2-weighted axial rectal MRI following long course chemoradiotherapy. The tumor shows regression and is now clear of the mesorectal fascia (*arrow*).

T-Stage

The CT criteria for identifying the T Stage of colonic tumors are outlined below:

T1 – Intraluminal projection of a colonic lesion without any visible distortion of the bowel wall layers
T2 – Asymmetrical thickening projecting intraluminally without disrupting the muscularis propria and clear adjacent pericolonic fat
T3 – Tumor extending beyond the muscularis propria with a smooth or nodular extension of a discrete mass of tumor tissue extending into pericolic fat
T4a – Irregular advancing edge of tumor penetrating adjacent organs with loss of well-defined plane between the colon and adjacent structures
T4b – Breach of the peritonealized surface covering the colon by tumor
T4c – Perforated tumors with evidence of pericolonic gas and free fluid in the abdomen

The T stage of the tumor is one of the main independent prognostic factors that determine survival in colorectal cancers *(23,24)*. Tumors confined to the bowel wall (TNM stage T1 and T2 tumors-5-year survival of 80–95%) have a better prognosis compared to tumors invading the muscularis propria or peritonealized surface (TNM stage T3 and T4) *(18,25,26)*. While earlier studies using CT for predicting T stage showed a sensitivity of about 55–60% and a specificity of 78–81%, *(27,28)* a recent study by Kanamoto et al, *(29)* with the benefit of MDCT, has shown a sensitivity and a specificity of 94% for T staging. The largest study, analyzing 365 patients, *(30)* achieved an accuracy rate of 74% for predicting the invasion of tumor beyond the muscularis propria.

The use of water enema CT for imaging colon cancers was first described by Angelelli in 1988 *(31)* and later by Gossios *(32)* in 1992. Amin et al *(33)*, in 1996, replaced water with air for rectal insufflation and performed abdominal spiral CT after cleansing the colon using a smooth muscle relaxant. This technique is increasing in popularity as rectal insufflation with air is required for CT colonography and studies using this technique have consistently achieved better accuracy rates *(29,34,35)*.

The overall accuracy of T-staging with CT using multiplanar formatting is around 86–87% *(36,37)*. Studies have shown that conventional CT has a high specificity for predicting positive CRM at around 92% although the sensitivity is low (47%), thus making it unsuitable for clinical use in the preoperative assessment of a potentially involved CRM in primary rectal cancer *(38)*. MDCT along with multiplanar image reconstruction provides more accurate prediction of CRM involvement in mid-lying and high-lying rectal tumors, but its accuracy drops significantly in low-lying tumors *(39)*.

Lymph Nodes

The criteria for defining a lymph node as metastatic on CT are inconsistent. The common definition applied in most of the studies evaluating the identification of metastatic lymph nodes is any node greater than 1 cm or a cluster of three or more nodes of less than 1 cm *(27,28,40–45)*. A few studies have used a size of 1.5 cm as the cutoff point, *(46,47)*. while a few others also added contrast enhancement above 100 Hounsfield units *(48)* or visible enhancement *(49)* as a variable, in order to help identify malignant nodes.

The detection of malignant nodes has always been a challenge in CT imaging due to the frequent occurrence of microscopic deposits in lymph nodes and enlargement of benign lymph nodes due to inflammatory processes. A large comparative study reported by the Radiology Diagnostic Oncology Group *(30)* found that the sensitivity for detecting lymph node metastases in 322 patients be 38% for rectal cancer and 56% for colon cancer; the overall accuracy in all patients studied was only 62%. A study utilizing MDCT has documented accuracy rates of 59% on observing axial images but improved detection rates to 83% on multiplanar reconstruction of the images *(50)*. A study by Kanamato et al analyzed each lymph node visible on CT and measured its longest and shortest diameter. They concluded that a short/long-axis diameter ratio of 0.8 or greater was the best index for the diagnosis of metastatic lymph nodes and achieved an accuracy index of 80% per node *(29)* Studies that have looked at the degree of node enhancement on CT and defined nodes that are more than 1 cm in size with contrast enhancement of >100 HU as malignant *(48,51)* have achieved accuracy rates of 61–81% in detection of malignant lymph nodes. Therefore, with the evidence so far, CT is unable to sufficiently identify malignant nodes with reliable accuracy and good interobserver variability, and hence its use as a prognostic factor is not indicated at this point.

Extramural Venous Invasion (EMVI)

The identification of EMVI on CT is even more challenging and is characterized by extension of tumor "tongue" along peritumoral veins. The classification of EMVI on CT is often documented as no EMVI, minimal stranding of veins, nodular enlargement of veins, or definite EMVI. The first two features are considered as negative for EMVI, while the last two are considered positive. Using the above criteria, Burton et al *(17)* achieved an accuracy rate of up to 61%, but had a very poor interobserver variability between the two observers.

MRI STAGING

Many studies have shown that depth of extramural invasion, nodal involvement, and involvement of the CRM are independent markers for poor prognosis. It has also been shown that these features can be accurately identified by MRI *(2,11,13,52–57)*.

T-STAGE

MRI is able to interpret the depth of tumor invasion and the relationship of the tumor to the surrounding structures. The layers of the bowel wall can usually be clearly identified (Figs. 2 and 3):

- On T2-weighted images, the muscularis mucosal layer is demonstrated as a fine low signal intensity line with the thicker, high signal submucosal layer seen beneath it.
- The muscularis propria can often be visualized as two distinct layers – the inner circular layer and the outer longitudinal layer. The outer muscle layer has an irregular, grooved appearance with interruptions due to vessels entering the rectal wall.
- The perirectal fat appears as high signal intensity line surrounding the low signal intensity line of the muscularis propria and contains signal void vessels. The mesorectal fascia is seen as a fine low signal layer enveloping the perirectal fat and rectum, and it is this layer that defines the surgical excision plane in TME anterior resections *(58)*.

Previous studies have described staging failures due to overstaging of T2 lesions *(59,60)* with difficulty in the distinction of spiculation in the perirectal fat caused by fibrosis alone versus that caused by fibrosis containing tumor cells. However, in most cases, peritumoral

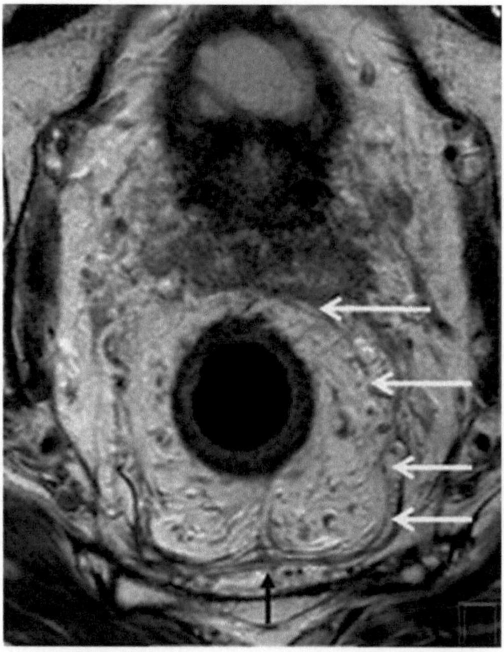

Fig. 2. T2-weighted axial MRI of the rectum in a 65-year-old male. The *arrows* depict the mesorectal fascia that forms the surgical resection margin. The presacral fascia covering the presacral space is highlighted by the *black arrow* posteriorly.

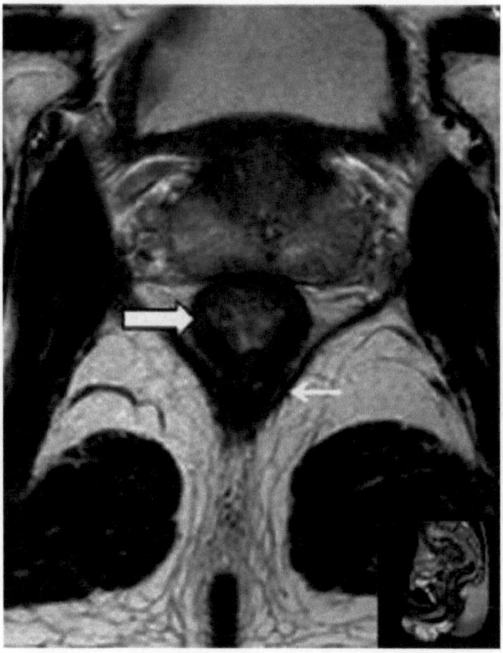

Fig. 3. T2-weighted axial rectal MRI in a 67-year-old male. The walls of the rectum are shown by the *white blocked arrow*, while the *white arrow* depicts the puborectalis muscle.

fibrosis can be seen as spiculation with low signal intensity compared with the broad based or nodular appearance of an advancing tumor margin *(54)*.

MRI diagnosis of a T3 lesion is based upon the presence of tumor signal extending into the perirectal fat with a broad-based bulging or nodular configuration in continuity with the intramural portion of the tumor. This is important to note, as there can be disruption in the outer longitudinal muscularis layer as a result of small vessels penetrating the wall, which are not necessarily invaded by tumor (Figs. 1 and 4).

The MERCURY study (Magnetic Resonance Imaging in Rectal Cancer European Equivalence Study) *(61)* demonstrated that MRI staging is feasible and reproducible in a multicentre setting and showed accurate prediction of involvement of the surgical CRM. The study also demonstrated that MRI can accurately measure the depth of extramural spread and showed equivalence with histopathological staging *(53)*.

Brown et al *(58)* compared the accuracy of high-resolution MRI with DRE and EUS in identifying favorable, unfavorable, and locally advanced rectal cancers in 98 patients undergoing TME. They demonstrated the superiority of MRI on cost and clinical effectiveness by selecting appropriate patients for neo-adjuvant therapy.

Margins

MRI can clearly visualize the mesorectal fascia and therefore is very good at predicting involvement of the CRM *(53,61,62)*. Wieder et al *(63)* retrospectively evaluated the prognostic importance of involvement of the CRM predicted using MRI before neo-adjuvant treatment in patients with rectal cancer. They concluded that patients with a tumor involved margin as predicted with the use of MRI before neo-adjuvant therapy had a substantially worse prognosis than patients without such involvement.

The MERCURY study was able to show that MRI accurately predicts the surgical resection margins, in a reproducible manner (Fig. 1). This has been confirmed with a recent meta-analysis *(64)* comparing preoperative MRI with histology after TME. This established that high-resolution

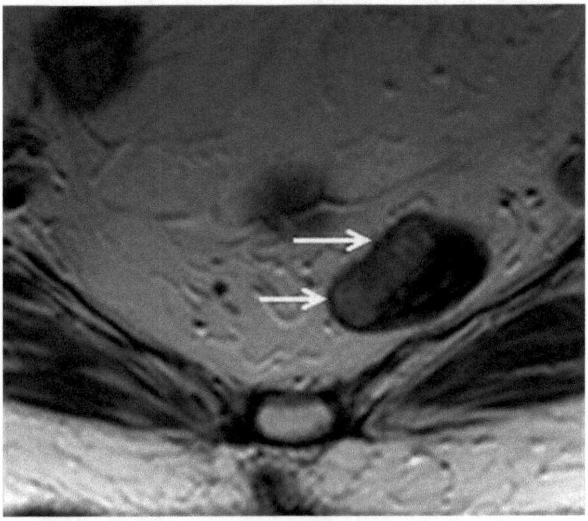

Fig. 4. T2-weighted axial rectal MRI in a 70-year-old female shows tumor in the lumen of the rectum. There is substantial presentation of muscularis propria seen as low signal intensity deep to tumor, indicating that the primary is a T2.

MRI can accurately predict tumor involvement of the CRM with a sensitivity and specificity of 94 and 85% respectively and concluded that this is reproducible across different centers. Birbeck in 2002 *(9)* showed that CRM status may be used as an immediate predictor of survival after rectal cancer surgery and serves as a useful indicator of the quality of surgery. They concluded that CRM involvement by tumor in rectal cancer is the only pathological variable that independently influences both survival and local recurrence. Ultimately, CRM involvement confers poorer prognosis, doubling the risk of death and increasing by 3.5 times the risk of local recurrence compared to patients with uninvolved margins.

Mesorectal Lymph Nodes

Nodal staging has traditionally relied upon the size of the nodes by MRI criteria. Nevertheless, several studies have indicated the inaccuracy of this technique, and we know from pathological studies of lymph node metastases that the size of the lymph node does not consistently correlate with the pathological findings *(65,66)*. Indeed, Andreola et al *(67)* examined 50 consecutive cases of rectal cancer using a manual histological method for the detection of lymph nodes less than 5 mm in diameter and confirmed that metastases in small lymph nodes are important in the accurate staging of rectal tumors. Similarly, involved nodes may well contain microscopic tumor foci and remain in normal size, and enlarged nodes are not always involved *(68)*. Criteria based upon the outline of the node and the features of signal intensity have been shown to be more reliable *(2,69)*. It is recognized that nodal replacement by tumor will cause gross distortion, and extranodal tumor extension will cause irregularity of the surrounding capsule, thus accounting for the appearances seen on MRI. Brown et al *(70)* showed that intranodal signal heterogeneity was a highly specific discriminator, and it gave a sensitivity of 85% and a specificity of 97% when using this technique. They also demonstrated that nodes with mixed signal intensity were likely to contain areas of necrosis or extracellular mucin corresponding to metastatic adenocarcinoma (Fig. 5). It has also

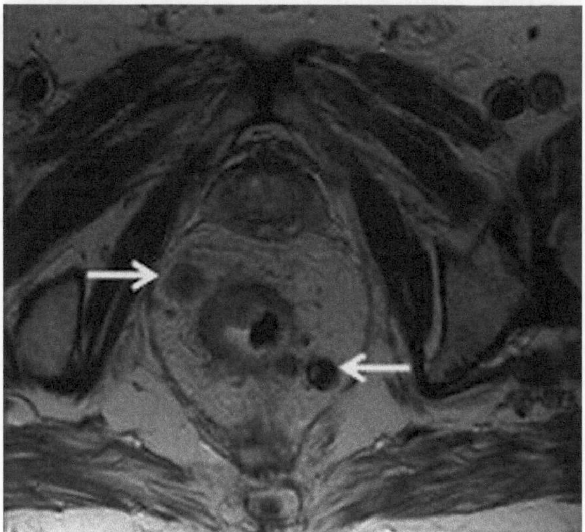

Fig. 5. T2-weighted axial rectal MRI in a 55-year-old female showing lymph nodes in the mesorectum which contain mixed signal intensity and have irregular borders indicating features of malignancy (*arrows*).

been shown that lymph node capsular invasion, as determined histologically, is a strong prognostic factor associated with recurrence. It may well be that noting the outline of the lymph node on MRI is equivalent to noting capsular invasion and if this can be seen preoperatively, then this may be an indicator that neo-adjuvant therapy is appropriate *(71)*.

It is possible that in the future lymph node staging will be augmented by using unique contrast agents. Early results have been quite promising *(72)*. Physiological imaging of lymph nodes using iron oxide contrast material works based on the fact that different cells show differential uptake of iron oxide particles. Lymph nodes involved with tumor contain less macrophages, and when compared to normal nodes, show less uptake and therefore give higher signal intensity *(73–75)*.

Extramural Vascular Invasion (EMVI)

EMVI has been shown to be associated with a higher risk of local recurrence, distant metastases, and death *(16,76,77)*. Smith et al *(3)* showed that that the presence of EMVI on a preoperative MRI scan was associated with a fourfold higher risk of distant metastases and a reduction in relapse-free survival at 3 years from 74 to 35% (Fig. 6).

Pelvic Sidewall Lymph Nodes

The presence of pelvic sidewall nodes is worth noting. In the UK, pelvic sidewall nodal dissection is not routinely performed; however, these nodes are generally included in preoperative radiation fields. In Japan, pelvic side wall dissection has been used since the late 1970s and a recent publication has suggested that positive lateral lymph nodes are the strongest predictor of both survival and local recurrence *(78)* (Fig. 7).

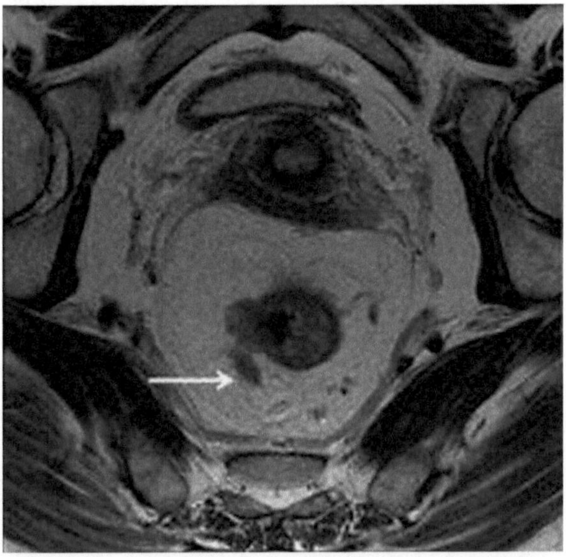

Fig. 6. T2-weighted axial rectal MRI in a 56-year-old female with tumor in the middle of the rectum. The *arrow* shows a tongue of tumor tissue extending along an extramural vein. The mesorectal fascia, however, is not threatened by tumor.

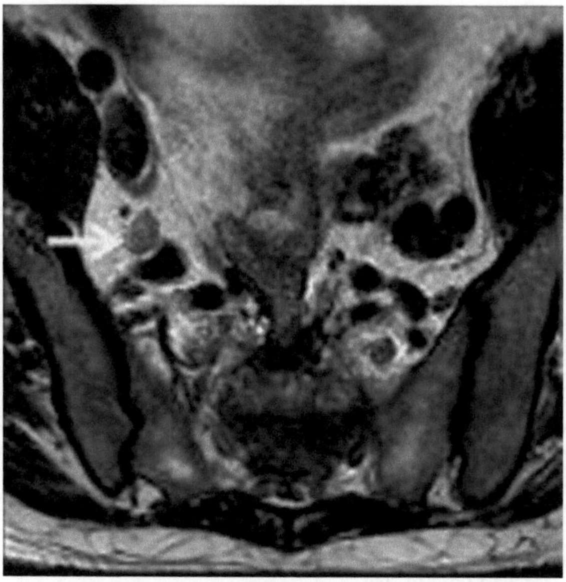

Fig. 7. T2-weighted axial rectal MRI in an 80-year-old male demonstrating a malignant node in the pelvic side wall.

Table 2
MRI staging system for low lying rectal cancers

MRI Low Rectal Stage 1	Tumour on MRI images appears confined to bowel wall but not through full thickness (intact muscularis propria of the internal sphincter)
MRI Low Rectal Stage 2	Tumour on MRI replaces the muscle coat of the internal sphincter but does not extend into the intersphincteric plane. Above the level of the sphincter it is confined to the mesorectum
MRI Low Rectal Stage 3	Tumour on MRI invading into the intersphincteric plane or lying within 1 mm of levator muscle above the level of the sphincter complex
MRI Low Rectal Stage 4	Tumour invading into the external anal sphincter and infiltrating/ extending beyond the levators +/– invading adjacent organ. Above the sphincter tumour invades the levator muscles

Post Chemoradiotherapy Images and Low-Lying Rectal Cancer

For those patients who received preoperative chemoradiotherapy, there is frequently tumor regression grade, which can be classified (Grade 1–5) according to the criteria modified from Dworak et al *(79)*. This has been shown to be a better predictor for post-treatment outcomes compared with T-stage *(80)* (Fig. 1).

Low-lying rectal tumors deserve special consideration since conventional staging systems are insufficient in these cases. We have devised a specific staging system that enables the identification of tumors with CRM at risk if a traditional abdomino-perineal excision is being performed. This staging is based upon axial and coronal images (Table 2).

REFERENCES

1. Fishman EK, Spiral CT. Clinical applications in the gastrointestinal tract. *Clin Imaging.* 1997;21(2):111–121.
2. Brown G, Radcliffe AG, Newcombe RG, Dallimore NS, Bourne MW, Williams GT. Preoperative assessment of prognostic factors in rectal cancer using high-resolution magnetic resonance imaging. *Br J Surg.* 2003;90(3):355–364.
3. Smith NJ, Barbachano Y, Norman AR, Swift RI, Abulafi AM, Brown G. Prognostic significance of magnetic resonance imaging-detected extramural vascular invasion in rectal cancer. *Br J Surg.* 2008;95(2):229–236.
4. Blomqvist L, Holm T, Rubio C, Hindmarsh T. Rectal tumours – MR imaging with endorectal and/or phased-array coils, and histopathological staging on giant sections. A comparative study. *Acta Radiol.* 1997;38(3):437–444.
5. Blomqvist L, Machado M, Rubio C, et al. Rectal tumour staging: MR imaging using pelvic phased-array and endorectal coils vs endoscopic ultrasonography. *Eur Radiol.* 2000;10(4):653–660.
6. Wang C, Zhou ZG, Yu YY, et al. Occurrence and prognostic value of circumferential resection margin involvement for patients with rectal cancer. *Int J Colorectal Dis.* 2009;24(4):385–390.
7. Wibe A, Rendedal PR, Svensson E, et al. Prognostic significance of the circumferential resection margin following total mesorectal excision for rectal cancer. *Br J Surg.* 2002;89(3):327–334.
8. Baik SH, Kim NK, Lee YC, et al. Prognostic significance of circumferential resection margin following total mesorectal excision and adjuvant chemoradiotherapy in patients with rectal cancer. *Ann Surg Oncol.* 2007;14(2):462–469.
9. Birbeck KF, Macklin CP, Tiffin NJ, et al. Rates of circumferential resection margin involvement vary between surgeons and predict outcomes in rectal cancer surgery. *Ann Surg.* 2002;235(4):449–457.
10. Quirke P, Durdey P, Dixon MF, Williams NS. Local recurrence of rectal adenocarcinoma due to inadequate surgical resection. Histopathological study of lateral tumour spread and surgical excision. *Lancet.* 1986;2(8514):996–999.
11. Cawthorn SJ, Parums DV, Gibbs NM, et al. Extent of mesorectal spread and involvement of lateral resection margin as prognostic factors after surgery for rectal cancer. *Lancet.* 1990;335(8697):1055–1059.
12. Lindmark G, Gerdin B, Pahlman L, Bergstrom R, Glimelius B. Prognostic predictors in colorectal cancer. *Dis Colon Rectum.* 1994;37(12):1219–1227.
13. Hall NR, Finan PJ, al-Jaberi T, et al. Circumferential margin involvement after mesorectal excision of rectal cancer with curative intent. Predictor of survival but not local recurrence? *Dis Colon Rectum.* 1998;41(8):979–983.
14. Nagtegaal ID, van de Velde CJ, van der Worp E, Kapiteijn E, Quirke P, van Krieken JH. Macroscopic evaluation of rectal cancer resection specimen: clinical significance of the pathologist in quality control. *J Clin Oncol.* 2002;20(7):1729–1734.
15. Wolmark N, Fisher B, Wieand HS. The prognostic value of the modifications of the Dukes' C class of colorectal cancer. An analysis of the NSABP clinical trials. *Ann Surg.* 1986;203(2):115–122.
16. Chapuis PH, Dent OF, Fisher R, et al. A multivariate analysis of clinical and pathological variables in prognosis after resection of large bowel cancer. *Br J Surg.* 1985;72(9):698–702.
17. Burton S, Brown G, Bees N, et al. Accuracy of CT prediction of poor prognostic features in colonic cancer. *Br J Radiol.* 2008;81(961):10–19.
18. Shepherd NA, Baxter KJ, Love SB. The prognostic importance of peritoneal involvement in colonic cancer: a prospective evaluation. *Gastroenterology.* 1997;112(4):1096–1102.
19. Thoeni RF. Colorectal cancer. Radiologic staging. *Radiol Clin North Am.* 1997;35(2):457–485.
20. Potter KC, Husband JE, Houghton SL, Thomas K, Brown G. Diagnostic accuracy of serial CT/magnetic resonance imaging review vs. positron emission tomography/CT in colorectal cancer patients with suspected and known recurrence. *Dis Colon Rectum.* 2009;52(2):253–259.
21. Wong LS, Morris AG, Fraser IA. The exfoliation of free malignant cells in the peritoneal cavity during resection of colorectal cancer. *Surg Oncol.* 1996;5(3):115–121.
22. Sobin LH, Fleming ID. TNM Classification of Malignant Tumors, fifth edition. Union Internationale Contre le Cancer and the American Joint Committee on Cancer. *Cancer.* 1997;80(9):1803–1804.

23. Moreaux J. Cancer of the colon. Survival and prognosis after surgical treatment in a series of 1000 patients. *Bull Acad Natl Med.* 989;173(6):777–780; discussion 81–82.
24. Gardner B, Feldman J, Spivak Y, et al. Investigations of factors influencing the prognosis of colon cancer. *Am J Surg.* 1987;153(6):541–544.
25. Hojo K. TNM staging of cancer of the colon. *Gan No Rinsho.* 1986;32(10):1373–1377.
26. Greene FL, Stewart AK, Norton HJ. A new TNM staging strategy for node-positive (stage III) colon cancer: an analysis of 50,042 patients. *Ann Surg.* 2002;236(4):416–421; discussion 21.
27. Freeny PC, Marks WM, Ryan JA, Bolen JW. Colorectal carcinoma evaluation with CT: preoperative staging and detection of postoperative recurrence. *Radiology.* 1986;158(2):347–353.
28. Balthazar EJ, Megibow AJ, Hulnick D, Naidich DP. Carcinoma of the colon: detection and preoperative staging by CT. *AJR Am J Roentgenol.* 1988;150(2):301–306.
29. Kanamoto T, Matsuki M, Okuda J, et al. Preoperative evaluation of local invasion and metastatic lymph nodes of colorectal cancer and mesenteric vascular variations using multidetector-row computed tomography before laparoscopic surgery. *J Comput Assist Tomogr.* 2007;31(6):831–839.
30. Zerhouni EA, Rutter C, Hamilton SR, et al. CT and MR imaging in the staging of colorectal carcinoma: report of the Radiology Diagnostic Oncology Group II. *Radiology.* 1996;200(2):443–451.
31. Angelelli G, Macarini L. CT of the bowel: use of water to enhance depiction. *Radiology.* 1988;169(3):848–849.
32. Gossios KJ, Tsianos EV, Kontogiannis DS, et al. Water as contrast medium for computed tomography study of colonic wall lesions. *Gastrointest Radiol.* 1992;17(2):125–128.
33. Amin Z, Boulos PB, Lees WR. Technical report: spiral CT pneumocolon for suspected colonic neoplasms. *Clin Radiol.* 1996;51(1):56–61.
34. Laghi A, Iannaccone R, Trenna S, et al. Multislice spiral CT colonography in the evaluation of colorectal neoplasms. *Radiol Med (Torino).* 2002;104(5–6):394–403.
35. Chung DJ, Huh KC, Choi WJ, Kim JK. CT colonography using 16-MDCT in the evaluation of colorectal cancer. *AJR Am J Roentgenol.* 2005;184(1):98–103.
36. Sinha R, Verma R, Rajesh A, Richards CJ. Diagnostic value of multidetector row CT in rectal cancer staging: comparison of multiplanar and axial images with histopathology. *Clin Radiol.* 2006;61(11):924–931.
37. Kulinna C, Scheidler J, Strauss T, et al. Local staging of rectal cancer: assessment with double-contrast multislice computed tomography and transrectal ultrasound. *J Comput Assist Tomogr.* 2004;28(1):123–130.
38. Wolberink SV, Beets-Tan RG, de Haas-Kock DF, et al. Conventional CT for the prediction of an involved circumferential resection margin in primary rectal cancer. *Dig Dis.* 2007;25(1):80–85.
39. Vliegen R, Dresen R, Beets G, et al. The accuracy of Multi-detector row CT for the assessment of tumor invasion of the mesorectal fascia in primary rectal cancer. *Abdom Imaging.* 2008;33(5):604–610.
40. Acunas B, Rozanes I, Acunas G, Celik L, Sayi I, Gokmen E. Preoperative CT staging of colon carcinoma (excluding the recto-sigmoid region). *Eur J Radiol.* 1990;11(2):150–153.
41. Gazelle GS, Gaa J, Saini S, Shellito P. Staging of colon carcinoma using water enema CT. *J Comput Assist Tomogr.* 1995;19(1):87–91.
42. Harvey CJ, Amin Z, Hare CM, et al. Helical CT pneumocolon to assess colonic tumors: radiologic-pathologic correlation. *AJR Am J Roentgenol.* 1998;170(6):1439–1443.
43. Ashraf K, Ashraf O, Haider Z, Rafique Z. Colorectal carcinoma, preoperative evaluation by spiral computed tomography. *J Pak Med Assoc.* 2006;56(4):149–153.
44. Cademartiri F, Luccichenti G, Rossi A, Pavone P. Spiral hydro-CT in the evaluation of colo-sigmoideal cancer. *Radiol Med (Torino).* 2002;104(4):295–306.
45. Gomille T, Aleksic M, Ulrich B, Christ F. Significance of CT in the detection of regional lymph node metastases in colorectal carcinoma. *Radiologe.* 1998;38(12):1077–1082.
46. Keeney G, Jafri SZ, Mezwa DG. Computed tomographic evaluation and staging of cecal carcinoma. *Gastrointest Radiol.* 1989;14(1):65–69.
47. Thompson WM, Halvorsen RA, Foster WL Jr, Roberts L, Gibbons R. Preoperative and postoperative CT staging of rectosigmoid carcinoma. *AJR Am J Roentgenol.* 1986;146(4):703–710.
48. Hundt W, Braunschweig R, Reiser M. Evaluation of spiral CT in staging of colon and rectum carcinoma. *Eur Radiol.* 1999;9(1):78–84.

49. Sun CH, Li ZP, Meng QF, Yu SP, Xu DS. Assessment of spiral CT pneumocolon in preoperative colorectal carcinoma. *World J Gastroenterol.* 2005;11(25):3866–3870.
50. Filippone A, Ambrosini R, Fuschi M, Marinelli T, Genovesi D, Bonomo L. Preoperative T and N staging of colorectal cancer: accuracy of contrast-enhanced multi-detector row CT colonography – initial experience. *Radiology.* 2004;231(1):83–90.
51. Smith NJ, Bees N, Barbachano Y, Norman AR, Swift RI, Brown G. Preoperative computed tomography staging of nonmetastatic colon cancer predicts outcome: implications for clinical trials. *Br J Cancer.* 2007;96(7):1030–1036.
52. Jass JR, Love SB. Prognostic value of direct spread in Dukes' C cases of rectal cancer. *Dis Colon Rectum.* 1989;32(6):477–480.
53. MERCURY Study Group. Extramural depth of tumor invasion at thin-section MR in patients with rectal cancer: results of the MERCURY study. *Radiology.* 2007;24(1):132–139.
54. Brown G, Richards CJ, Newcombe RG, et al. Rectal carcinoma: thin-section MR imaging for staging in 28 patients. *Radiology.* 1999;211(1):215–222.
55. Martling A, Holm T, Bremmer S, Lindholm J, Cedermark B, Blomqvist L. Prognostic value of preoperative magnetic resonance imaging of the pelvis in rectal cancer. *Br J Surg.* 2003;90(11):1422–1428.
56. Adam IJ, Mohamdee MO, Martin IG, et al. Role of circumferential margin involvement in the local recurrence of rectal cancer. *Lancet.* 1994;344(8924):707–711.
57. Cawthorn SJ, Gibbs NM, Marks CG. Clearance technique for the detection of lymph nodes in colorectal cancer. *Br J Surg.* 1986;73(1):58–60.
58. Brown G, Davies S, Williams GT, et al. Effectiveness of preoperative staging in rectal cancer: digital rectal examination, endoluminal ultrasound or magnetic resonance imaging? *Br J Cancer.* 2004;91(1):23–29.
59. Laghi A, Ferri M, Catalano C, et al. Local staging of rectal cancer with MRI using a phased array body coil. *Abdom Imaging.* 2002;27(4):425–431.
60. Beets-Tan RG, Beets GL, Vliegen RF, et al. Accuracy of magnetic resonance imaging in prediction of tumour-free resection margin in rectal cancer surgery. *Lancet.* 2001;357(9255):497–504.
61. MERCURY Study Group. Diagnostic accuracy of preoperative magnetic resonance imaging in predicting curative resection of rectal cancer: prospective observational study. *BMJ.* 2006;333(7572):779.
62. Blomqvist L, Rubio C, Holm T, Machado M, Hindmarsh T. Rectal adenocarcinoma: assessment of tumour involvement of the lateral resection margin by MRI of resected specimen. *Br J Radiol.* 1999;72(853):18–23.
63. Wieder HA, Rosenberg R, Lordick F, et al. Rectal cancer: MR imaging before neoadjuvant chemotherapy and radiation therapy for prediction of tumor-free circumferential resection margins and long-term survival. *Radiology.* 2007;243(3):744–751.
64. Purkayastha S, Tekkis PP, Athanasiou T, Tilney HS, Darzi AW, Heriot AG. Diagnostic precision of magnetic resonance imaging for preoperative prediction of the circumferential margin involvement in patients with rectal cancer. *Colorectal Dis.* 2007;9(5):402–411.
65. Herrera L, Villarreal JR. Incidence of metastases from rectal adenocarcinoma in small lymph nodes detected by a clearing technique. *Dis Colon Rectum.* 1992;35(8):783–788.
66. Kotanagi H, Fukuoka T, Shibata Y, et al. The size of regional lymph nodes does not correlate with the presence or absence of metastasis in lymph nodes in rectal cancer. *J Surg Oncol.* 1993;54(4):252–254.
67. Andreola S, Leo E, Belli F, et al. Manual dissection of adenocarcinoma of the lower third of the rectum specimens for detection of lymph node metastases smaller than 5 mm. *Cancer.* 1996;77(4):607–612.
68. Gunther K, Dworak O, Remke S, et al. Prediction of distant metastases after curative surgery for rectal cancer. *J Surg Res.* 2002;103(1):68–78.
69. Kim JH, Beets GL, Kim MJ, Kessels AG, Beets-Tan RG. High-resolution MR imaging for nodal staging in rectal cancer: are there any criteria in addition to the size? *Eur J Radiol.* 2004;52(1):78–83.
70. Brown G, Richards CJ, Bourne MW, et al. Morphologic predictors of lymph node status in rectal cancer with use of high-spatial-resolution MR imaging with histopathologic comparison. *Radiology.* 2003;227(2):371–377.

71. Yano H, Saito Y, Kirihara Y, Takashima J. Tumor invasion of lymph node capsules in patients with Dukes C colorectal adenocarcinoma. *Dis Colon Rectum.* 2006;49(12):1867–1877.
72. Koh DM, Brown G, Temple L, et al. Rectal cancer: mesorectal lymph nodes at MR imaging with USPIO versus histopathologic findings – initial observations. *Radiology.* 2004;231(1):91–99.
73. Rich T, Gunderson LL, Lew R, Galdibini JJ, Cohen AM, Donaldson G. Patterns of recurrence of rectal cancer after potentially curative surgery. *Cancer.* 1983;52(7):1317–1329.
74. Vassallo P, Matei C, Heston WD, McLachlan SJ, Koutcher JA, Castellino RA. AMI-227-enhanced MR lymphography: usefulness for differentiating reactive from tumor-bearing lymph nodes. *Radiology.* 1994;193(2):501–506.
75. Weissleder R, Elizondo G, Wittenberg J, Lee AS, Josephson L, Brady TJ. Ultrasmall superparamagnetic iron oxide: an intravenous contrast agent for assessing lymph nodes with MR imaging. *Radiology.* 1990;175(2):494–498.
76. Krasna MJ, Flancbaum L, Cody RP, Shneibaum S, Ben Ari G. Vascular and neural invasion in colorectal carcinoma. Incidence and prognostic significance. *Cancer.* 1988;61(5):1018–1023.
77. Ouchi K, Sugawara T, Ono H, et al. Histologic features and clinical significance of venous invasion in colorectal carcinoma with hepatic metastasis. *Cancer.* 1996;78(11):2313–2317.
78. Sugihara K, Kobayashi H, Kato T, et al. Indication and benefit of pelvic sidewall dissection for rectal cancer. *Dis Colon Rectum.* 2006;49(11):1663–1672.
79. Dworak O, Keilholz L, Hoffmann A. Pathological features of rectal cancer after preoperative radiochemotherapy. *Int J Colorectal Dis.* 1997;12(1):19–23.
80. Bouzourene H, Bosman FT, Seelentag W, Matter M, Coucke P. Importance of tumor regression assessment in predicting the outcome in patients with locally advanced rectal carcinoma who are treated with preoperative radiotherapy. *Cancer.* 2002;94(4):1121–1130.

73. Yano H, Saito Y, Kirihara Y, Takashima J. Tumor invasion of lymph node capsules in patients with Dukes C colorectal adenocarcinoma. Dis Colon Rectum [illegible]
74. Koh DM, Brown G, Temple L, [illegible]
[illegible]

3 Local Excision

Y. Nancy You and Heidi Nelson

INTRODUCTION

Key outcome measures of successful management of rectal cancer involve maximizing survival benefit, minimizing disease recurrence in the pelvis, and preserving preoperative bowel function and health-related quality of life. To achieve these goals, surgical options range from local excision (LE) of tumor to extended multivisceral resections. In addition, adjuvant radiation therapy (RT) and chemotherapy can be combined with surgical resection. Tailoring the optimal treatment regimen for an individual patient involves matching the patient's disease burden to the extent of surgical resection and additional therapies, in order to achieve the best balance of all aforementioned treatment goals. With increasing interest in sphincter-preservation, local management of rectal cancer has gained appeal in recent years, particularly for patients with early-stage rectal cancer. A critical examination of the advantages and pitfalls of LE is therefore relevant today.

The most common local management option is transanal tumor excision, either via conventional technique or via an operating microscope (transanal endoscopic microsurgery, TEMS). Other LE approaches, such as the posterior trans-sacral proctotomy of Kraske, are infrequently seen in practice today and will not be the focus of subsequent discussion. Standard resection (SR) techniques, as referred to in this chapter, will be defined to include abdominal perineal resection (APR), coloanal anastomosis, and/or low anterior resection (LAR). This chapter aims to summarize the current controversies, the technical details, and relevant evidence surrounding the use of LE as potentially curative therapy for stage I rectal cancer.

HISTORICAL PERSPECTIVE AND RELEVANCE TO CLINICAL PRACTICE TODAY

Historically, LE was performed to palliate patients who were unfit candidates for SR procedures, either because of age or because of medical comorbidities; alternatively, it was performed for patients who adamantly refused SR and the risk of a permanent colostomy.

From: *Current Clinical Oncology: Rectal Cancer*,
Edited by: B.G. Czito and C.G. Willett, DOI: 10.1007/978-1-60761-567-5_3,

In 1977, Morson et al reported results from patients treated under a policy of LE or "total biopsy" for early rectal cancer as long as it was deemed technically feasible. Among 91 patients with R0 resection, the crude 5-year overall survival (OS) rate was 82% and disease recurred in only three patients. This study encouraged surgeons to perform LE for technically accessable low rectal cancers as long as its histology was not poorly differentiated. In the meantime, it cautioned that, if positive resection margin or unfavorable histology were found on pathology, further transabdominal resections should be performed *(1)*. Since then, experience with LE has accumulated. Today, LE is being increasingly offered as a potentially curative resection for patients with stage I rectal cancer. A recent query of the United States National Cancer Database (NCDB) data sampled patients treated for American Joint Commission on Cancer (AJCC) stage I (T1N0 and T2N0). The rates of LE increased significantly between January 1, 1989 and December 31, 2003, for both T1 lesions (27% in 1989 vs. 44% in 2003; $p<0.001$) and T2 lesions (6% in 1989 vs. 17% in 2003; $p<0.001$) *(2)*. Thus, an evidence-based review of LE is highly relevant today.

CURRENT CONTROVERSIES SURROUNDING LE

While LE has gained appeal as a treatment strategy for early-stage rectal cancer, its oncologic adequacy has remained highly controversial, with three key areas of concern.

First, the preoperative staging of rectal adenocarcinoma is currently imperfect. The most commonly used imaging modalities include the endoscopic ultrasound (EUS) or magnetic resonance imaging (MRI). The accuracy of T staging ranges between 63–91% for EUS and 66–91% for MRI. The corresponding accuracies of N staging are 64–83% by EUS and 65–88% by MRI, respectively *(3)*. Therefore, at present, precise and accurate selection of patients with clinical stage I (T1N0 or T2N0) rectal cancer as appropriate candidates for LE is not possible.

Second, the adequacy of LE to manage the nodal basin draining the rectal cancer remains problematic. SR for potentially curable rectal cancer demands total mesorectal excision with removal of nodal tissue en bloc with primary tumor. The incidence of occult nodal involvement in even T1 tumors is 10–13%. The rate increases to at least 17–22% for T2 tumors *(4–6)*. Recently, the St Mark's Lymph Node Positivity Model has been developed to predict nodal involvement based on patient age, T stage, and other histological features *(7)*. However, to date, no method can predict the nodal status of a patient with complete accuracy preoperatively. Because LE does not remove nodal tissue, there is a significant risk of under-treatment and/or under-staging of nodal disease, when LE rather than SR is chosen as therapy for rectal cancer.

Third is the debate as to the effectiveness of salvage following LE: either immediate or delayed. For patients who undergo LE but later develop a recurrence in the pelvis, salvage operations typically involve multivisceral pelvic resections, with morbidity rates of 34% and R0 resection rates between 79 and 94%. The 5-year disease-free survival after salvage surgery ranges between 53 and 59% at best *(8,9)*. On the other hand, for patients who undergo LE but were found to have either T3 lesion, evidence of lymphovascular invasion, or gross residual disease on pathology, proceeding to immediate salvage resection does not appear to compromise long-term outcomes, with one series describing a 5-year OS of 79% *(10)* Thus, the risk of delayed failure after LE may be costly.

TECHNICAL ASPECTS OF LE

The most common approach to LE in practice is transanal. Transanal excision can be performed using the conventional technique or through an operating rectoscope, and will form the focus of subsequent discussions. Alternative approaches *(11)* include: the posterior proctotomy approach of Kraske, first described in 1885 *(12)*, and the posterior transsphincteric approach of York-Mason, first described in the early 1900s and reintroduced in the 1970s *(13)*. Additionally, transanal fulguration or electrocoagulation of rectal tumor should be regarded as palliative procedures only *(14)*. These latter techniques will not be discussed further.

Preoperative Preparation

Depending on surgeon's preference and practice, patients undergo either a full mechanical bowel preparation or simply distal enemas preoperatively. Prophylactic intravenous antibiotics are administered. For anterior and lateral lesions, prone jackknife position is used, while lithotomy position with candy cane stirrups may be more suitable for posterior lesions. The rectum may be irrigated with either saline or betadine solution. A Foley catheter is typically inserted.

Conventional Transanal Excision

From only the technical standpoint, there is general agreement that the most ideal tumors for transanal LE are less than 4 cm in greatest diameter, located below the middle rectal valve or within 8 cm from the dentate line, comprising no more than 40% of the rectal circumference, and exhibit favorable histology.

Exposure of the low rectum can be achieved using a Pratt speculum, a Parks retractor, or the Lone Star retractor (Lone Star Medical Products, Stafford, TX) *(15)*. With the lesion well-visualized, electrocautery is used to mark the line of excision. It is critical that at least a 1 cm circumferential margin of normal tissue is taken with the specimen. Excision is typically started distally and completed using electrocautery. Allis clamps and/or stay sutures around the lesion can be used for retraction during the dissection, but care must be taken to avoid fragmenting the specimen. A full-thickness disk of tissue should be excised, allowing visualization of perirectal fat after removal of higher lesions. For very distal tumors, a perianorectal plane (deeper than the internal sphincter) is entered. Next, the specimen should be diligently oriented as right, left, caudad, and cephalad, for proper pathological assessment of margins. It has been the preference of the authors to transversely reapproximate the wound edges using absorbable suture, but extraperitoneal rectal wounds may also be left open to heal (Fig. 1). Complete rigid proctoscopy may be performed to ensure a patent rectal lumen.

Transanal Endoscopic Microsurgery

Originally described by Buess et al, *(64)* TEM is a minimally invasive technique that utilizes a lighted rectoscope, carbon dioxide insufflation, and special instruments. A four-port working unit, containing a stereoscopic rectoscope and a maximum of three working instruments, is inserted transanally and secured to the operating table. The rectoscope has a diameter of 40 mm, and a length of either 12 or 20 cm. An airtight seal is created to allow gas insufflation for a pneumorectum. Electrocautery instruments are used to mark the line of excision, ensuring

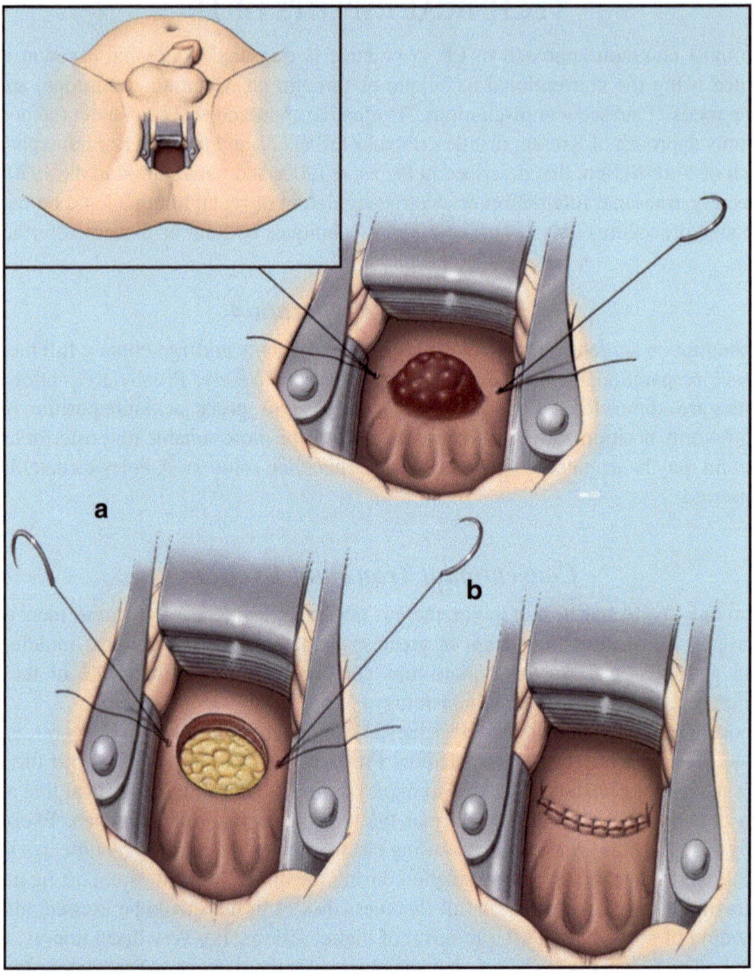

Fig. 1. Conventional transanal LE.

at least 1 cm margin clearance in a fashion similar to conventional LE. Although lesions in the upper rectum (up to 18 cm from anal verge) are technically accessible by TEM, in practice, application of TEM has remained for lesions in the extraperitoneal rectum because of the need to obtain a full-thickness rectal excision and the risk of intraperitoneal perforation *(15,16)*. The specimen should be properly oriented for pathological examination. Overall, the main advantage of TEM is that a magnified, stereoscopic view of the tumor in an insufflated rectum provides excellent technical conditions to the operating surgeon and therefore affords a higher chance of obtaining adequate negative margins, nonfragmented samples, and full-thickness rectal excision, when compared to conventional transanal LE *(17,18)*. However, widespread adoption of this technique has been limited by the steep learning curve, the expensive and specialized equipment and the limited applications of the technique to tumors with suitable anatomy.

OUTCOMES OF LE FOR EARLY-STAGE RECTAL CANCER

Studies Containing Tumors of Differing T Stages

CONSECUTIVE AND NONCONSECUTIVE CASE SERIES

Since the late 1970s, numerous single-institutions have reported their experiences with LE for rectal cancer *(11,19)*. The majority of the studies were retrospective in design. These studies confirmed favorable peri-operative morbidity rates of LE. However, the oncologic outcomes of LE reported in these series were difficult to interpret. Nearly all studies contained relatively small patient numbers, and a heterogeneous mix of tumors of differing pathological stages (i.e., T1, T2, and/or T3) *(20–23)*. Preoperative patient selection not only differed among studies but also differed by the staging modalities used and time periods studied *(24,25)*. Additionally, some studies included patients who received postoperative RT either as an institutional policy, or due to various reasons such as positive resection margin or unfavorable histology *(26–35)*. Final analyses of oncologic outcomes were typically not stratified by tumor stage, selection factors, or RT use, thereby making it difficult to draw any conclusions to influence clinical practice. Nonetheless, as experience with LE accumulated, it appeared that LE does benefit patients by sparing them the major morbidities of SR and may afford acceptable long-term survival and local control outcomes in a select subgroup of patients. Newer studies have allowed a more detailed study of LE and SR in the treatment of T1 vs. T2 tumors, as outlined below.

T1 Tumors

CONSECUTIVE CASE SERIES

Proper selection of rectal tumors for LE vs. SR was brought into focus in an early study by Willett et al *(36)*. Comparing 56 patients treated with LE vs. 69 patients treated with APR, 5-year recurrence-free survival of 87% and local control rate of 96% were achieved after LE. These results compared favorably with corresponding rates of 91% achieved after SR, suggesting that LE may be an acceptable alternative to SR when tumors with favorable histology were selected. Further analysis also demonstrated that significantly worse outcomes were seen if LE was performed for poorly differentiated tumors with venous/lymph vessel involvement. Subsequent single institutional studies compared oncologic outcomes of LE vs. SR (Table 1). Studies from the University of Minnesota first bought attention to the alarmingly high rates of local failure after LE *(37,38)* Other studies largely substantiated significantly higher local recurrence rates of 7–18% after LE vs. 0–3% after SR (Table 1) *(17,37–41)*. However, there was no agreement on whether LE and SR differentially impact on 5-year OS. While some reported disturbingly lower OS after LE *(37,38,41)*, no significant difference was found in the largest study *(39)*. Furthermore, investigators were unable to identify any consistent clinical or pathological predictors of local failure *(17)*. Nonetheless, there emerged a general agreement that LE should be reserved for low-risk T1 tumors only, as initially suggested by Willett et al *(36)*.

POPULATION-BASED CASE SERIES

Recently, oncologic outcomes of patients treated with LE vs. SR have been captured by several nationwide cancer registries (Table 2). These registries have allowed examination of substantially larger sample sizes of patients treated contemporaneously by LE and SR (Table 2). The data contained in these national cancer registries were collected on an ongoing

Table 1
Oncologic outcomes after local excision (LE) and standard resection (SR) for T1 rectal tumors: summary of consecutive case series

	No. of patients		*5-Year overall survival (%)*		*5-Year local recurrence (%)*		
Author, year	*LE*	*SR*	*LE*	*SR*	*LE*	*SR*	*Follow-up (years)*
Mellgren, 2000 *(38)*	69	30	72	80[a]	18	0[a]	4.4–4.8, mean
Nascimbeni, 2004 *(41)*	70	74	72	90[a]	6.6	2.8	8.1, median
Madbouly, 2005 *(40)*	52	–	75	–	17	–	4.6, median
Bentrem, 2005 *(39)*	152	168	89	93	15	3[a]	4.3, median

[a]Denotes statistically significant difference

Table 2
Oncologic outcomes after local excision (LE) and standard resection (SR) for T1 rectal tumors: summary of population-based case series

	No. of patients		*5-Year overall survival (%)*		*5-Year local recurrence (%)*		
Author, year	*LE*	*SR*	*LE*	*SR*	*LE*	*SR*	*Follow-up (years)*
Endreseth, Norwegian Rectal Cancer Group, 2005 *(43)*	35	256	70	80[a]	12	6[a]	Not reported
You, National Cancer Database, 2007 *(2)*	601	493	77	82	12.5	6.9[a]	6.3, median
Ptok, German Colon/ Rectal Cancer Study Group, 2007 *(42)*	85	359	84	92	5.1	1.4[a]	3.5, mean
Folkesson, Swedish Rectal Cancer Registry, 2007 (mix of T1 and T2) *(44)*	256	1,141	87	93	7	2[a]	Not reported

[a]Denotes statistically significant difference

basis through well-described methodologies, and were subject to rigorous quality-validation measures to ensure data quality. While comparisons of outcomes after LE vs. SR reported in these studies remain subject to the selection biases and follow-up practices of the individual surgeons, remarkably consistent trends were reported. On the one hand, significantly higher rates of local failure were observed after LE vs. SR in all studies: 5–13% vs. 1–7% (Table 2). Even in studies where patients with positive resection margin (non-R0 resection) were excluded, local failure was more frequent after LE *(2,42)*. Importantly, the local failure rate continued to increase even through 8 years of follow-up (Fig. 2: NCDB) *(2)*. On the other hand, 5-year OS ranged between 70–87% after LE and 80–93% after SR; only a borderline difference was demonstrated in one of the four studies *(2,42–44)*. Based on data from the NCDB, where long-term follow-up was available, estimated OS did not significantly diverge even at 8 years after LE vs. SR: 62 vs. 66%, after adjusting for patient and tumor variables ($p=0.09$; Fig. 3) *(2)*. In multivariate analyses, LE was an independent predictor of local failure *(2,42)*, and the risk was as high as threefold in one study *(2)*. On the other hand, OS was not influenced by the type of procedure, but was independently predicted by patient-related

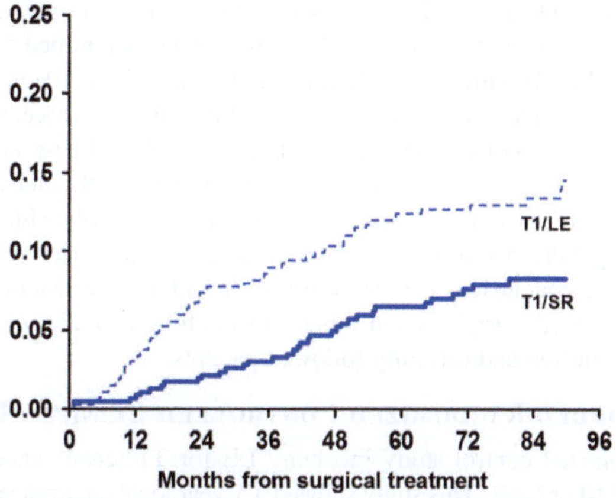

Fig. 2. Cumulative hazard of local disease recurrence in patients with T1 tumors treated by local excision (LE) and standard resections (SR) National Cancer Database. Reprinted with permission.

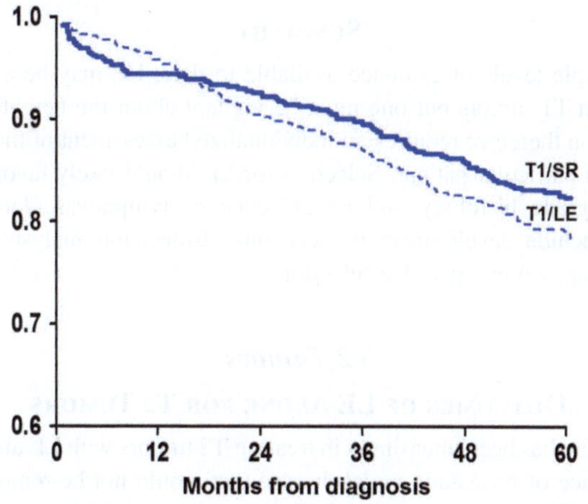

Fig. 3. Overall survival of patients with T1 tumors treated by local excision (LE) and standard resections (SR) National Cancer Database. Reprinted with permission.

factors including: age *(2,42,43)*, gender *(43)*, American Society of Anesthesiology class *(42)*, and number of comorbidities (*2*). These findings reveal that patients face increased risk of local failure after LE but other factors, relating more to the patient rather than the surgical procedure, may exert stronger influences on OS.

Nonrandomized Controlled Clinical Trials

A few prospective, single-institution registry studies of LE have been reported *(35,45–47)*. These prospective series contained well-defined inclusion and exclusion criteria and several included a mixture of tumors (T1, T2, and/or T3) treated with or without adjuvant RT, making reported outcomes difficult to interpret. To date, two prospective multi-institutional trials have been published: RTOG 89-02 and CALBG 8984 *(48–50)*. Twenty-seven patients with T1 rectal cancer undergoing LE were registered to the RTOG trial and followed. Their local failure rate was 4% *(49)*. Similarly, the CALBG 8984 trial enrolled 59 patients with T1 tumor resected with LE. The inclusion criteria were tumors within 10 cm of the anal verge, measuring ≤4 cm in diameter and involving ≤ 40% of the circumference, and resection with negative margins. After a median follow-up of 7.1 years, the 6- and 10-year local failure rates were 6.8 and 8%, while the corresponding rates for OS were 87 and 84%, respectively *(48,50)*. The authors suggest that these outcomes compared favorably with historical controls of patients treated by APR: 5-year OS of 94% according to data queried from NCDB in 1997 *(48)*. While definitive conclusions cannot be drawn from historical comparisons, data from these single-arm prospective trials establish benchmarks for oncologic outcomes when LE is performed in well-selected and carefully followed patients.

Nonblinded Randomized Controlled Clinical Trials

The only randomized control study involving LE for T1 rectal cancer randomized 50 patients to either TEM or LAR. This study showed a 5-year local recurrence rate of 4.1% after TEM and 0% after LAR with a median follow-up of 3.5 years. There was no difference in 5-year OS (96 vs. 96%) *(51)*. These favorable findings highlight technical advantages offered by TEM where better exposure, dissection, and specimen retrieval are possible. A definitive, randomized comparison between TEM and LAR would require upwards of a 1,000 patients and 5-year follow-up data on at least 900 patients.

Summary

Based on multiple levels of evidence available to date, LE may be a viable option for select patients with T1 tumors but one must be vigilant about the heightened risk of local failure. The decision therefore requires an individualized assessment of the risk and benefits of LE vs. SR for a particular patient. Selection for LE should likely favor low-lying, small tumors with low-grade histology and no evidence of lymphovascular invasion. Future research should include development of decision-aids/decision-analysis, or molecular or imaging tools to improve preoperative selection.

T2 Tumors

Outcomes of LE Alone for T2 Tumors

Historically, there has been uneasiness in treating T2 tumors with LE alone, primarily due to the high incidence of metastatic nodal disease that would not be removed by LE alone. Data pertaining to T2 tumors treated by LE alone without additional therapy vs. SR are therefore limited. The University of Minnesota reported outcomes of 39 patients with T2 tumors treated with LE without postoperative therapy, as well as outcomes of 123 patients who underwent SR. The 5-year local recurrence rate was as high as 47% after LE, significantly more than a rate of 6% after SR. Similarly, 5-year OS was only 65% after LE, significantly compromised from 81% seen after SR *(38)*. These differences were further corroborated by data from the NCDB *(2)*, where patients who received additional chemotherapy or RT were excluded from the analysis. A significantly higher rate of local failure: 22 vs. 15% occurred after LE vs. SR. Additionally, lower OS rates were seen: 68 vs. 77% (Figs. 4 and 5). However, a strong selection bias is likely present as the type of surgery did not emerge as an independent predictor of local failure or of poor OS *(2)*. Thus, in practice, LE may be chosen as the sole therapy for T2 lesions only when patients are elderly, have multiple comorbidities, or otherwise carry a compromised life expectancy.

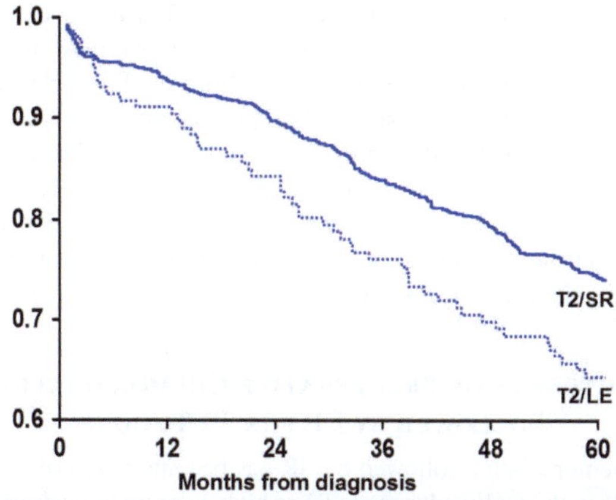

Fig. 4. Overall survival of patients with T2 tumors treated by local excision (LE) and standard resections (SR) National Cancer Database. Reprinted with permission.

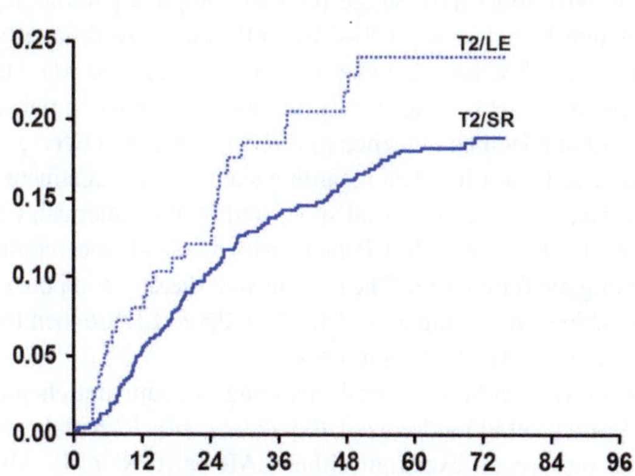

Fig. 5. Cumulative hazard of local disease recurrence in patients with T2 tumors treated by local excision (LE) and standard resections (SR) National Cancer Database. Reprinted with permission.

Outcomes of LE and Postoperative Chemotherapy and/or RT for T2 Tumors

While LE alone appears to be inadequate therapy for potentially curable T2 lesions, the concept of combining LE with external beam RT to maximize local control has existed since the early 1980s. Several institutions accumulated experience with this strategy, but reported case series contained few patients, a mix of tumors at different T stages, and oncologic outcomes were not specific to T2 tumors. Minsky et al reported an encouraging 14% local failure rate among seven patients with T2 tumors treated with LE, 5-fluorouracil (5-FU) and RT *(52)*. Additionally, authors reported higher 5-year local failure rates of 20–24%, with lymphovascular invasion, positive resection margins and tumor fragmentation the most commonly identified predictors of local failure *(53–56)*. Only one study has attempted to isolate the impact of postoperative RT on oncologic outcomes: comparing eight patients treated with LE alone vs. 33 patients treated with LE and RT, the 5-year actuarial local control rates were 33 and 85%, suggesting that postoperative adjuvant RT may improve local control ($p = 0.004$) *(57)*. However, this single study suffered from small sample sizes.

Prospectively collected outcomes data of LE as the sole treatment for T2 tumors are lacking *(48,58)*. The CALGB 8984 trial enrolled 51 patients who underwent LE and postoperative RT (5,400 cGy in 30 fractions) with radiosensitizing 5-FU. The 10-year estimated local recurrence was 18% and the 10-year survival is 66%. The only independent predictor of recurrence was lymphovascular invasion *(48)*. Thus, LE and postoperative chemoradiation has been practiced, although rigorous proof of its oncologic advantage over LE alone remains ill-defined.

Outcomes of Preoperative Chemoradiation Followed by LE for T2 Tumors

Neoadjuvant chemoradiation followed by SR has become a part of a standard treatment regimen for patients with locally advanced (T3 or higher) or node-positive rectal cancer, due to a local control and survival advantage *(3)*. An extension of this concept led several investigators to use neoadjuvant chemoradiation in combination with LE, with hopes of improved outcomes when compared to LE alone *(59)*. Small institutional series including a mixture of T2N0, T3N0, and T3N1 tumors have suggested that complete pathologic response (CR) to neoadjuvant therapy may be achieved in 30–73% of the cases. Additionally, local and distant tumor recurrence rates are low among those who achieve CR *(60,61)*. However, with relatively small numbers of patients with T2N0 tumors and highly variable outcomes, these studies did not constitute adequate evidence to direct clinical practice.

Recognizing the need for further data regarding such a novel treatment approach, there is an ongoing prospective phase II clinical trial sponsored by the American College of Surgeons Oncology Group (ACOSOG Z6041) *(62)*. Patients with rectal adenocarcinoma staged as T2N0 by EUS or MRI are eligible for the trial. The neoadjuvant therapy component consists of external beam RT, capecitabine, and oxaliplatin. Patients undergo LE are then followed for disease recurrence, survival, and quality of life outcomes.

Recently, a prospective randomized trial involving neoadjuvant chemoradiation therapy has been reported. Lezoche et al randomized 70 patients with T2 rectal cancer to either TEM or laparoscopic total mesorectal excision (either LAR or APR) *(63)*. All patients received neoadjuvant radiation (5,040 cGy) with 5-FU. After a median of 7 years of follow-up, no statistically significant difference was seen in either 5-year local failure rate (TEM vs. laparoscopic resection: 5.7 vs. 2.8%), or OS rate (94 vs. 94%). These results await further confirmation by other studies with larger sample sizes.

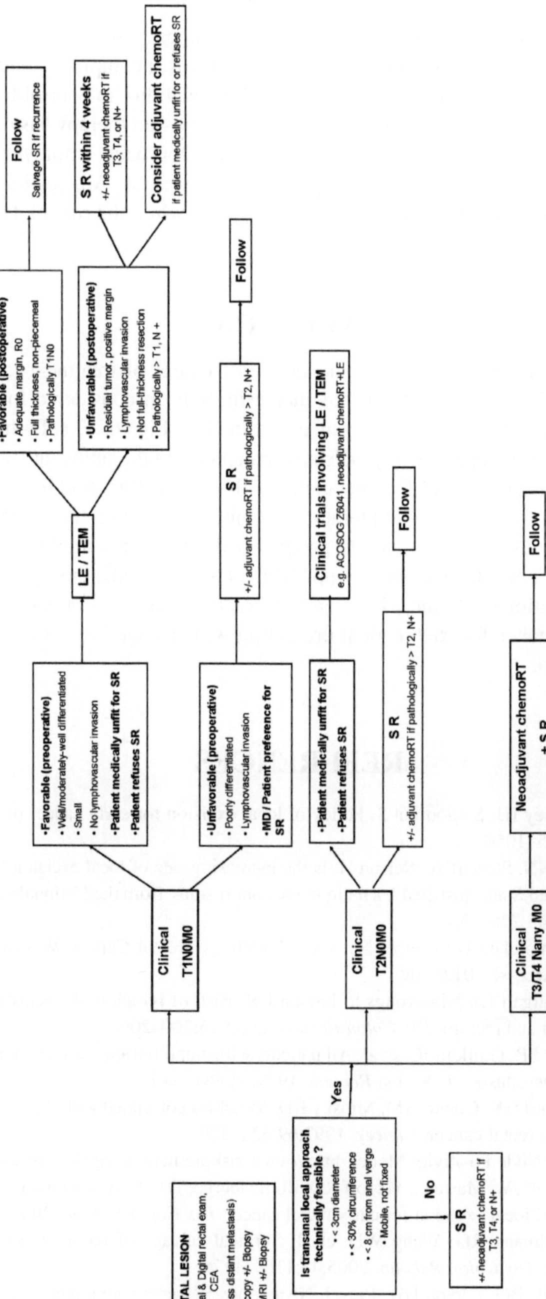

Fig. 6. A clinical algorithm for considering LE for early-stage rectal cancer.

Summary

Conventional LE alone appears to compromise oncologic outcomes if used to treat T2 tumors. However, oncologic outcomes of LE alone remains incompletely understood based on currently available retrospective data, because of the inability to control for preoperative selection biases based on patient factors. The benefit of adjuvant therapy has not been definitively demonstrated in a comparative study, while an approach employing neoadjuvant therapy is under investigation through prospective clinical trials. Application of LE for T2 tumors should be limited to these trial settings at present, while the role of TEM remains to be confirmed in larger trials.

CONCLUSIONS

With an increasing desire to refine and tailor the extent of treatment to the extent of disease for each individual patient, LE has increasingly been considered for patients with stage I rectal cancer. A clinical algorithm is outlined in Fig. 6. For T1 tumors, current evidence suggests that appropriately selected patients should enjoy an acceptable OS. However, existing data suggests LE is associated with a nearly threefold increase in the local failure rate. For T2 tumors, available literature is limited by the presence of strong selection biases that favor the use of LE in elderly patients with multiple comorbidities. Until long-term oncologic data become available to support LE for T2 lesions, this approach should be considered investigational. On the whole, an individualized analysis of benefits and risks of LE should be undertaken for each patient presenting with a stage I rectal cancer amendable to transanal excision.

REFERENCES

1. Morson BC, Bussey HJ, Samoorian S. Policy of local excision for early cancer of the colorectum. *Gut.* 1977;18:1045–1050.
2. You YN, Baxter NN, Stewart A, Nelson H. Is the increasing rate of local excision for stage I rectal cancer in the United States justified?: a nationwide cohort study from the National Cancer Database. *Ann Surg.* 2007;245:726–733.
3. The National Comprehensive Cancer Network Guidelines. Rectal Cancer. Version 4. http://www.nccn.org/; 2008 Accessed 01.01.09.
4. Nascimbeni R, Burgart LJ, Nivatvongs S, Larson DR. Risk of lymph node metastasis in T1 carcinoma of the colon and rectum. *Dis Colon Rectum.* 2002;45:200–206.
5. Blumberg D, Paty PB, Guillem JG, et al. All patients with small intramural rectal cancers are at risk for lymph node metastasis. *Dis Colon Rectum.* 1999;42:881–885.
6. Brodsky JT, Richard GK, Cohen AM, Minsky BD. Variables correlated with the risk of lymph node metastasis in early rectal cancer. *Cancer.* 1992;69:322–326.
7. St Mark's Lymph Node Positivity Model. http://www.riskprediction.org.uk/; Accessed 15.12.08.
8. Friel CM, Cromwell JW, Marra C, Madoff RD, Rothenberger DA, Garcia-Aguilar J. Salvage radical surgery after failed local excision for early rectal cancer. *Dis Colon Rectum.* 2002;45:875–879.
9. Weiser MR, Landmann RG, Wong WD, et al. Surgical salvage of recurrent rectal cancer after transanal excision. *Dis Colon Rectum.* 2005;48:1169–1175.
10. Hahnloser D, Wolff BG, Larson DW, Ping J, Nivatvongs S. Immediate radical resection after local excision of rectal cancer: an oncologic compromise? *Dis Colon Rectum.* 2005;48:429–437.
11. Bleday R. Local excision of rectal cancer. *World J Surg.* 1997;21:706–714.
12. Kraske P, Perry EG, Hinrichs B. A new translation of professor Dr P. Kraske's Zur Exstirpation Hochsitzender Mastdarmkrebse. 1885. *Aust N Z J Surg.* 1989;59:421–424.

13. Mason AY. Transsphincteric approach to rectal lesions. *Surg Annu*. 1977;9:171–194.
14. Madden JL, Kandalaft S. Electrocoagulation. A primary and preferred method of treatment for cancer of the rectum. *Ann Surg*. 1967;166:413–419.
15. Touzios J, Ludwig KA. Local management of rectal neoplasia. *Clin Colon Rectal Surg*. 2008;21: 291–299.
16. Tytherleigh MG, Warren BF, Mortensen NJ. Management of early rectal cancer. *Br J Surg*. 2008;95:409–423.
17. Paty PB, Nash GM, Baron P, et al. Long-term results of local excision for rectal cancer. *Ann Surg*. 2002;236:522–529; discussion 529–530.
18. Moore JS, Cataldo PA, Osler T, Hyman NH. Transanal endoscopic microsurgery is more effective than traditional transanal excision for resection of rectal masses. *Dis Colon Rectum*. 2008;51:1026–1030; discussion 1030–1021.
19. Sengupta S, Tjandra JJ. Local excision of rectal cancer: what is the evidence? *Dis Colon Rectum*. 2001;44:1345–1361.
20. Varma MG, Rogers SJ, Schrock TR, Welton ML. Local excision of rectal carcinoma. *Arch Surg*. 1999;134:863–867; discussion 867–868.
21. Faivre J, Chaume J, Pigot F, Trojani M, Bonichon F. Transanal electroresection of small rectal cancer: a sole treatment? *Dis Colon Rectum*. 1996;39:270–278.
22. Frazee RC, Patel R, Belew M, Roberts JW, Hendricks JC. Transanal excision of rectal carcinoma. *Am Surg*. 1995;61:714–717.
23. Wong CS, Stern H, Cummings BJ. Local excision and post-operative radiation therapy for rectal carcinoma. *Int J Radiat Oncol Biol Phys*. 1993;25:669–675.
24. Whiteway J, Nicholls RJ, Morson BC. The role of surgical local excision in the treatment of rectal cancer. *Br J Surg*. 1985;72:694–697.
25. DeCosse JJ, Wong RJ, Quan SH, Friedman NB, Sternberg SS. Conservative treatment of distal rectal cancer by local excision. *Cancer*. 1989;63:219–223.
26. Lamont JP, McCarty TM, Digan RD, Jacobson R, Tulanon P, Lichliter WE. Should locally excised T1 rectal cancer receive adjuvant chemoradiation? *Am J Surg*. 2000;180:402–405; discussion 405–406.
27. Gonzalez QH, Heslin MJ, Shore G, Vickers SM, Urist MM, Bland KI. Results of long-term follow-up for transanal excision for rectal cancer. *Am Surg*. 2003;69:675–678; discussion 678.
28. Chorost MI, Petrelli NJ, McKenna M, Kraybill WG, Rodriguez-Bigas MA. Local excision of rectal carcinoma. *Am Surg*. 2001;67:774–779.
29. Ellis LM, Mendenhall WM, Bland KI, Copeland EM 3rd. Local excision and radiation therapy for early rectal cancer. *Am Surg*. 1988;54:217–220.
30. Hershman MJ, Myint AS, Makin CA. Multi-modality approach in curative local treatment of early rectal carcinomas. *Colorectal Dis*. 2003;5:445–450.
31. Le Voyer TE, Hoffman JP, Cooper H, Ross E, Sigurdson E, Eisenberg B. Local excision and chemoradiation for low rectal T1 and T2 cancers is an effective treatment. *Am Surg*. 1999;65:625–630; discussion 630–621.
32. Rouanet P, Saint Aubert B, Fabre JM, et al. Conservative treatment for low rectal carcinoma by local excision with or without radiotherapy. *Br J Surg*. 1993;80:1452–1456.
33. Read DR, Sokil S, Ruiz-Salas G. Transanal local excision of rectal cancer. *Int J Colorectal Dis*. 1995;10:73–76.
34. Romano G, Rotondano G, Esposito P, Novi A, Santangelo ML. Transanal excision and postoperative radiation therapy in selected patients with cancer of the low rectum. *Int Surg*. 1996;81:40–44.
35. Taylor RH, Hay JH, Larsson SN. Transanal local excision of selected low rectal cancers. *Am J Surg*. 1998;175:360–363.
36. Willett CG, Compton CC, Shellito PC, Efird JT. Selection factors for local excision or abdominoperineal resection of early stage rectal cancer. *Cancer*. 1994;73:2716–2720.
37. Garcia-Aguilar J, Mellgren A, Sirivongs P, Buie D, Madoff RD, Rothenberger DA. Local excision of rectal cancer without adjuvant therapy: a word of caution. *Ann Surg*. 2000;231:345–351.
38. Mellgren A, Sirivongs P, Rothenberger DA, Madoff RD, Garcia-Aguilar J. Is local excision adequate therapy for early rectal cancer? *Dis Colon Rectum*. 2000;43:1064–1071; discussion 1071–1064.

39. Bentrem DJ, Okabe S, Wong WD, et al. T1 adenocarcinoma of the rectum: transanal excision or radical surgery? *Ann Surg*. 2005;242:472–477; discussion 477–479.
40. Madbouly KM, Remzi FH, Erkek BA, et al. Recurrence after transanal excision of T1 rectal cancer: should we be concerned? *Dis Colon Rectum*. 2005;48:711–719; discussion 719–721.
41. Nascimbeni R, Nivatvongs S, Larson DR, Burgart LJ. Long-term survival after local excision for T1 carcinoma of the rectum. *Dis Colon Rectum*. 2004;47:1773–1779.
42. Ptok H, Marusch F, Meyer F, et al. Oncological outcome of local vs radical resection of low-risk pT1 rectal cancer. *Arch Surg*. 2007;142:649–655; discussion 656.
43. Endreseth BH, Myrvold HE, Romundstad P, Hestvik UE, Bjerkeset T, Wibe A. Transanal excision vs. major surgery for T1 rectal cancer. *Dis Colon Rectum*. 2005;48:1380–1388.
44. Folkesson J, Johansson R, Pahlman L, Gunnarsson U. Population-based study of local surgery for rectal cancer. *Br J Surg*. 2007;94:1421–1426.
45. Bleday R, Breen E, Jessup JM, Burgess A, Sentovich SM, Steele G Jr. Prospective evaluation of local excision for small rectal cancers. *Dis Colon Rectum*. 1997;40:388–392.
46. Coco C, Magistrelli P, Granone P, Roncolini G, Picciocchi A. Conservative surgery for early cancer of the distal rectum. *Dis Colon Rectum*. 1992;35:131–136.
47. Fortunato L, Ahmad NR, Yeung RS, et al. Long-term follow-up of local excision and radiation therapy for invasive rectal cancer. *Dis Colon Rectum*. 1995;38:1193–1199.
48. Greenberg JA, Shibata D, Herndon JE 2nd, Steele GD Jr, Mayer R, Bleday R. Local excision of distal rectal cancer: an update of cancer and leukemia group B 8984. *Dis Colon Rectum*. 2008;51:1185–1191; discussion 1191–1184.
49. Russell AH, Harris J, Rosenberg PJ, et al. Anal sphincter conservation for patients with adenocarcinoma of the distal rectum: long-term results of radiation therapy oncology group protocol 89–02. *Int J Radiat Oncol Biol Phys*. 2000;46:313–322.
50. Steele GD Jr, Herndon JE, Bleday R, et al. Sphincter-sparing treatment for distal rectal adenocarcinoma. *Ann Surg Oncol*. 1999;6:433–441.
51. Winde G, Nottberg H, Keller R, Schmid KW, Bunte H. Surgical cure for early rectal carcinomas (T1). Transanal endoscopic microsurgery vs. anterior resection. *Dis Colon Rectum*. 1996;39:969–976.
52. Minsky BD, Cohen AM, Enker WE, Mies C. Sphincter preservation in rectal cancer by local excision and postoperative radiation therapy. *Cancer*. 1991;67:908–914.
53. Benson R, Wong CS, Cummings BJ, et al. Local excision and postoperative radiotherapy for distal rectal cancer. *Int J Radiat Oncol Biol Phys*. 2001;50:1309–1316.
54. Rich TA, Weiss DR, Mies C, Fitzgerald TJ, Chaffey JT. Sphincter preservation in patients with low rectal cancer treated with radiation therapy with or without local excision or fulguration. *Radiology*. 1985;156:527–531.
55. Wagman R, Minsky BD, Cohen AM, Saltz L, Paty PB, Guillem JG. Conservative management of rectal cancer with local excision and postoperative adjuvant therapy. *Int J Radiat Oncol Biol Phys*. 1999;44:841–846.
56. Bouvet M, Milas M, Giacco GG, Cleary KR, Janjan NA, Skibber JM. Predictors of recurrence after local excision and postoperative chemoradiation therapy of adenocarcinoma of the rectum. *Ann Surg Oncol*. 1999;6:26–32.
57. Chakravarti A, Compton CC, Shellito PC, et al. Long-term follow-up of patients with rectal cancer managed by local excision with and without adjuvant irradiation. *Ann Surg*. 1999;230:49–54.
58. Marks G, Mohiuddin MM, Masoni L, Pecchioli L. High-dose preoperative radiation and full-thickness local excision. A new option for patients with select cancers of the rectum. *Dis Colon Rectum*. 1990;33:735–739.
59. Borschitz T, Wachtlin D, Mohler M, Schmidberger H, Junginger T. Neoadjuvant chemoradiation and local excision for T2-3 rectal cancer. *Ann Surg Oncol*. 2008;15:712–720.
60. Kim CJ, Yeatman TJ, Coppola D, et al. Local excision of T2 and T3 rectal cancers after downstaging chemoradiation. *Ann Surg*. 2001;234:352–358; discussion 358–359.

61. Ruo L, Guillem JG, Minsky BD, Quan SH, Paty PB, Cohen AM. Preoperative radiation with or without chemotherapy and full-thickness transanal excision for selected T2 and T3 distal rectal cancers. *Int J Colorectal Dis*. 2002;17:54–58.
62. American College of Surgeons Oncology Group Z 6041. http://www.acosog.org/; Accessed 15.12.2008.
63. Lezoche G, Baldarelli M, Guerrieri M, et al. A prospective randomized study with a 5-year minimum follow-up evaluation of transanal endoscopic microsurgery versus laparoscopic total mesorectal excision after neoadjuvant therapy. *Surg Endosc*. 2008;22:352–358.
64. Buess G. Transanal endoscopic microsurgery. *J R Coll Surg Edinb*. 1993;38:239–245.

4 Total Mesorectal Excision and Lateral Pelvic Lymph Node Dissection

Miranda Kusters, Yoshihiro Moriya, Harm J.T. Rutten, and Cornelis J.H. van de Velde

TOTAL MESORECTAL EXCISION

Introduction

For rectal cancer, surgery is the principal treatment for cure. The main goal of surgical treatment is en bloc excision of the primary tumor with its locoregional lymph nodes. Furthermore, the focus of surgery is not only radical resection of the distal margin, but even more importantly at the circumferential margin. If the rectum is not removed within its envelope of mesorectal fascia, a subtotal resection with persistence of tumor cells and subsequent high chance for local recurrence is likely to occur.

In preoperative preparation, two aspects are essential in deciding whether, and which surgery, should be performed. First, the extent of spread of the tumor both locally and systemically needs to be established. This is achieved by physical examination, endoscopy, and preoperative imaging. Ideally, patients with rectal cancer are evaluated and discussed in a multidisciplinary setting and decisions as to whether neoadjuvant (chemo)radiation therapy can be made, especially in the setting of possible circumferential resection margin (CRM) involvement and/or nodal status. Tumors invading surrounding structures require en bloc resection with the primary tumor in order to prevent tumor spill. In unresectable, obstructive disease, palliative surgery may be required in the form of stoma construction.

Second is the evaluation of the fitness of the patient, as elderly patients often present with comorbidities, predisposing them to a higher likelihood of perioperative complications and associated higher risk of perioperative mortality. Postoperative mortality is at least

From: *Current Clinical Oncology: Rectal Cancer*,
Edited by: B.G. Czito and C.G. Willett, DOI: 10.1007/978-1-60761-567-5_4,

double in elderly patients following resection compared to their younger counterparts (*1*). Further, in addition to oncological outcomes, postoperative quality of life is an objective in clinical decision making. Thus, good physical and mental condition is a prerequisite for major surgery.

History

The surgical treatment of rectal cancer has undergone significant evolution over several centuries. In the eighteenth century, the only resolution of obstructing colorectal cancer was a diverting colostomy. The first successful perineal excision of the rectum was performed by Lisfranc from Paris in 1826, (*2*) although the long-term results were poor. Czerny from Heidelberg first used a combined abdominal and anal approach in 1879, (*3*) because the tumor was too large for a perineal-only approach. By 1908, this combined abdominoperineal approach was perfected by Miles, through which curative surgery of rectal cancer became reality. Miles is to be credited for having introduced rectal cancer surgery based on the primary zones of lymphatic spread (*4*). The initial operative mortality rate was 42%, although the principles of resection of the zone of upward spread and a wide perineal approach are still important in rectal surgery today. In 1939, Lloyd-Davies (*5*) performed an abdominoperineal resection in which two surgeons operated simultaneously; one on the abdominal side, while the other performed the perineal phase of the resection.

While the abdominoperineal approach was performed for low lying rectal tumors, a solely abdominal approach was used for upper rectal cancer by Hartmann in 1921 (*6*). However, restoration of continuity of the colostomy was not an objective of this procedure. In 1939, Dixon (*7*) described a primary anastomosis after anterior resection. He believed that the distal margins had to be at least 5 cm in order to completely resect intramural disease spread and that the anastomosis had to be at least 6 cm from the anal verge to maintain continence. Thus, in the first half of the twentieth century, anterior resections were only performed in sigmoid lesions and the majority of rectal surgery was through an abdominoperineal approach. When pathologic studies demonstrated that there was generally a maximum of 2 cm of intramural disease spread and the construction of a low anastomosis became technically feasible through the introduction of mechanical staplers, the anterior resection began to gradually replace the abdominoperineal approach in mid-rectal tumors during the second half of the twentieth century. However, recurrence rates following low anterior resection were disappointing. Locoregional recurrence was reported to be between 25 and 50% after "curative" surgery.

The term total mesorectal excision (TME) was first introduced in a report by Heald in 1982 (*8*). He described the "holy plane," an avascular interface between the mesorectal fascia and the parietal dorsolateral pelvic fascia. He also stated that the rectum and mesorectum are an embryologically distinct lymphovascular entity. In TME surgery, dissection is along this "holy plane" through sharp dissection, in contrast to the more conventional blunt approach. Heald reported local recurrence rates well below 10% and survival rates of up to 87%.

The pathological basis of lateral tumor spread in the mesorectum was detailed by Quirke in 1986 (*9*). In contrast to routine sampling methods in which blocks are taken only from the distal surface, he developed a method in which tumor and mesorectum were sliced in the transverse plane. On an early analysis, the lateral resection margin involvement by tumor was present in 14 of 52 curatively operated patients, of which 85% developed local recurrence as a result of incomplete surgical resection. Quirke advocated that a TME might improve the results of the anterior resection.

Nowadays, the principle of TME has been accepted worldwide. An additional advantage of TME surgery is the excellent exposure of the pelvic floor and relative ease with which the surgeon is able to perform an anastomosis at this level. This fact has resulted in a steady decrease in rates of abdominoperineal resection in parallel to the increasing implementation of TME surgery.

Anatomical Considerations

The pelvis can be divided into two distinct anatomical compartments: the visceral and the parietal. The rectum and the anterior organs are the visceral organs, enveloped in the visceral fascia. The rectum is surrounded by a layer of fatty tissue, which contains lymph nodes and the superior and middle rectal vessels. The parietal compartment is the muscular and bony pelvic wall, covered by the parietal fascia.

Posterior to the rectum, the visceral and parietal fascia are separated by a layer of loose connective tissue. At the level of the third or fourth sacral vertebrae, a double layer of visceral fascia is present, the rectosacral fascia, which is firmly attached to the parietal fascia on the sacrum.

Anteriorly, between the visceral fascia covering the mesorectum and the seminal vessels and prostate in males, or the vagina in females, is Denonvilliers' fascia. More cranially, the peritoneum covering the pelvic organs reaches its deepest fold at the peritoneal reflection.

Laterally, the visceral fascia is attached to the pelvic side wall in the upper rectum. At the level of the mid-rectum, the attachment consists of thicker connective tissue, often referred to as the lateral ligament. This ligament contains the relatively small middle rectal vessels, lymphatic tissue and neurologic structures.

The pelvic nervous system is an intricate network of sympathetic and parasympathetic nerves (Fig. 1) *(10)*. The preaortic hypogastric plexus originates from ventral roots of T12 through L2. These sympathetic fibers extend downward to the sacral promontory behind the pelvic fascia, where they divide into two hypogastric nerves. The parasympathetic nerves originate from the roots of S2–S4, which enter the pelvis through the sacral foramina. Laterally, the hypogastric nerves blend with these sacral nerves to form the inferior hypogastric plexus. This plexus lies in close proximity to the lateral part of the mesorectum. At this level, some branches of the plexus penetrate the mesorectal fascia for innervation of the rectum. The majority of the hypogastric plexus branches travel more anteriorly to innervate the urogenitary organs.

Technique

After a midline incision and retraction of the omentum and small intestine, the peritoneum is opened to the left of the sigmoid. The sigmoid is mobilized in an avascular plane between the mesocolon and the retroperitoneal fascia. The ureter and the ovarian (or spermatic) vessels lie just below this fascia. At the level of the sigmoid artery distal to the left colic branch, the superior rectal artery can be ligated and divided. In case of a high tie of the inferior mesenteric artery, it is important to identify the superior hypogastric plexus. Damage to this plexus might result in ejaculation disorders and urinary incontinence. The mesenteric vein can be ligated at the level of the artery. However, a tie just inferior to the pancreatic border enables maximal mobilization of the left colon, which may facilitate a low anastomosis in a later stage of the procedure. The mesosigmoid is divided and the sigmoid colon or distal colon is transsected with a considerable proximal margin from the tumor, at a level where good vascular supply is guaranteed.

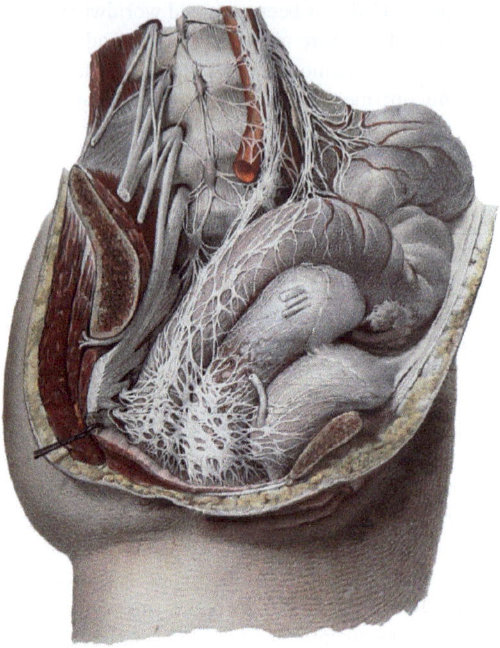

Fig. 1. Anatomic drawing of autonomic nervous system in a female pelvis *(10)*.

In the phase that follows, an undisturbed view and adequate lightning is essential. As the rectosigmoid is lifted anteriorly, the plane between the visceral and parietal fascia is identified. The presacral plane is opened sharply by diathermy or scissors. At the lateral side, the hypogastric nerves can be identified. Extending downward, the fascia on the piriform muscle, which is continuous with the rectosacral fascia, is uncovered. At the inferior margin of the piriform muscle, the pelvic splanchnic nerves are located. By meticulous sharp cuts of the parietal fascia, the roots of these nerves are exposed.

Subsequently, the rectosigmoid is moved posteriorly and the peritoneum is incised just anterior to the peritoneal reflection. Continuing the dissection between the rectum and the seminal vesicles or the posterior vaginal wall, Denonvilliers' fascia is identified. It serves as the reference plane, on which sharp dissection is carried downward and laterally. At the lateral edges of Denonvilliers' fascia the inferior hypogastric plexus divides into branches to the rectum (lateral ligament) and the genitourinary organs. By pushing the rectum contralaterally and dorsally, the branch to the rectum can easily be divided. Electrocautery should not be used to avoid damage to the inferior hypogastric plexus. Denonvilliers' fascia ends distal to the prostate in males and proximal to the perineal body in females. At this level, further dissection is possible only in the thin ventral mesorectum. After transsection of the lateral ligament, the lateral mesorectum can be followed down to the pelvic floor.

Then, the rectum is only attached to the pelvic floor. Dependent on tumor location, the next step is either the perineal phase in the case of an abdominoperineal resection, or cross-clamping, washing out, dividing and stapling of the rectum in the case of a low anterior resection.

Nerve-Sparing Surgery

Deliberate tracking and preservation of the autonomic nerves combined with TME was introduced in Western countries and performed in 246 patients with Dukes B or C rectal cancer by Enker, beginning in 1991 *(11)*. The 5-year local recurrence and survival rates were 7.3 and 74.2%, respectively. Functional results in a group of 136 patients showed that 73% of the males and 64% of the females had no urinary complaints. In male patients, sexual function was related to age and to the type of surgery. All 33 patients who were younger than 60 years and who underwent low anterior resection maintained erection and sexual function. After APR and in older patients, however, spontaneous erection was diminished in 19–29% and ejaculation disturbed in two-thirds of the patients. In female patients, 86% of sexually active patients remained sexually active after the operation *(12)*. Since these reports, functional results have been further studied extensively.

Urinary Function

The sympathetic nervous system plays a major role in urinary continence, while the parasympathetic nervous system is essential for normal voiding *(13)*. Symptoms associated with injury include difficulty in bladder emptying, overflow incontinence, and loss of sensation of bladder fullness. However, it is still unclear exactly what injury and to which autonomic nerves or plexuses causes urinary dysfunction.

Currently, the incidence of urinary dysfunction after TME surgery varies between 30 and 70% *(14–17)*. In the Dutch TME trial, in which 785 patients were questioned about urinary function, incontinence was reported in 38% of patients and voiding difficulties in 31% *(18)*. Preoperative incontinence and female gender were risk factors for incontinence, while preoperative voiding dysfunction, intraoperative blood loss, and autonomic nerve damage were associated with voiding difficulties.

Thus, damage to the autonomic nerves during surgery is still a major problem. Adequate autonomic nerve identification is influenced by patient gender, the learning curve of the surgeon, and T-stage *(15)*. Intraoperative blood loss and obesity also make identification difficult, and nerve sparing virtually impossible *(18,19)*.

Causes of urinary dysfunction other than pelvic nerve damage have also been identified. Previous hysterectomy in females and posterior tilting of the bladder during an abdominoperineal resection may weaken the pelvic floor, aggravating incontinence *(20)*. Further, surgical interruption of the levator ani muscle innervation during abdominoperineal surgery may result in loss of support of the bladder, which can be associated with incontinence *(21)*. Radiotherapy seems to have less influence on urinary function.

Sexual Function

Sacrifice of the superior hypogastric plexus in males is associated with ejaculation dysfunction. Impotence is probably the result of damage to the inferior hypogastric plexus *(13)*. In females the sympathetic nerves are considered responsible for the rhythmic contraction of the genital ducts and organs during an orgasm. The parasympathetic nerves are associated with increased blood flow to the vagina and vulva, causing vaginal lubrication and swelling of the labia and the clitoris *(22)*. However, reports on sexual function in women are scarce and many aspects are still unknown.

The largest study published about autonomic nerve preservation with TME is the Dutch TME trial. Four hundred ninety-three patients received no neoadjuvant therapy. Before treatment 78% male patients and 50% of female patients were sexually active. Two years after surgery, 76% of the males who were previously active were still active; for females this was 90%. In males, erection and ejaculation disorders occurred in 47 and 32%, respectively.

Vaginal dryness occurred in 35% of the females and pain during intercourse was present in 20%. Radiotherapy had a negative influence on sexual activity and functioning *(23)*.

Therefore, even after preservation of the autonomic nerves, sexual functioning frequently declines after TME surgery. As most patients are older, one factor of influence might be a physiological decline in sexual function, as well as a higher prevalence of cardiovascular disease with associated medications that may impact sexual functioning *(24)*. Further, nerve preservation is more difficult during APR-surgery compared to low anterior resection, as determination of the correct surgical plane and visibility in the perineal phase is challenging. In addition, as the results of the TME trial show, the addition of radiotherapy influences sexual functioning considerably *(23)*. A short- or long course of radiotherapy is the standard neoadjuvant treatment in most Western countries, adding further morbidity.

Defecation Function

Normal defecation function is dependent on adequate defecation reflexes, which are an interaction between reservoir and sphincteric functions. Sphincter-saving surgery has become increasingly common since the introduction of stapling devices and better assessment of the extent of intramural tumor growth. However, a portion of the patients having undergone a low anterior resection suffer from defecation dysfunction, such as soiling, incontinence, and urgency. This is referred to as the low anterior syndrome.

Incontinence is reported to be present in 20–40% of patients undergoing sphincter-saving procedures *(25,26)*. The exact mechanism of incontinence is unknown, but poor functional outcomes are associated with low anastomoses or anastomotic leakage *(27)*. Lower anastomoses may cause more injury to structures in the sphincter complex, causing a deterioration of reservoir function and loss of the defecation reflex. To improve continence in very low anterior resection, the construction of a colonic J-pouch has been suggested *(28)*. Reduction of capacity of the neorectum following an anastomotic leak might underlie the increased incidence of defecation dysfunction *(29)*. Radiotherapy also has been described as reducing fecal continence, causing incontinence in 50–60% of patients *(23,25–27)*. The anal function is probably maintained after radiotherapy, although rectal compliance might be compromised *(27)*. The avoidance of a permanent stoma by sphincter-saving surgery is generally seen as the best strategy. However, patients having undergone an abdominoperineal resection have been reported to have fewer physical and psychological difficulties compared to patients undergoing low anterior resection *(23)*.

Besides the role of parasymphathetic and symphathetic nerve supply in fecal and urinary continence, recently the role of a previously neglected nerve, the levator ani nerve, has been described *(30)*. Common knowledge is that the pudendal nerve innervates the levator ani muscle, but the levator ani nerve is a separate nerve, which arises from the sacral nerves S3 and/or S4. It lies in the field of TME surgery and can be disrupted during the operation, when the parietal fascia is accidentally entered during posterior dissection. The risk of levator ani nerve disruption is substantial, especially in low lying tumors, which could contribute to an increased risk of urinary and fecal incontinence. Adhering to the surgical plane, refraining from blunt dissection and improving rectal traction may lower the risk of levator ani nerve disruption *(30)*.

Anastomotic Leakage

Anastomotic leakage is one of the most serious and potentially life-threatening complications in colorectal surgery. Since the introduction of TME the risk for symptomatic anastomotic leakage has increased *(31)*. This can probably be explained by the increase in sphincter-saving procedures and subsequent lower anastomoses since the introduction of TME.

Other explanations might be compromised blood supply to the remaining rectum by TME and accumulation of hematoma in the large pelvic space after removal of the mesorectum, leading to pelvic sepsis *(32)*.

Currently the incidence of anastomotic leakage in patients undergoing a low anterior resection with the TME technique is around 10–18% *(32–35)*. However, comparison of studies is difficult due to a lack of standardized definitions. Anastomotic leakage may present as generalized peritonitis requiring abdominal reoperation; however, pelvic abscesses, discharge of pus per rectum or a rectovaginal fistula are defined as anastomotic leakage in some reports. Sometimes a subclinical leak is only incidentally detected on contrasted radiographic studies. This wide spectrum of presentations of anastomotic leakage thus not only makes it difficult to accurately report the incidence, but also hinders adequate detection of this life-threatening condition in individual cases.

In retrospective studies with uni- and multivariate analysis, several risk factors are associated with anastomotic leakage in rectal cancer. There is common agreement that male gender and low anastomoses are important risk factors *(34,36)*. Other technical factors have been reported as factors of influence, including bowel preparation, pelvic haemostasis, anastomotic tension, complete doughnuts, and intraoperative testing of the anastomosis *(34)*. Whether the operation was performed in an emergency setting and whether the anastomosis was hand-sewn or stapled also seems to affect the incidence of anastomotic leakage *(37,38)*. In the Dutch TME trial the absence of pelvic drainage and the absence of a covering stoma were associated with an anastomotic leakage *(32)*. Lastly, preoperative radiotherapy is mentioned as a predisposing factor in some studies, *(35,39–41)* while this was not found in large randomized studies *(42–44)*.

The 30-day postoperative mortality rate after anastomotic leakage is generally between 10 and 20% *(32,33,45,46)*. However, even if postoperative deaths are excluded, patients with an anastomotic leak have a poorer prognosis. Anastomotic leakage is even reported to be associated with oncologic outcomes following rectal cancer surgery. Local recurrence rates are higher in patients with anastomotic leakage, *(33,46,47)* although this is not confirmed in all studies *(48)*. There are a few theories explaining the mechanisms by which anastomotic leakage may adversely affect oncologic results. First, there is some evidence that local tumor recurrence after anastomotic leakage can be caused by a "wash-out" of exfoliated tumor cells from the bowel lumen into the wound cavity, *(49,50)* resulting in disease upstaging and reducing survival. Secondly, the inflammatory response to anastomotic leakage might play a role. The release of proinflammatory cytokines and growth factors as part of the systemic inflammatory response secondary to intra-abdominal sepsis, and the associated immunosuppression, may have a direct effect on the growth of residual tumor cells *(51,52)*. Thirdly, there is a possibility that leaks occur as a consequence of other conditions, which themselves lead to local recurrence and reduced survival. We recently speculated that transit tumor cells from the lateral lymph nodes might "leak" back into the surgical wound after TME, causing local recurrence *(53)*. This tumor containing lymph fluid, collected presacrally in a seroma, could induce an inflammatory reaction which also affects the anastomosis. This theory would suggest that anastomotic leakage is not affecting tumor progression, but that tumor cells themselves indirectly cause anastomotic leakage and local recurrence. This theory remains speculative and requires further study.

Independent of what the cause of anastomotic leakage is, the best approach is prevention. Of the aforementioned risk factors, some cannot be prevented, but the specific technical factors can be influenced. Special staplers might also strengthen the anastomosis and by early identification of symptoms of anastomotic leakage, emergency situations might be prevented. Further, a construction of a diverting stoma decreases the rate of symptomatic anastomotic leakage *(35,48)*. As the fecal stream is diverted, the anastomosis can heal appropriately, although restoration of intestinal continuity by a second operation with associated morbidity and mortality must be considered. Further, it is unknown whether diversion reduces local recurrence or improves survival. Thus it can be concluded that anastomotic leakage is a severe complication of rectal surgery whose pathophysiologic mechanism remains unknown.

Possible Causes of Local Recurrence: The Dutch TME Trial

The TME trial is a large prospective randomized multicenter study in which 1,861 patients (of which 1,530 were Dutch), were enrolled between January 1996 and December 1999. This trial analyzed the effect of short-term preoperative radiotherapy (5×5 Gy) in patients operated with a TME (RT+TME), compared to patients with TME alone (TME) *(43)*. Inclusion criteria were the presence of a primary adenocarcinoma of the rectum, without evidence of metastatic disease at the time of surgery and tumor location within 15 cm from the anal verge. Patients with other malignant diseases or with fixed tumors were excluded. Standardized techniques for surgery, radiotherapy, and pathology were used *(54)*.

The 5-year local recurrence rate of patients having undergone a macroscopically complete resection was 5.6% in case of preoperative radiotherapy, compared with 10.9% in patients undergoing TME alone ($p<0.001$). Overall survival at 5 years was 64.2 and 63.5%, respectively ($p=0.902$). In multivariate analyses a significant effect of radiotherapy in reducing local recurrence risk for patients with nodal involvement, for patients with lesions between 5 and 10 cm from the anal verge, and for patients with uninvolved CRM was seen *(55)*.

In a recently conducted study, the patterns of local recurrence in the Dutch patients of the TME trial were analyzed in efforts to reconstruct the most likely mechanisms of local recurrence and the effect of preoperative radiotherapy *(56)*. All patients with a local recurrence, defined as any rectal cancer recurrence in the small pelvis, were identified. Available images of the primary tumor, the images at the time of discovery of the local recurrence and the prospective data were reviewed case by case by a team consisting of two radiologists, one radiation oncologist and one surgeon. Examining the images and data, the location of the recurrence was classified into one of the following subsites: presacral, anterior, anastomotic, lateral, or perineal. The results showed that at a median follow-up of 7.0 years, 114 of the 1417 patients developed a local recurrence; 36 patients in the RT+TME group (5-year 4.6% LR-rate) and 78 patients in the TME group (5-year 11.0% LR-rate).

The subsites of local recurrence are presented in Table 1. Presacral local recurrences occurred most in both randomisation groups (5-year local recurrence rate RT+TME: 2.0% and

Table 1
Subsites of local recurrence

	RT+TME N=713	*TME N*=704
Presacral	15 (2.0)	25 (3.6)
Lateral	9 (1.1)	14 (1.9)
Anterior	6 (0.7)	14 (1.9)
Anastomosis	5 (0.7)	19 (2.7)
Perineum	0 (0)	4 (0.6)
Unknown	1 (0.1)	2 (0.3)
Total	36 (4.6)	78 (11.0)

Values in parenthesis are 5-year LR-rates, by competing risks analysis

TME: 3.6%). There was a significant difference between the two randomisation arms in the anastomotic subsite, with 0.7% 5-year local recurrence in the RT+TME group and 2.7% in the TME group (p = 0.003). Lateral local recurrences comprised about 20% of all local recurrences.

Since this trial, preoperative imaging, preoperative therapy, surgery and adjuvant treatment modalities have changed; nonetheless, these new data give insight into the genesis of local recurrence and help in the understanding of how to prevent local relapse in current rectal cancer treatment.

ADVANCED DISEASE

In the Dutch TME trial, surgeons were trained in TME-surgery by workshops and tutorials in order to achieve optimal surgical quality. Although locally advanced tumors were supposed to be excluded, only fixed tumors at rectal examination could be identified, since routine imaging was not mandatory at that time *(43)*. However, histological evaluation of the circumferential resection margins (CRM) suggested that a substantial proportion of advanced tumors had been included *(57)*. In the TME trial CRM-positivity was 17% and even as much as 30% after an abdominoperineal resection. Our hypothesis is that this advanced disease is the main cause of the high rate of presacral local recurrences *(58)*.

An involved or close circumferential resection margin (CRM) has repeatedly been confirmed as one of the most important risk factors for local recurrence *(57)*. Apart from the CRM, T4 tumors and massive lymph node involvement (N2 disease), all signs of advanced disease, can currently be identified by preoperative MR imaging *(59,60)*. In the Dutch TME study, at least 30% of the tumors could be defined as advanced, in retrospect *(56)*. In most cases, a long course of neo-adjuvant (chemo)radiation, rather than a short-course of radiotherapy, can probably downstage these tumors and lead to better results *(61)*. Thus, nowadays, with good imaging and preoperative discussion in a multidisciplinary setting, a positive margin is probably more a sign of inadequate surgical technique rather than unrecognized advanced disease *(62)*.

LOW ANTERIOR RESECTION

In the TME trial, apart from presacral recurrences, anastomotic recurrences were relatively frequent, especially in non-irradiated LAR patients *(56)*. Most of the anastomotic recurrences following sphincter-saving surgery in limited disease could probably have been prevented by a longer distal margin. TME alone in node-positive tumors resulted in considerable local recurrence rates when distal margins were 2 cm or less. The addition of radiotherapy resulted in few local recurrences, except when distal margins were less than 5 mm.

This suggests that TME without radiotherapy in node-positive disease requires a longer distal margin than in node-negative disease. Without preoperative irradiation, a short distal margin of 1 cm can be accepted in node-negative patients, whereas in node-positive patients, a margin longer than 2 cm is required. Radiotherapy can prevent anastomotic recurrences, except when distal margins are < 5 mm. MRI techniques and lymph node specific contrast agents may allow reliable assessment of lymph node status in the near future, so that customized surgery can be applied according to preoperative staging *(60,63)*.

A complicating factor in analyzing the sphincter-saving procedures in the TME trial is that a total mesorectal excision down to the pelvic floor was not mandatory and surgeons were allowed to transect the mesorectum 5 cm below the tumor. Unfortunately, it is unclear what proportion of the patients received a partial mesorectal excision instead of a TME. It has been reported that distal mesorectal spread is documented in 10-15% of rectal cancer patients, usually within 2-3 cm of primary disease and more often in the form of small mesorectal deposits than involved nodes *(64–66)*. Koh et al *(67)*, examining the distribution of mesorectal lymph nodes based on imaging and histopathology, found very few lymph nodes distal to the tumor. This in contrast to an anatomical cadaver study of Perez et al *(68)*, who found lymph nodes up to the distal third of the mesorectum.

Thus, data are conflicting, but surgeons should be aware that in node positive patients a transection of the mesorectum closer to the tumor carries a risk of leaving small tumor deposits behind. This should be kept in mind when, for whatever reason, a patient is not receiving preoperative radiotherapy. In these situations, a mesorectal transection of 5 cm below the tumor is a wise precaution.

Abdominoperineal Resection

APR-surgery has shown poor results in several reports, with higher local recurrence rates compared to low anterior resections *(69)*. In the TME trial, APR-surgery mainly resulted in presacral local recurrences *(56)*. It is known from previous studies that APR is associated with higher CRM involvement *(57)*. Anatomical and radiological studies show that in the lowest part of the rectum the mesorectum tapers and terminates at the pelvic floor *(70)*. If a tumor is located in the distal third of the rectum, the surrounding mesorectum is very thin, especially on the ventral side. Near the anal margin the visceral fascia (covering the mesorectum) blends with the parietal fascia (covering the levator ani muscle), forming the corrugator muscle, which separates the internal from the external sphincter. At this level a tumor that extends only a few millimeters beyond the muscular bowel wall is at risk for a positive margin when following the normal resection plane.

Even when negative margins are achieved, these low tumors seem to behave differently compared to proximal tumors. In studying the patterns of recurrence, as much as 18% of the CRM-negative N+ tumors operated by APR developed a local recurrence *(56)*. Apparently, in these low tumors, tumor particles still seem to be left behind, even when the circumferential margin seems sufficient, causing local recurrences at various subsites.

A wide APR, resecting the complete levator ani muscle, might provide better local control of low tumors *(58,72)*. Japanese surgeons advocate the lateral lymph node dissection (LLND), as distal tumors are known to metastasize to lateral lymph nodes, as discussed below. This can be combined with chemoradiation prior to surgery in low T3 tumors, as if they are true locally advanced disease *(73)*. This has been reported to result in downstaging and even the possibility of sphincter-saving surgery in some instances *(73)*.

Lateral Disease

Although the main lymphatic flow is upward in the mesorectum, involvement of lateral nodes outside the mesorectum does occur. In the TME trial lateral local recurrences represent about 20% of all local recurrences, a figure in accordance with an overview of Roels et al *(74)*. We can conclude that lateral disease is responsible for a considerable amount of local relapse. When analyzing only low rectal tumors, where lateral lymph node spread is especially present, the lateral recurrence rate in the nonirradiated TME group of the Dutch TME study was 2.7%, comprising 24% of all local recurrences. The difference in lateral recurrence in the RT+TME group (0.8%) vs. the TME group was significant, suggesting that radiotherapy plays a significant role in the reduction of local recurrence in the lateral pelvic subsite. Thus, radiotherapy can probably sterilize lateral tumor particles in most of the cases *(58)*.

A problem, however, arises if positive lateral lymph nodes are not included in the radiation target volume, as can occur where more accurate delineation of pertinent nodal basins are required (i.e. in intensity modulated radiation therapy (IMRT) planning). In contrast to the TME trial, in which the lateral lymph nodes were probably always irradiated, some nodal basins have the potential to be underirradiated or excluded with advanced radiation therapy planning techniques, emphasizing the importance of knowledge of patterns of spread and careful radiation planning when adopting these techniques.

The question remains, however, whether tumor cells in the lateral lymph flow routes are responsible for only lateral local recurrences, or whether they also result in recurrences in other pelvic subsites. Comparing the LLND in Japanese patients with TME in Dutch patients, the number of presacral local recurrences was higher in the Dutch group *(58)*. However, it is unclear whether this difference is caused by removal of the lateral lymph flow routes or by a wider APR practiced in Japan, resulting in less CRM involvement. We will discuss this subject further in the next section of this chapter.

Future Perspectives

The introduction of TME surgery in combination with neoadjuvant treatment has reduced the local recurrence rate considerably *(55,75)*. On a population level it seems that even survival of rectal cancer patients is steadily improving *(76)*. However, surgical treatment also carries a relative high morbidity rate *(18,23,77,78)*. It is probable that only a minority of patients benefit from the addition of neoadjuvant treatment. Improved preoperative evaluation will allow a more tailor-made approach. MRI has proven to be very accurate in visualizing the relation of the tumor with the mesorectal fascia *(60,79)*. Promising data have been published about the capability of identifying lymph node metastases with special contrast agents *(80)*. Furthermore, translational research will help to identify those patients with a high local recurrence risk and therefore benefiting from neoadjuvant treatment versus those at low risk *(81)*. It is to be expected that for the near future the quality of surgery *(71)* and the presence of lymph nodes *(82)* will remain important variables to base such a decision on. Appropriate staging of lymph nodes may open the door to more organ preserving treatments like proposed by Habr-Gama *(83)*. The best treatment for involved lymph nodes still remains uncertain: neoadjuvant treatment with its inherent toxicity or selected lymph node dissection of the lateral zones of spread. In the next part of this chapter, the role of the LLND will be explored.

LATERAL LYMPH NODE DISSECTION

From anatomic studies it has been shown that lymph node drainage occurs retrograde along the arterial vessels of the rectum. The complex network of lymphatic channels can be divided into three lymphatic flow routes. The upper route is along the superior rectal artery in the direction of the inferior mesenteric artery. The lateral route reaches from the middle rectal artery to the internal iliac and obturator basins. And the third, downward, route extends to the inguinal lymph nodes. The downward route is only involved when tumor growth has infiltrated into the anterior organs. The upper route is enveloped in the mesorectum and is thus removed in standard TME. The lateral route has been shown to be involved, especially in low and more advanced rectal cancer.

History

The treatment of lymph node metastases in the lateral lymph flow route has been controversial and has undergone different development in the East and the West.

West

The division of the rectum in two main lymphatic zones has been known since 1895, when Gerota described these from anatomic studies *(84)*. Nevertheless, the description of Miles *(4)*, of solely up- and downward spread, was generally accepted. He stated that the zones of "lateral spread" were located between the levators ani and the pelvic fascia, thus promoting a wide abdominoperineal resection as the method to resect these lymphatic networks.

Results, however, differed between lower and higher rectal carcinomas, with 5-year survival rates between 25 and 45% in lesions up to 6 cm from the anal verge and 30–80% in lesions at least 6 cm from the anal verge *(85,86)*. This difference between high and low lesions was also apparent when lesions were treated by abdominoperineal resection alone, with a similar worse outcome in local recurrence rates between high and low lesions *(87)*. Meanwhile, the significance of the peritoneal reflection and the middle valve of Houston as a landmark in low and high lesions was described by Villemin and Oliveira *(88,89)*. According to these authors, this level was the border between two lymphatic areas of the rectum.

In 1940, Coller described that in 7 of 19 very low lying rectal cancers, there was nodal involvement up to the margin of the excision of the levator ani muscle *(90)*. Dukes suggested in 1943 that growth might be laterally along the lymphatics accompanying the middle rectal vessels *(91)*. Sauer et al *(92)* stated in 1951 that the "lateral spread" suggested by Miles was an anatomic misinterpretation. He quoted previous studies in which it was described that not all nodes are located over the levators ani, but rather on the pelvic walls and within the lateral ligaments. Lateral spread into these lateral lymph nodes would be responsible for the worse results seen in low rectal cancers as compared to higher disease. Waugh and Kirklin had a similar argument *(85)*. Sauer reported on 17 patients with low rectal carcinoma undergoing extended dissection of the iliac and sacral nodes, with two cases demonstrating metastases in the lateral nodes. In higher tumors, no lateral metastases were found. In later series he reported no increase in mortality or morbidity by LLND, although survival numbers were not given.

Stearns and Deddish *(93)* examined the role of abdominopelvic lymphadenectomy in the management of rectal cancer in 1959. One hundred twenty-two patients with high and low rectal carcinoma underwent resection, although lateral lymph node metastases occurred only in tumors located <10 cm from the anal verge. In Dukes C patients, the 5-year survival for the extended operation was 40%, while it was 23% in conventional surgery. Because this difference was not significant, and morbidity was significant, the authors suggested that LLND had no beneficial effect.

Enker et al *(94)* reported on LLND in 1986 in order to set objective definitions for LLND surgery. One hundred ninety-two of 412 patients underwent en bloc pelvic lymphadenectomy, mainly for low and middle rectal tumors, combined with abdominoperineal resection or low anterior resection. A difference with the method of Stears and Deddish was that obturator compartment remained undissected, only dissecting the para-iliac nodes. Enker observed a superior survival after extended dissections, when compared to conventional resections (63.8% vs. 54.3%) in Dukes C patients in particular. There was no added operative mortality and in terms of morbidity, only urinary function was mentioned as being temporarily compromised. Enker suggested LLND as appropriate therapy when preoperative examination suggests that the rectal cancer penetrates the bowel wall.

A group of patients having undergone LLND was retrospectively reviewed by Glass in 1985 *(95)*. Based upon vague indications, namely local extension or unfavorable histologic grade, 75 patients underwent LLND. These were compared to 2,266 patients who underwent conventional resection. No improvement in 5-year survival or local recurrence rate was observed in patients with the extended resection, thus the authors concluded that no patients would benefit from LLND.

In 1992, Michelassi reported on 73 patients who had conventional surgery and 64 who underwent wide pelvic lymphadenectomy *(96)*. The indications were dependent on the surgeons' preference. There was a reduction in local recurrence rate from 16.4% to 9.4%, but this was not significant. No numbers were given on survival or morbidity.

Following this, only few reports from Italy described outcomes of LLND in Western patients, as focus was more on TME and (neo)adjuvant regimens in the treatment of rectal cancer in the 1990s.

East

Reports on the LLND in the East mainly come from Japan. There, Senba *(97)* conducted a study of lymphatic system of the rectum in more than 200 fetuses. He found the same routes as Gerota in 1908, *(84)* but also found an additional route running along the inferior rectal artery, passing through the ischiorectal fossa, to the internal iliac artery.

In a report from 1940, Kuru *(98)* applied the knowledge of the lateral lymph flow route directly to the clinical setting. One hundred twenty-six patients underwent LLND; overall lymph node involvement was 42% and lateral lymph node involvement was approximately 9%. In low rectal cancer, lateral lymph node involvement was seen in 4 of 13 cases (31%). In 1977, Koyama reported a 5-year survival of 45% in LLND patients vs. 30% in conventional surgery *(99)*.

The first English report on LLND surgery performed from 1962 to 1976 was from Hojo *(100)*. He reported better survival rates following the introduction of LLND at the National Cancer Center Hospital (NCCH) in 1969 (5-year survival rates of 71% vs. 59%). Local recurrence rate was significantly reduced in Dukes B lesions (25% to 7%). Lateral lymph node positivity was observed in 20% of low rectal cancer vs. 6% in higher cancers. In 1989, Hojo reported on urinary dysfunction and sexual dysfunction, occurring in 39 and 76%, respectively, of LLND patients *(101)*. He concluded pelvic nerves should be preserved in patients with lower rectal cancer without lymph node spread.

In 1991, Sato described the results of anatomic dissections of 45 cadavers, in which he observed that the lateral ligament could be divided into a medial part, primarily containing the middle rectal artery, and a lateral part in which the pelvic plexus was located *(102)*. To reduce urinary and sexual dysfunction Hojo reported how injury to this plexus could be avoided through nerve-sparing techniques *(103)*. Moriya described several nerve-sparing techniques in 1995 *(104,105)*. Dependent on tumor extent, total or partial nerve preserving techniques were applied. In total nerve preservation, urinary function was preserved in 98% of the cases and erection was preserved in 90%, although ejaculation was possible in only 68%. Operative time was 90 min longer as compared to more limited operations. Oncologic outcomes did not seem to be compromised by autonomic preservation *(106)*.

In 1998, Mori *(107)* reported on 803 patients in which he found lateral lymph node metastases in 25.5% of 157 patients with Dukes C stage low rectal carcinoma. The mean 5-year survival rate of patients with lateral lymph node metastases was 37.5%. Sexual function was reported to be poor in unilateral autonomic nerve preservation. In bilateral preservation erection could be achieved in 75% and ejaculation in about 50%.

In 2005, Matsumoto *(108)* analyzed 387 lymph nodes after bilateral LLND and found that 15.5% of histologically negative lymph nodes were shown by RT-PCR to harbor micrometastases. The possible survival benefit of resection of micrometastases by LLND was described by Sugihara, *(109)* who reviewed 2,916 patients from various centers. Stage II disease patients undergoing LLND had a better (87.1%) 5-year survival relative to patients without LLND (78.0%). He concluded that these results may be due to resection of micrometastases by LLND, which would not be considered to be involved in standard histopathology.

West vs. East

Comparing data on LLND is difficult, not only because of nonrandomization and selection-bias, but also because of the following differences between the East and the West, which further hinder reliable comparison.

First, the definition of rectum and low rectal cancer differs between the continents. In the West, distance from the anal verge is often measured by rigid endoscopy and the rectum is mostly defined as 15–16 cm from the anal verge *(54,110)*. The distance of a rectal carcinoma from the anal verge is the distance between the lower edge of the tumor and the anal verge. The definition of low rectal carcinoma differs per publication, but mostly between 5–6 cm from the anus, as measured by endoscopy. In the East, in particular in Japan, definitions are related to anatomy rather than endoscopic measurement. The rectum is located below the lower border of the second sacral vertebral body and the rectosigmoid is located more proximal, up to the level of the promontory *(111)*. "Low" rectal cancer is defined as a tumor of which the major part is located at or below the peritoneal reflection, as seen on preoperative imaging or as palpated intraoperatively. Due to anatomic variations and differences in sex, the distance of the peritoneal reflection to the anal verge can differ from 6 to 9 cm *(112)*. Thus, cohorts of patients with low rectal carcinoma in Japan probably also contain tumors which would be defined as "middle" in Western terms.

Secondly, pathologic techniques differ between the East and the West. In the West, the resected specimen is first fixated and then sliced in order to perform CRM measurement according to the method of Quirke *(113)*. During this process, the number of resected lymph nodes are counted. In Japan, lymph nodes are harvested from the fresh specimen by the surgeons, directly after surgery *(111)*. This immediate harvesting of lymph nodes precludes assessment of the CRM at a later stage. Thus, the focus of pathology is on CRM-management in the West and lymph node harvesting in the East. The difference in average number of lymph nodes harvested might be a result of these differences in technique, as the number of mesorectal lymph nodes (without LLND) is generally at least 20 in Japan, rarely reaching that amount in the West. Further, removal of lymph nodes might be more difficult in Western patients, as only a low number of lymph nodes could be removed from Dutch patients by Japanese clearing methods in one series *(114)*. It is well known that removal of higher numbers of lymph nodes results in better staging, or maybe even upstaging, referred to as the Will-Rogers phenomenon *(115)*. This automatically changes prognostic outcomes and therefore can be responsible for differences between various groups.

Lastly, consideration of differences in body mass index is crucial in comparing the feasibility of LLND in Japanese and Western patients. Japanese patients, particularly males, are significantly thinner than Western patients *(116)*. Obesity makes LLND with nerve-sparing techniques considerably more difficult, which might result in more complications and morbidity. These might overshadow oncologic outcomes and worsen results of LLND in Western patients, as compared to Japanese patients.

Technique

When the rectum is removed via low anterior resection or abdominoperineal resection, TME is followed by LLND. As in the TME procedure, the inferior hypogastric plexuses have been identified and separated from the proper rectal fascia; in the lateral ligament, only the lateral part is left. The lateral dissection is started along the inner side of the internal iliac vessels and proceeds down to the stump of the middle rectal artery. The vessels are cleared of lymphatics and fatty tissue by sharp dissection using electrocautery, avoiding damage to the pelvic plexus. Next, the paravesical and obturator spaces are opened between the lateral

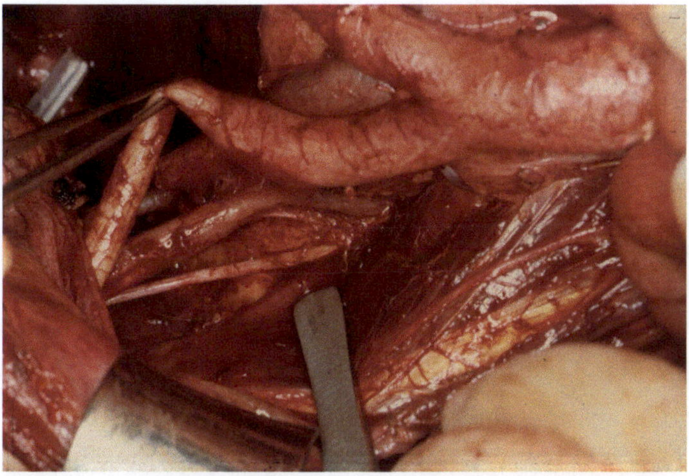

Fig. 2. Photo after a lateral lymph node dissection (LLND) with autonomic nerve preservation.

border of the internal iliac vessels and the external iliac artery. The lymphatic tissue next to the urinary bladder is cleared, sparing the vesical vessels and the distal branches of the plexus running to the anterior organs. Above the obturator channel, the obturator nerves and vessels are identified and cleared of all lymphatic tissue. After completion of the LLND, the following structures can be well identified in each lateral compartment (Fig. 2): the internal and external iliac vessels, the obturator nerve, the vesical arteries, and the pelvic nerve plexus.

According to Japanese guidelines, when involved lateral lymph nodes are suspected on preoperative evaluation or intraoperative findings, extended lateral dissection is recommended *(110,117)*. This encompasses en bloc excision of the internal iliac vessels and resection of the autonomic nervous system.

Nerve-Sparing Surgery and LLND

Various types of nerve-sparing surgery exist, even differing by institution. Total automatic nerve preservation encompasses preservation of the superior hypogastric plexus, the bilateral pelvic nerves and the inferior hypogastric plexuses (Figs. 3 and 4). Other forms include uni- and bilateral pelvic nerve and plexus preservation, with dissection of the superior hypogastric plexus. When lateral lymph nodes are suspected to be involved, no autonomic nerve preservation is conducted.

It is established that damage to the autonomic nervous system is associated with urinary and sexual function disturbance. Moreover, the psychological effects of surgery itself, having a serious disease and sometimes a stoma, have effects of functional well-being. Although there are good questionnaires, functional results are liable to subjectivity and variations in terminology. Table 2 shows functional results of Japanese studies in which total autonomic nerve preservation combined with LLND are reported. Also, results of partial preservation techniques and autonomic nerve preservation without LLND are mentioned. Generally, urinary dysfunction can be prevented by nerve preservation, except in the report by Matsuoka et al. In this study, however, many patients with partial preservation were included in the

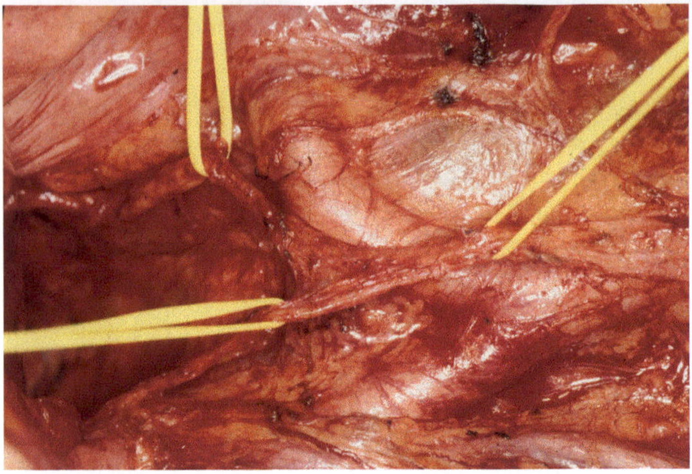

Fig. 3. Photo after nerve preservation of the superior hypogastric plexus.

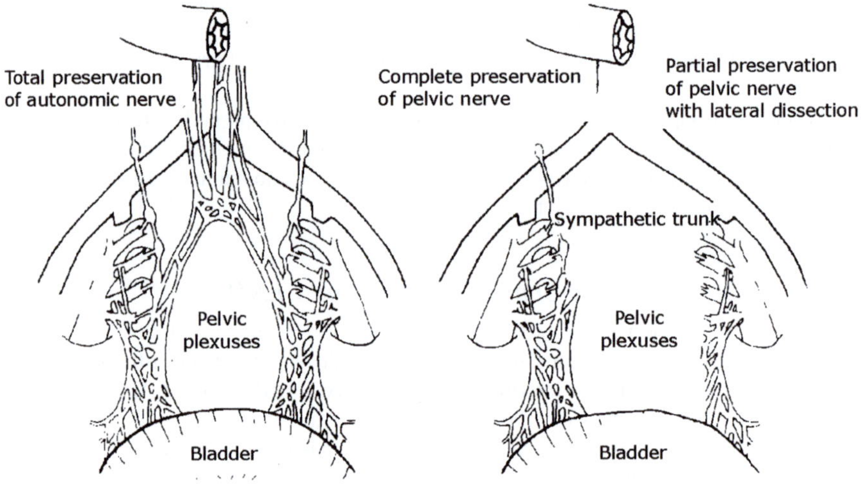

Fig. 4. Scheme of types of LLND with autonomic nerve preservation.

calculations. Sexual dysfunction varies greatly, with erectile dysfunction ranging from 10 to 83%. Ejaculatory dysfunction remains a major problem, ranging from 18 to 90%, even after nerve preservation. Unfortunately, the number of published results is too limited to make any definitive conclusions regarding outcomes comparing LLND to standard TME.

Table 2
Functional results of LLND with ANP, LLND with partial ANP and TME with ANP

			LLND with total ANP				*LLND with partial ANP*		
Name author	Year	No	UD	ErD	EjD	No	UD	ErD	EjD
Hojo *103*	1991	10	NS	28%	40%	18	NS	77%	100%
Moriya *104*	1995	31	2%	10%	32%	30	29%	73%	93%
Masui *129*	1996	98	NS	10%	18%	17	NS	47%	53%
Mori *107*	1998	45	0%	>45%	45%	64	6%	>45%	75%
Ameda *130*	2005	27	0%	83%	75%	25	8%	92%	92%
			LLND with total ANP				*TME with total ANP*		
Maeda *131*	2003	65	15%	27%	38%	12	25%	20%	40%
Matsuoka *132*	2005	15	47%	NS	NS	42	24%	NS	NS
Kyo *118*	2006	15	27%	50%	90%	22	18%	10%	30%

UD urinary dysfunction, *ErD* erectile dysfunction, *EjD* ejaculatory dysfunction, *NS* not stated

The explanation of urinary and sexual dysfunction following nerve-sparing surgery is ascribed to traction and injury to the nerves during mobilization and electrocautery required for LLND *(118)*. Although care is taken during mobilization and manipulation of the rectum in order to reach the lateral compartments, the risk of injury remains.

Patterns of Local Recurrence

In the many decades of LLND surgery in Japan, constant evaluation has been undertaken with the intent of preventing over-treatment and minimizing morbidity *(119)*. Nowadays the policy in many Japanese hospitals is case-oriented, adapting the degree of surgical resection and autonomic nerve preservation to the extent of cancer spread *(120)*. Whereas the standard procedure was to perform bilateral LLND in case of advanced rectal cancer during the 1970s and 1980s at the NCCH in Tokyo, unilateral LLND has been performed more recently.

In a recent study, we evaluated the treatment at the NCCH for rectal carcinoma at or below the peritoneal reflection between 1993 and 2002, evaluating patterns of local recurrence and risk factors for local recurrence *(53)*. Preoperative evaluation consisted of CT-imaging and endoscopic ultrasonography for all patients. Based on preoperative imaging and intraoperative findings, standard TME was performed in T1 or T2 disease without suspected lymph nodes. LLND was added to TME in stage T3 or T4 rectal cancer at or below the peritoneal reflection, or when positive mesorectal lymph nodes were suspected. Unilateral LLND was performed when the tumor was located laterally in the low rectum and bilateral LLND when the tumor was located centrally. When the lateral lymph nodes were 1 cm or larger on preoperative imaging or intraoperative findings, bilateral extended lymph node dissection was performed, consisting of dissection of the complete internal iliac arteries and the autonomic nerve system. When there was no suspicion on positive lateral lymph nodes, autonomic nerve preservation was carried out.

Of the 351 patients studied, 145 had standard TME surgery without LLND, 73 unilateral LLND and 133 patients bilateral LLND. LLND was performed in significantly younger patients and more often in combination with a nonsphincter-saving procedure, compared to patients who had not undergone LLND. The tumors in the LLND patients had higher T- and N-stages and were significantly larger. Comparing the clinicopathological characteristics

Table 3
Sites of local recurrence

	All patients			*Only N+ patients*		
Site of local recurrence	*Unilateral LLND (n=73)*	*Bilateral LLND (n=133)*	*P*	*Unilateral LLND (n=32)*	*Bilateral LLND (n=74)*	*P*
Lateral	5 (5.6)	4 (3.3)		4 (13.2)	3 (4.6)	
Ipsilateral	3 (4.5)			3 (9.9)		
Contralateral	2 (2.2)			1 (3.3)		
Presacral	2 (2.8)	0 (0)		2 (6.7)	0 (0)	
Perineal	2 (2.8)	2 (1.7)		1 (3.1)	2 (3.4)	
Anterior	0 (0)	1 (0.9)		0 (0)	1 (1.8)	
Anastomotic	3 (4.2)	2 (1.6)		3 (9.8)	2 (3.0)	
Unknown	0 (0)	1 (0.8)		0 (0)	1 (1.4)	
Total	**12**	**10**		**10**	**9**	
5-Year LR-rate	**15.4%**	**8.3%**	**0.06**	**32.8%**	**14.2%**	**0.04**

Values in parenthesis are the 5-year local recurrence rates per subsite

between the unilateral and the bilateral LLND, no significant differences were found, except that unilateral LLND was combined with autonomic nerve preservation more often.

The mean lymph node harvest was 21 lymph nodes following standard TME. After unilateral LLND, the mean number of recovered lymph nodes was 38 and following bilateral LLND, this was 45 ($p=0.004$). Overall lymph node involvement was 42% and lateral lymph node involvement was 10%. Jump metastases (negative mesorectal lymph nodes and positive lateral lymph nodes) occurred in 3% (7/207) of the patients with a LLND.

The results of this study showed a 5-year local recurrence rate of 6.6% in rectal cancer at or below the peritoneal reflection by Japanese surgery. This primarily surgical approach compares favorably to the results in Western countries, where neoadjuvant therapy is adopted as the standard treatment in order to reduce local recurrence rates. Therefore, the Japanese concept of removing the lateral basins of lymph node spread can be considered successful. Patterns of local recurrence are shown in Table 3.

This study, although retrospective, provides further evidence of disease outside the TME envelope in higher stage tumors. Bilateral LLND (5-year local recurrence rate of 14%) resulted in improved local control versus unilateral LLND (5-year local recurrence rate of 33%) in *N*+ patients (Table 3). Persistent disease in lateral lymph nodes that is left behind may account for some local recurrences, as would occur in standard TME surgery. However, if that was the case, it would be expected that most recurrences would originate in this lateral basin. In this study, we noted that not all local recurrences involved the lateral side walls. In fact, most recurrences could not be explained by the anatomical position of the lateral lymph nodes. One can only speculate about other mechanisms, including how tumor cells seed into the surgical resection bed. It is possible that removal of the lateral lymph nodes also removes (microscopic) tumor cells which are in transit in the lateral lymph flow route, which could otherwise leak back into the surgical wound. This would explain why results of unilateral dissection is inferior to bilateral dissection, resulting in more local recurrence in not only the lateral subsite, but in the presacral, perineal, and anastomotic subsites as well.

The rationale behind unilateral LLND is that the contra-lateral autonomic nervous system remains intact, as urinary and sexual dysfunction following nerve-sparing surgery is often ascribed to traction and injury to the nerves during mobilization and electrocautery required for LLND *(118)*. Unfortunately, we have no data on urinary and sexual function of this cohort and are unable to report on the results after unilateral LLND with nerve preservation. Therefore, the question whether functional results are truly better remains unanswered.

The tumors of the patients who underwent TME without LLND were smaller and less advanced compared to LLND patients. This lower staging is reflected in better survival. The fact that only one patient who had standard TME surgery had local relapse (5-year local recurrence rate of 0.8%) is striking. The selection of low-risk disease by pre- and intraoperative evaluation therefore appears accurate. Interestingly, however, pathologic evaluation showed that about 30% of patients undergoing TME had T3 or N-positive disease. Pathology appears to reveal more metastatic lymph nodes than preoperative imaging, but these (micro) metastases do not appear to impact local control. "Jump" metastases occurred in only 3% of LLND patients, thus, when mesorectal lymph nodes are unsuspected, the risk of lateral lymph node recurrence is very low.

Current Practice in Japan

Since 2003, the NCCH in Tokyo has coordinated a national multicenter randomized clinical trial comparing TME with or without LLND, with autonomic nerve preservation. The preoperative evaluation consists of endoscopic ultrasonography and MRI-imaging. Patients with histologically confirmed adenocarcinoma below the peritoneal reflection and clinical stage II or III disease are included. Patients with lymph nodes larger than 10 mm or with tumor invasion into other organs are not in included in the trial. Final accrual of 600 patients was estimated to be completed in 2009.

For patients with T1 or T2 disease without suspected lymph node involvement, TME without (neo)adjuvant therapy is the standard treatment in Japan. For T4-disease and disease with overt lateral metastases, there is currently a debate whether neoadjuvant (chemo)radiation needs to be added to TME plus LLND.

Lymphoscintigraphy

Sentinel node mapping is still in an experimental phase in colorectal cancer *(121,122)*. With this approach, visibility is compromised, especially in the rectum which is mainly located retroperitoneally. Ex vivo procedures make injection of blue dye and identification of the blue nodes possible. However, in order to identify extramesorectal lymph node drainage patterns, lymphoscintigraphy might be the most promising method. Although lymphoscintigraphic localization of sentinel nodes seems reliable in early colorectal cancers, the method might not be as accurate for the indication of lateral lymph node spread in advanced disease. Studies have shown inferior results in large rectal tumors, tumors with extensive metastases, tumors invading adjacent organs and patients receiving preoperative chemoradiation therapy *(123)*. Nonetheless, recent studies have revealed interesting results.

Funahashi et al *(124)*. injected 99 m Tc-colloid around the tumor preoperatively using a fiberscope or rectoscope. Following tumor resection by TME, "hot" nodes were identified in the pelvis using a radioactive tracer and the area of the highest nodal emission defined as the draining lymph node basin of the tumor. Following this, LLND was performed and all lymph nodes were examined histologically and immunologically. From the distribution of the hot nodes, a lateral type and a mesorectal type of lymph node basin could be identified. Seventeen of the 39 tumors (44%) drained mainly laterally and of these 17, 8 had involved lymph nodes (4 positive lateral nodes). In the 22 patients with mesorectal draining lymph node basins, one false-negative was found, which demonstrated a lateral lymph node metastasis. The authors concluded that the concordance between lymph node metastases and the draining lymph node basin was good.

Another study was performed by Kawahara et al *(125)* in order to identify the first lateral draining lymph node. Indocyanine green was injected into the rectum in 14 patients with T3 lower rectal cancer. A LLND was performed with usage of infrared ray electronic endoscopy to identify the lymph nodes. Drainage of indocyanine green into the lateral lymph nodes was seen in 6 of 14 patients (43%), which were all detected intraoperatively with the infrared endoscopy. Lymph node drainage was limited exclusively to the peri-internal iliac artery nodes.

Thus, although further studies are needed to assess its accuracy, lymphoscintigraphy may play a future role in detecting the presence of lateral lymph basins in individual patients in the East. In the absence of lateral involvement, patients might be spared from LLND. In the West, this method should also be considered in the management of lateral nodes.

Locally Advanced Disease: (Chemo)Radiation or LLND?

To date, there are no randomized studies comparing preoperative (chemo)radiotherapy and TME with LLND in similar patients, making it difficult to make a statement about which regimen is preferred in advanced rectal carcinoma. In a few nonrandomized studies, an attempt has been made to compare (neo)adjuvant treatment with LLND.

Watanabe et al *(126)* divided 115 patients into four subgroups; Rad+LLND–, Rad+LLND+, Rad–LLND+, and Rad–LLND–. Local recurrence rates, disease-free survival and overall survival were not significantly different between Rad+LLND– and Rad–LLND+. The authors suggested that preoperative radiotherapy could be an alternative for LLND in patients with low rectal carcinoma.

Kim et al *(127)* compared 176 patients with TME and postoperative chemoradiotherapy or TME combined with a LLND. The 5-year overall survival and disease-free survival rates did not differ significantly. In patients in the LLND-group with stage III low rectal cancer, local recurrence rate was 16.7%, which is higher than 7.5% in the postoperative CRT group ($p=0.044$). However, the LLND group may have contained "very low" rectal cancers *(128)*.

In our recent study, we analyzed the differences between Japan and the Netherlands in the treatment of low rectal cancer, with focus on the patterns of local recurrence *(58)*. The Dutch group consisted of patients of the TME trial; 376 patients underwent TME for low rectal cancer and 379 received preoperative radiotherapy (RT+TME). Three hundred twenty-four patients were analyzed in the Japanese group, who received extended surgery consisting of LLND and a wider abdominoperineal excision. The majority received no (neo)adjuvant therapy. The Dutch and Japanese patients were matched as closely as possible by selecting only tumors up to 7 cm from the anal verge, which was considered the level of the peritoneal reflection. Five-year local recurrence rates were 6.9% for the Japanese NCCH group, 5.8% in the Dutch RT+TME group and 12.1% in the Dutch TME group. It could be concluded that Japanese extended surgery and RT+TME result in good local control, as compared to TME alone.

Because of the differences in patient groups mentioned previously, it remains difficult to compare Japanese and Western series. A trial currently being conducted in Japan will show whether a LLND can truly prevent local recurrence, and is designed to study the effect of a "preventive" LLND, as patients with definite lateral metastases are not included. Modern MRI may allow identification of patients with clearly involved or suspected lateral lymph nodes. In these cases, LLND is probably not enough and it is uncertain whether the nodal metastases can be fully sterilized by preoperative chemoradiation. Additionally, the risk for disseminated disease is high and prognosis unfavorable for lateral lymph node-positive patients. For these patients, it may be wise to consider a combination of treatments: neoadjuvant chemoradiation therapy, LLND and possibly adjuvant systemic therapy.

REFERENCES

1. Rutten HJ, den Dulk M, Lemmens VE, van de Velde CJ, Marijnen CA. Controversies of total mesorectal excision for rectal cancer in elderly patients. *Lancet Oncol.* 2008;9((5):494–501.
2. Lisfranc J. Mémoire sur l'excision de la partie inférieure du rectum devenue carcinomateuse. [Observation on a cancerous condition of the rectum treated by excision.]. *Rev Méd Franc.* 1826;2:380; Translated in Dis Colon Rectum 1983;26:694.
3. Czerny V. Casuistische Mittheilungen aus der Chirurg. Klin zu Heidelberg 1894; 11.
4. Miles WE. A method of performing abdomino-perineal excision for carcinoma of the rectum and of the terminal portion of the pelvic colon. *Lancet.* 1908;2:1812–1813.
5. Lloyd-Davies OV. Lithotomy-Trendelenburg position for resection of rectum and lower pelvic colon. *Lancet.* 2008;237:74–76.
6. Hartmann H. *Nouveau procédé d'ablation des cancers de la partie terminale du colon pelvien.* Strasbourg: Trentieme Congres de Chirurgie; 1921:411.
7. Dixon CF. Surgical removal of lesions occurring in sigmoid and rectosigmoid. *Am J Surg.* 1939;46:12–17.
8. Heald RJ, Husband EM, Ryall RD. The mesorectum in rectal cancer surgery – the clue to pelvic recurrence? *Br J Surg.* 1982;69(10):613–616.
9. Quirke P, Durdey P, Dixon MF, Williams NS. Local recurrence of rectal adenocarcinoma due to inadequate surgical resection. Histopathological study of lateral tumour spread and surgical excision. *Lancet.* 1986;2(8514):996–999.
10. Hirschfeld L, Leveillé J-B. *Néurologie. Description et iconographie du systeme nerveux et des organes des sens de l'homme avec leur mode de preparation.* 1st ed. Paris: Baillière; 1853.
11. Enker WE, Thaler HT, Cranor ML, Polyak T. Total mesorectal excision in the operative treatment of carcinoma of the rectum. *J Am Coll Surg.* 1995;181(4):335–346.
12. Havenga K, Enker WE, McDermott K, Cohen AM, Minsky BD, Guillem J. Male and female sexual and urinary function after total mesorectal excision with autonomic nerve preservation for carcinoma of the rectum. *J Am Coll Surg.* 1996;182(6):495–502.
13. Maas CP, Moriya Y, Steup WH, Kiebert GM, Kranenbarg WM, van de Velde CJ. Radical and nerve-preserving surgery for rectal cancer in The Netherlands: a prospective study on morbidity and functional outcome. *Br J Surg.* 1998;85(1):92–97.
14. Leveckis J, Boucher NR, Parys BT, Reed MW, Shorthouse AJ, Anderson JB. Bladder and erectile dysfunction before and after rectal surgery for cancer. *Br J Urol.* 1995;76(6):752–756.
15. Junginger T, Kneist W, Heintz A. Influence of identification and preservation of pelvic autonomic nerves in rectal cancer surgery on bladder dysfunction after total mesorectal excision. *Dis Colon Rectum.* 2003;46(5):621–628.
16. Vironen JH, Kairaluoma M, Aalto AM, Kellokumpu IH. Impact of functional results on quality of life after rectal cancer surgery. *Dis Colon Rectum.* 2006;49(5):568–578.
17. Pollack J, Holm T, Cedermark B, et al. Late adverse effects of short-course preoperative radiotherapy in rectal cancer. *Br J Surg.* 2006;93(12):1519–1525.
18. Lange MM, Maas CP, Marijnen CA, et al. Urinary dysfunction after rectal cancer treatment is mainly caused by surgery. *Br J Surg.* 2008;95(8):1020–1028.
19. Moriya Y. Function preservation in rectal cancer surgery. *Int J Clin Oncol.* 2006;11(5):339–343.
20. Daniels IR, Woodward S, Taylor FG, Raja A, Toomey P. Female urogenital dysfunction following total mesorectal excision for rectal cancer. *World J Surg Oncol.* 2006;4:6.

21. Wallner C, Maas CP, Dabhoiwala NF, Lamers WH, DeRuiter MC. Innervation of the pelvic floor muscles: a reappraisal for the levator ani nerve. *Obstet Gynecol.* 2006;108(3 Pt 1):529–534.
22. Hendren SK, O'Connor BI, Liu M, et al. Prevalence of male and female sexual dysfunction is high following surgery for rectal cancer. *Ann Surg.* 2005;242(2):212–223.
23. Marijnen CA, van de Velde CJ, Putter H, et al. Impact of short-term preoperative radiotherapy on health-related quality of life and sexual functioning in primary rectal cancer: report of a multicenter randomized trial. *J Clin Oncol.* 2005;23(9):1847–1858.
24. Havenga K, Enker WE. Autonomic nerve preserving total mesorectal excision. *Surg Clin North Am.* 2002;82(5):1009–1018.
25. Dahlberg M, Glimelius B, Graf W, Pahlman L. Preoperative irradiation affects functional results after surgery for rectal cancer: results from a randomized study. *Dis Colon Rectum.* 1998;41(5): 543–549.
26. Peeters KC, van de Velde CJH, Leer JW, et al. Late side effects of short-course preoperative radiotherapy combined with total mesorectal excision for rectal cancer: increased bowel dysfunction in irradiated patients – a Dutch colorectal cancer group study. *J Clin Oncol.* 2005;23(25): 6199–6206.
27. Welsh FK, McFall M, Mitchell G, Miles WF, Woods WG. Pre-operative short-course radiotherapy is associated with faecal incontinence after anterior resection. *Colorectal Dis.* 2003;5(6): 563–568.
28. Williams N, Seow-Choen F. Physiological and functional outcome following ultra-low anterior resection with colon pouch-anal anastomosis. *Br J Surg.* 1998;85(8):1029–1035.
29. Nesbakken A, Nygaard K, Lunde OC. Outcome and late functional results after anastomotic leakage following mesorectal excision for rectal cancer. *Br J Surg.* 2001;88(3):400–404.
30. Wallner C, Lange MM, Bonsing BA, et al. Causes of fecal and urinary incontinence after total mesorectal excision for rectal cancer based on cadaveric surgery: a study from the Cooperative Clinical Investigators of the Dutch total mesorectal excision trial. *J Clin Oncol.* 2008;26(27): 4466–4472.
31. Carlsen E, Schlichting E, Guldvog I, Johnson E, Heald RJ. Effect of the introduction of total mesorectal excision for the treatment of rectal cancer. *Br J Surg.* 1998;85(4):526–529.
32. Peeters KC, Tollenaar RA, Marijnen CA, et al. Risk factors for anastomotic failure after total mesorectal excision of rectal cancer. *Br J Surg.* 2005;92(2):211–216.
33. Law WL, Choi HK, Lee YM, Ho JW, Seto CL. Anastomotic leakage is associated with poor long-term outcome in patients after curative colorectal resection for malignancy. *J Gastrointest Surg.* 2007;11(1):8–15.
34. Rullier E, Laurent C, Garrelon JL, Michel P, Saric J, Parneix M. Risk factors for anastomotic leakage after resection of rectal cancer. *Br J Surg.* 1998;85(3):355–358.
35. Matthiessen P, Hallbook O, Rutegard J, Simert G, Sjodahl R. Defunctioning stoma reduces symptomatic anastomotic leakage after low anterior resection of the rectum for cancer: a randomized multicenter trial. *Ann Surg.* 2007;246(2):207–214.
36. Vignali A, Fazio VW, Lavery IC, et al. Factors associated with the occurrence of leaks in stapled rectal anastomoses: a review of 1,014 patients. *J Am Coll Surg.* 1997;185(2):105–113.
37. Bokey EL, Chapuis PH, Fung C, et al. Postoperative morbidity and mortality following resection of the colon and rectum for cancer. *Dis Colon Rectum.* 1995;38(5):480–486.
38. Folkesson J, Nilsson J, Pahlman L, Glimelius B, Gunnarsson U. The circular stapling device as a risk factor for anastomotic leakage. *Colorectal Dis.* 2004;6(4):275–279.
39. Poon RT, Chu KW, Ho JW, Chan CW, Law WL, Wong J. Prospective evaluation of selective defunctioning stoma for low anterior resection with total mesorectal excision. *World J Surg.* 1999;23(5):463–467.
40. Graf W, Ekstrom K, Glimelius B, Pahlman L. A pilot study of factors influencing bowel function after colorectal anastomosis. *Dis Colon Rectum.* 1996;39(7):744–749.
41. Eriksen MT, Wibe A, Norstein J, Haffner J, Wiig JN. Anastomotic leakage following routine mesorectal excision for rectal cancer in a national cohort of patients. *Colorectal Dis.* 2005;7(1):51–57.
42. Swedish Rectal Cancer Trial. Improved survival with preoperative radiotherapy in resectable rectal cancer. *N Engl J Med.* 1997;336(14):980–987.

43. Kapiteijn E, Marijnen CA, Nagtegaal ID, et al. Preoperative radiotherapy combined with total mesorectal excision for resectable rectal cancer. *N Engl J Med.* 2001;345(9):638–646.
44. Stockholm Colorectal Cancer Study Group. Randomized study on preoperative radiotherapy in rectal carcinoma. *Ann Surg Oncol.* 1996;3(5):423–430.
45. McArdle CS, McMillan DC, Hole DJ. Impact of anastomotic leakage on long-term survival of patients undergoing curative resection for colorectal cancer. *Br J Surg.* 2005;92(9):1150–1154.
46. Branagan G, Finnis D. Prognosis after anastomotic leakage in colorectal surgery. *Dis Colon Rectum.* 2005;48(5):1021–1026.
47. Petersen S, Freitag M, Hellmich G, Ludwig K. Anastomotic leakage: impact on local recurrence and survival in surgery of colorectal cancer. *Int J Colorectal Dis.* 1998;13(4):160–163.
48. den Dulk M, Marijnen CA, Colette L, Putter H, Pahlman L, Folkesson J et al. Anastomotic leakage associated with long-term reduced overall survival: the results of a pooled analysis of five European randomized clinical trials on rectal cancer. Submitted 2008.
49. Umpleby HC, Fermor B, Symes MO, Williamson RC. Viability of exfoliated colorectal carcinoma cells. *Br J Surg.* 1984;71(9):659–663.
50. Skipper D, Cooper AJ, Marston JE, Taylor I. Exfoliated cells and in vitro growth in colorectal cancer. *Br J Surg.* 1987;74(11):1049–1052.
51. Abramovitch R, Marikovsky M, Meir G, Neeman M. Stimulation of tumour growth by wound-derived growth factors. *Br J Cancer.* 1999;79(9–10):1392–1398.
52. Balkwill F, Mantovani A. Inflammation and cancer: back to Virchow? *Lancet.* 2001;357(9255): 539–545.
53. Kusters M, van de Velde CJ, Beets-Tan RG, et al. Patterns of local recurrence in rectal cancer at or below the peritoneal reflection: a single-center experience. *Ann Surg Oncol.* 2008;16(2): 289–296.
54. Kapiteijn E, Kranenbarg EK, Steup WH, et al. Total mesorectal excision (TME) with or without preoperative radiotherapy in the treatment of primary rectal cancer. Prospective randomised trial with standard operative and histopathological techniques. Dutch ColoRectal Cancer Group. *Eur J Surg.* 1999;165(5):410–420.
55. Peeters KC, Marijnen CA, Nagtegaal ID, et al. The TME trial after a median follow-up of 6 years: increased local control but no survival benefit in irradiated patients with resectable rectal carcinoma. *Ann Surg.* 2007;246(5):693–701.
56. Kusters M, Marijnen CA, van de Velde CJ, Rutten HJ, Lahaye MJ, Kim JH, Beets-Tan RG, Beets GL. Patterns of local recurrence in rectal cancer; a study of the Dutch TME trial. Eur J Surg Oncl. 2010 Jan 20. [Epub ahead of print].
57. Nagtegaal ID, Quirke P. What is the role for the circumferential margin in the modern treatment of rectal cancer? *J Clin Oncol.* 2008;26(2):303–312.
58. Kusters M, Beets GL, van de Velde CJ, et al. A comparison between the treatment of low rectal cancer in Japan and the Netherlands, with focus on the patterns of local recurrence. *Ann Surg.* 2009;249(2):229–235.
59. Beets-Tan RG, Beets GL. Rectal cancer: review with emphasis on MR imaging. *Radiology.* 2004;232(2):335–346.
60. Brown G. Thin section MRI in multidisciplinary pre-operative decision making for patients with rectal cancer. *Br J Radiol.* 2005;78(Spec No 2):S117-S127.
61. Bosset JF, Calais G, Mineur L, et al. Enhanced tumorocidal effect of chemotherapy with preoperative radiotherapy for rectal cancer: preliminary results – EORTC 22921. *J Clin Oncol.* 2005;23(24): 5620–5627.
62. Burton S, Brown G, Daniels IR, Norman AR, Mason B, Cunningham D. MRI directed multidisciplinary team preoperative treatment strategy: the way to eliminate positive circumferential margins? *Br J Cancer.* 2006;94(3):351–357.
63. Kim JH, Beets GL, Kim MJ, Kessels AG, Beets-Tan RG. High-resolution MR imaging for nodal staging in rectal cancer: are there any criteria in addition to the size? *Eur J Radiol.* 2004;52(1): 78–83.
64. Zhao GP, Zhou ZG, Lei WZ, et al. Pathological study of distal mesorectal cancer spread to determine a proper distal resection margin. *World J Gastroenterol.* 2005;11(3):319–322.

65. Wang Z, Zhou Z, Wang C, et al. Microscopic spread of low rectal cancer in regions of the mesorectum: detailed pathological assessment with whole-mount sections. *Int J Colorectal Dis*. 2005;20 (3):231–237.
66. Chen W, Shen W, Chen M, Cai G, Liu X. Study on the relationship between lymphatic vessel density and distal intramural spread of rectal cancer. *Eur Surg Res*. 2007;39(6):332–339.
67. Koh DM, Brown G, Temple L, et al. Distribution of mesorectal lymph nodes in rectal cancer: in vivo MR imaging compared with histopathological examination. Initial observations. *Eur Radiol*. 2005;15(8):1650–1657.
68. Perez RO, Seid VE, Bresciani EH, et al. Distribution of lymph nodes in the mesorectum: how deep is TME necessary? *Tech Coloproctol*. 2008;12(1):39–43.
69. Heald RJ, Moran BJ, Ryall RD, Sexton R, MacFarlane JK. Rectal cancer: the Basingstoke experience of total mesorectal excision, 1978-1997. *Arch Surg*. 1998;133(8):894–899.
70. Salerno G, Sinnatamby C, Branagan G, Daniels IR, Heald RJ, Moran BJ. Defining the rectum: surgically, radiologically and anatomically. *Colorectal Dis*. 2006;8(Suppl 3):5–9.
71. den Dulk M, Marijnen CA, Putter H, et al. Risk factors for adverse outcome in patients with rectal cancer treated with an abdominoperineal resection in the total mesorectal excision trial. *Ann Surg*. 2007;246(1):83–90.
72. Holm T, Ljung A, Haggmark T, Jurell G, Lagergren J. Extended abdominoperineal resection with gluteus maximus flap reconstruction of the pelvic floor for rectal cancer. *Br J Surg*. 2007;94(2): 232–238.
73. Valentini V, Coco C, Cellini N, et al. Preoperative chemoradiation with cisplatin and 5-fluorouracil for extraperitoneal T3 rectal cancer: acute toxicity, tumor response, sphincter preservation. *Int J Radiat Oncol Biol Phys*. 1999;45(5):1175–1184.
74. Roels S, Duthoy W, Haustermans K, et al. Definition and delineation of the clinical target volume for rectal cancer. *Int J Radiat Oncol Biol Phys*. 2006;65(4):1129–1142.
75. Bosset JF, Collette L, Calais G, et al. Chemotherapy with preoperative radiotherapy in rectal cancer. *N Engl J Med*. 2006;355(11):1114–1123.
76. den Dulk M, Krijnen P, Marijnen CA, et al. Improved overall survival for patients with rectal cancer since 1990: the effects of TME surgery and pre-operative radiotherapy. *Eur J Cancer*. 2008;44(12):1710–1716.
77. Lange MM, den Dulk M, Bossema ER, et al. Risk factors for faecal incontinence after rectal cancer treatment. *Br J Surg*. 2007;94(10):1278–1284.
78. Rutten H, den Dulk M, Lemmens V, et al. Survival of elderly rectal cancer patients not improved: analysis of population based data on the impact of TME surgery. *Eur J Cancer*. 2007;43(15): 2295–2300.
79. Beets-Tan RG, Beets GL, Vliegen RF, et al. Accuracy of magnetic resonance imaging in prediction of tumour-free resection margin in rectal cancer surgery. *Lancet*. 2001;357(9255):497–504.
80. Lahaye MJ, Engelen SM, Kessels AG, et al. USPIO-enhanced MR imaging for nodal staging in patients with primary rectal cancer: predictive criteria. *Radiology*. 2008;246(3):804–811.
81. de Heer P, de Bruin EC, Klein-Kranenbarg E, et al. Caspase-3 activity predicts local recurrence in rectal cancer. *Clin Cancer Res*. 2007;13(19):5810–5815.
82. Nagtegaal ID, Gosens MJ, Marijnen CA, Rutten HJ, van de Velde CJH, van Krieken JH. Combinations of tumor and treatment parameters are more discriminative for prognosis than the present TNM system in rectal cancer. *J Clin Oncol*. 2007;25(13):1647–1650.
83. Habr-Gama A, Perez RO, Nadalin W, et al. Operative versus nonoperative treatment for stage 0 distal rectal cancer following chemoradiation therapy: long-term results. *Ann Surg*. 2004;240(4): 711–717.
84. Gerota D. Die lymphgefasse des rectums und des anus. *Arch Anat Physiol*. 1895;181:240.
85. Waugh JM, Kirklin JW. The importance of the level of the lesion in the prognosis and treatment of carcinoma of the rectum and low sigmoid colon. *Ann Surg*. 1949;129(1):22–33.
86. Sunderland DA. The significance of vein invasion by cancer of the rectum and sigmoid; a microscopic study of 210 cases. *Cancer*. 1949;2(3):429–437.
87. Wangsteen OH. Primary resection of the colon and rectum with particular reference to cancer and ulcerative colitis. *Am J Surg*. 1948;75:384.

88. Villemin F. Recherches anatomiques sur les lymphatiques du rectum et l'anus: leur applications dans le traitement chirurgical du cancer. *Rev Chir*. 1925;63:39–80.
89. Oliviera E. Observacao sobre os linfaticos anoretais. Tese Rio de Janeiro 1947;77.
90. Coller FA, Kay EB, Macintyre RS. Regional lymphatic metastases of carcinoma of the colon. *Ann Surg*. 1941;114(1):56–67.
91. Dukes WC. The surgical pathology of rectal cancer. *Proc R Soc Med*. 1943;37:131.
92. Sauer I, Bacon HE. Influence of lateral spread of cancer of the rectum on radicability of operation and prognosis. *Am J Surg*. 1951;81(1):111–120.
93. Stearns MW Jr, Deddish MR. Five-year results of abdominopelvic lymph node dissection for carcinoma of the rectum. *Dis Colon Rectum*. 1959;2(2):169–172.
94. Enker WE, Pilipshen SJ, Heilweil ML, et al. En bloc pelvic lymphadenectomy and sphincter preservation in the surgical management of rectal cancer. *Ann Surg*. 1986;203(4): 426–433.
95. Glass RE, Ritchie JK, Thompson HR, Mann CV. The results of surgical treatment of cancer of the rectum by radical resection and extended abdomino-iliac lymphadenectomy. *Br J Surg*. 1985;72(8):599–601.
96. Michelassi F, Block GE. Morbidity and mortality of wide pelvic lymphadenectomy for rectal adenocarcinoma. *Dis Colon Rectum*. 1992;35(12):1143–1147.
97. Senba Y. An anatomical study of the lymphatic system of the rectum. *J Hukuoka Med Coll*. 1927;20:1213–1268.
98. Kuru M. Cancer of the rectum. *J Jpn Surg Soc*. 1940;41:832–877.
99. Koyama Y. Extended surgery for rectal cancer. *Geka Chiryo*. 1977;36:41–45.
100. Hojo K, Koyama Y. Postoperative follow-up studies on cancer of the colon and rectum. *Am J Surg*. 1982;143(3):293.
101. Hojo K, Sawada T, Moriya Y. An analysis of survival and voiding, sexual function after wide iliopelvic lymphadenectomy in patients with carcinoma of the rectum, compared with conventional lymphadenectomy. *Dis Colon Rectum*. 1989;32(2):128–133.
102. Sato K, Sato T. The vascular and neuronal composition of the lateral ligament of the rectum and the rectosacral fascia. *Surg Radiol Anat*. 1991;13(1):17–22.
103. Hojo K, Vernava AM III, Sugihara K, Katumata K. Preservation of urine voiding and sexual function after rectal cancer surgery. *Dis Colon Rectum*. 1991;34(7):532–539.
104. Moriya Y, Sugihara K, Akasu T, Fujita S. Nerve-sparing surgery with lateral node dissection for advanced lower rectal cancer. *Eur J Cancer*. 1995;31A(7–8):1229–1232.
105. Moriya Y, Sugihara K, Akasu T, Fujita S. Patterns of recurrence after nerve-sparing surgery for rectal adenocarcinoma with special reference to loco-regional recurrence. *Dis Colon Rectum*. 1995;38(11):1162–1168.
106. Sugihara K, Moriya Y, Akasu T, Fujita S. Pelvic autonomic nerve preservation for patients with rectal carcinoma. Oncologic and functional outcome. *Cancer*. 1996;78(9):1871–1880.
107. Mori T, Takahashi K, Yasuno M. Radical resection with autonomic nerve preservation and lymph node dissection techniques in lower rectal cancer surgery and its results: the impact of lateral lymph node dissection. *Langenbecks Arch Surg*. 1998;383(6):409–415.
108. Matsumoto T, Ohue M, Sekimoto M, Yamamoto H, Ikeda M, Monden M. Feasibility of autonomic nerve-preserving surgery for advanced rectal cancer based on analysis of micrometastases. *Br J Surg*. 2005;92(11):1444–1448.
109. Sugihara K, Kobayashi H, Kato T, et al. Indication and benefit of pelvic sidewall dissection for rectal cancer. *Dis Colon Rectum*. 2006;49(11):1663–1672.
110. Martling A, Holm T, Johansson H, Rutqvist LE, Cedermark B. The Stockholm II trial on preoperative radiotherapy in rectal carcinoma: long-term follow-up of a population-based study. *Cancer*. 2001;92(4):896–902.
111. Japanese Research Society for Cancer of the Colon and Rectum. *General rules for clinical and pathological studies on cancer of the colon, rectum and anus*. 7th ed. Tokyo: Kanehira-Syuppan; 2006.
112. Najarian MM, Belzer GE, Cogbill TH, Mathiason MA. Determination of the peritoneal reflection using intraoperative proctoscopy. *Dis Colon Rectum*. 2004;47(12):2080–2085.

113. Quirke P. Training and quality assurance for rectal cancer: 20 years of data is enough. *Lancet Oncol.* 2003;4(11):695–702.
114. Maas CP, Moriya Y, Steup WH, Klein KE, van de Velde CJ. A prospective study on radical and nerve-preserving surgery for rectal cancer in the Netherlands. *Eur J Surg Oncol.* 2000;26(8):751–757.
115. Feinstein AR, Sosin DM, Wells CK. The Will Rogers phenomenon. Stage migration and new diagnostic techniques as a source of misleading statistics for survival in cancer. *N Engl J Med.* 1985;312(25):1604–1608.
116. Steup WH. Chapter 6: Historical comparison Japanese data NCCH; Comparison between Japan and the Netherlands. Thesis: Colorectal cancer surgery with emphasis on lymphadenectomy 1994;83–100.
117. Japanese Research Society for Cancer of the Colon and Rectum. General rules for clinical and pathological studies on cancer of the colon, rectum and anus. Part I. Clinical classification. *Jpn J Surg.* 1983;13(6):557–573.
118. Kyo K, Sameshima S, Takahashi M, Furugori T, Sawada T. Impact of autonomic nerve preservation and lateral node dissection on male urogenital function after total mesorectal excision for lower rectal cancer. *World J Surg.* 2006;30(6):1014–1019.
119. Yano H, Moran BJ. The incidence of lateral pelvic side-wall nodal involvement in low rectal cancer may be similar in Japan and the West. *Br J Surg.* 2008;95(1):33–49.
120. Moriya Y, Sugihara K, Akasu T, Fujita S. Importance of extended lymphadenectomy with lateral node dissection for advanced lower rectal cancer. *World J Surg.* 1997;21(7):728–732.
121. Saha S, Seghal R, Patel M, et al. A multicenter trial of sentinel lymph node mapping in colorectal cancer: prognostic implications for nodal staging and recurrence. *Am J Surg.* 2006;191(3):305–310.
122. Stojadinovic A, Nissan A, Protic M, et al. Prospective randomized study comparing sentinel lymph node evaluation with standard pathologic evaluation for the staging of colon carcinoma: results from the United States Military Cancer Institute Clinical Trials Group Study GI-01. *Ann Surg.* 2007;245(6):846–857.
123. Quadros CA, Lopes A, Araujo I, Fahel F, Bacellar MS, Dias CS. Retroperitoneal and lateral pelvic lymphadenectomy mapped by lymphoscintigraphy and blue dye for rectal adenocarcinoma staging: preliminary results. *Ann Surg Oncol.* 2006;13(12):1617–1621.
124. Funahashi K, Koike J, Shimada M, Okamoto K, Goto T, Teramoto T. A preliminary study of the draining lymph node basin in advanced lower rectal cancer using a radioactive tracer. *Dis Colon Rectum.* 2006;49(10 Suppl):S53-S58.
125. Kawahara H, Nimura H, Watanabe K, Kobayashi T, Kashiwagi H, Yanaga K. Where does the first lateral pelvic lymph node receive drainage from? *Dig Surg.* 2007;24(6):413–417.
126. Watanabe T, Tsurita G, Muto T, et al. Extended lymphadenectomy and preoperative radiotherapy for lower rectal cancers. *Surgery.* 2002;132(1):27–33.
127. Kim JC, Takahashi K, Yu CS, et al. Comparative outcome between chemoradiotherapy and lateral pelvic lymph node dissection following total mesorectal excision in rectal cancer. *Ann Surg.* 2007;246(5):754–762.
128. Watanabe T, Matsuda K, Nozawa K, Kobunai T. Lateral pelvic lymph node dissection or chemoradiotherapy: which is the procedure of choice to reduce local recurrence rate in lower rectal cancer? *Ann Surg.* 2008;248(2):342–343.
129. Masui H, Ike H, Yamaguchi S, Oki S, Shimada H. Male sexual function after autonomic nerve-preserving operation for rectal cancer. *Dis Colon Rectum.* 1996;39(10):1140–1145.
130. Ameda K, Kakizaki H, Koyanagi T, Hirakawa K, Kusumi T, Hosokawa M. The long-term voiding function and sexual function after pelvic nerve-sparing radical surgery for rectal cancer. *Int J Urol.* 2005;12(3):256–263.
131. Maeda K, Maruta M, Utsumi T, Sato H, Toyama K, Matsuoka H. Bladder and male sexual functions after autonomic nerve-sparing TME with or without lateral node dissection for rectal cancer. *Tech Coloproctol.* 2003;7(1):29–33.
132. Matsuoka H, Masaki T, Sugiyama M, Atomi Y. Impact of lateral pelvic lymph node dissection on evacuatory and urinary functions following low anterior resection for advanced rectal carcinoma. *Langenbecks Arch Surg.* 2005;390(6):517–522.

5 Abdominoperineal Resection, Low Anterior Resection, and Beyond

Kirk Ludwig, Lauren Kosinski, and Timothy Ridolfi

INTRODUCTION

Historically, the gold standard operation for rectal cancer was the abdominoperineal resection (APR) performed using blunt dissection. This operation, championed by Ernest Miles in the early 1900s, stood for decades as the benchmark treatment of rectal cancer *(1,2)*. This began to change in the middle part of the twentieth century when Claude Dixon reported a 64% 5-year survival in over 400 patients treated with low anterior resection (LAR) *(3)*. While there remains a role for APR in the treatment of rectal cancer, it has diminished substantially. The permanent colostomy rate for rectal cancer patients treated by experienced rectal cancer surgeons should be well below 30% *(4,5)*. During the last two decades, dramatic changes have taken place in the conduct of rectal cancer surgery and the results obtained using these techniques.

The current treatment of rectal cancer involves a multidisciplinary approach aimed at achieving two primary goals: (1) curing the cancer, or at least reducing the rate of local recurrence, and (2) optimizing the patient's quality of life, which in most cases translates into sphincter preservation. Despite the fact that combined modality, neoadjuvant therapy achieves pathologic complete response rates of 15–30% *(6,7)* and may change the management strategy for some patients, *(8)* surgery remains the cornerstone of curative treatment for the vast majority of patients.

From: *Current Clinical Oncology: Rectal Cancer*,
Edited by: B.G. Czito and C.G. Willett, DOI: 10.1007/978-1-60761-567-5_5,

TOTAL MESORECTAL EXCISION

The Holy Plane

One of the most significant advances in rectal cancer treatment is the principle of total mesorectal excision (TME). Bill Heald, from Basingstoke, England introduced this technique in 1982 and is credited with dramatically changing how the rectum is removed whether by APR or LAR. While curative treatment of rectal cancer had extirpative surgery as its primary modality, disappointing results, including local recurrence rates of 15–50%, were observed before the adoption of TME *(9,10)*. Previously, most surgeons learned and practiced blunt dissection of the rectum for cancer resection. When Heald first described the technique of TME, *(11)* he recognized that most local recurrences after rectal cancer resection were the result of inadequate resections, using imprecise, blunt dissection. He found that meticulous, sharp dissection, under direct vision, between the visceral and parietal pelvic fascia down to the level of the levator muscles (which define the upper aspect of the anal canal) enabled removal of the rectum and its mesentery as an intact unit and that this approach led to three very favorable outcomes. First, the lateral margin positivity rate was dramatically reduced and corresponded with astonishingly low local failure rates. Second, there was a sharp decline in the need for APR's. Third, the incidence of bladder and sexual dysfunction after surgery also decreased because dissection in the proper planes helped to avoid injury to the sympathetic and parasympathetic nerves in the pelvis *(12)*.

Historically, local failure rates of >30% were observed following resection of locally advanced, T3 or node-positive tumors *(13)*. In contrast, Heald reported a local recurrence rate of just 6% in 519 patients with rectal cancer <15 cm from the anal margin. In patients who had what he termed "curative" resections, the local failure rate was even better at only 3%. These results were achieved when only 49 patients (9.4%) were treated with neoadjuvant radiation therapy *(14)*. Soon others reported superior local recurrence rates after TME. The multicenter, multisurgeon Dutch TME Trial compared TME alone to TME combined with preoperative radiation; the overall local failure rate for TME alone was only 8.2% (10% for tumors <10 cm from the anal verge and 15% for Stage III cancers) *(15)*. Others have reported similarly impressive low local recurrence figures after adopting Heald's exacting surgical technique *(16–20)*. Likewise, the reduction of APR rate by surgeons skilled in TME mirrored Heald's experience. Heald's 1998 report included just 37 APRs (7.1%) Others have subsequently reported similarly low APR rates *(21–24)*.

Further evidence that adoption of the TME technique improves oncologic outcomes comes from Norway where decreased local recurrence rates and increased survival rates were found after a TME training program was introduced. A Norwegian national audit of rectal cancer resections performed between 1986 and 1988 identified a local recurrence rate of 28% and a survival rate of 55%. A TME training program was initiated in 1994, and by 1998, 96% of rectal cancer resections were conducted according to the principles of TME. The 1998 audit showed that even with a very low rate of neoadjuvant treatment (9% of patients underwent preoperative radiation therapy, and only 2% with concurrent chemotherapy), the local recurrence rate had dropped to 8% and the survival rate had improved to 71% *(9)*.

The "old style" proctectomy employing blunt dissection showed little appreciation for the fine points of pelvic anatomy and too often failed to preserve autonomic functions supplied by the sympathetic and parasympathetic pelvic nerves. Sexual dysfunction was seen in up to 75% of males and 40% of females, with bladder dysfunction seen in up to 80% of patients. In the TME era, these rates have improved substantially, and, while patient's age, tumor location, and preoperative functional status continue to influence outcomes, sexual dysfunction should be in the 10–30% range and bladder dysfunction should be 5% or less *(25)*.

The implementation of TME has spread throughout Europe, Asia and the United States. This technique of rectal dissection has been and can be taught on a broad scale. It is now clear that blunt dissection of the rectum should no longer be taught or practiced. TME has significantly influenced both the outcomes and surgical options for patients with rectal cancer.

One of the best descriptions of the TME remains Heald's Presidential Address to the Royal Society of Medicine, Surgery Section, in 1987, the publication of which has become known as the "Holy Plane" paper *(12)*. In his address, Heald described the three basic principles that one must understand and follow in order to perform a TME. First, one must recognize that there is mobility between tissues of different embryologic origins. The rectum and its mesentery, encased by the fascia propria of the mesorectum, are separate from those structures outside of this fascial envelope. The plane of dissection is just outside the fascia propria (i.e., the visceral endopelvic fascia) and just inside the parietal endopelvic fascia. This is the so-called Holy Plane. Second, the dissection must be performed sharply (no ripping, tearing, or blunt dissection) under direct vision, with good illumination. The sharp dissection is generally performed with either scissors, or more commonly, with the electrocautery. Good lighting can best be achieved by using fiberoptically lit pelvic retractors (Fig. 1). These retractors allow placement of light directly where it is needed and facilitates excellent visualization even in the depths of the pelvis. An alternative is a headlight worn by the surgeon or assistant. To perform precise dissection, one must know the anatomy as well as be able to see the

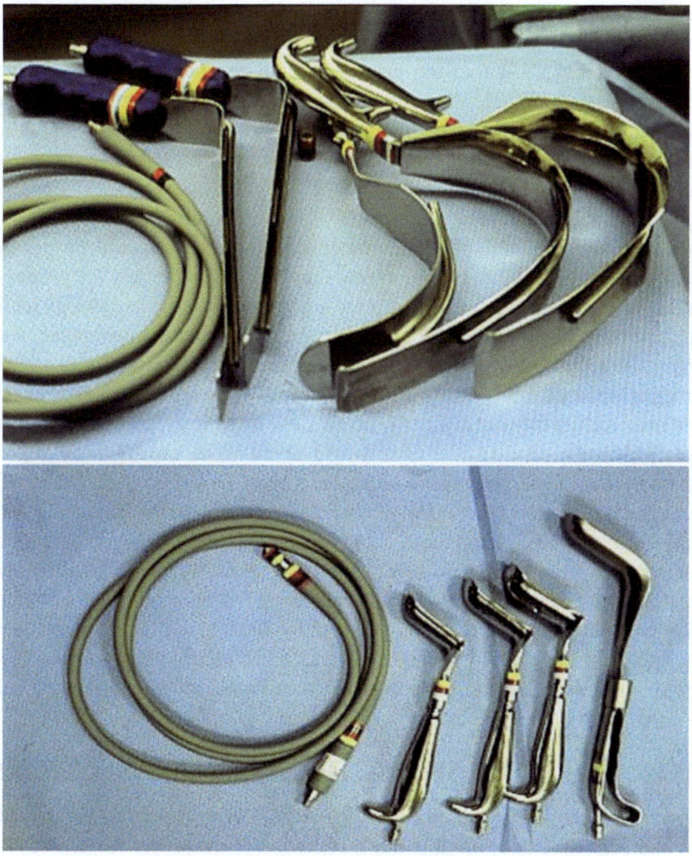

Fig. 1. Tools of the trade. These pelvic and anal retractors are equipped with fiber-optic light cords. These facilitate adequate visualization during TME.

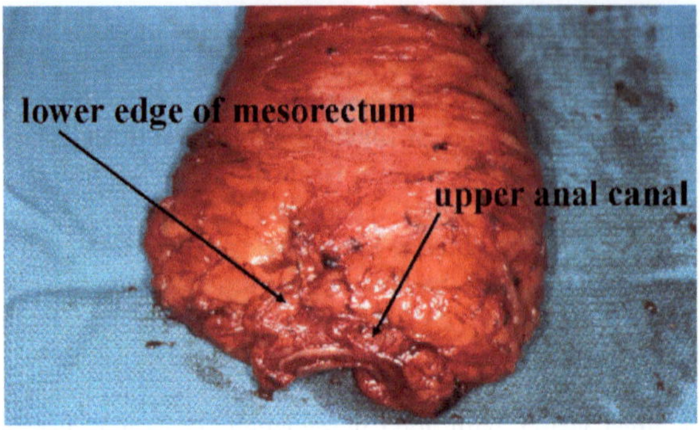

Fig. 2. A low anterior resection specimen. The mesorectum ends 1–2 cm above the top of the anal canal. Beneath the mesorectum, there is simply a muscular tube of bowel. It is in this bowel that the anastomosis takes place following a standard TME.

anatomy, i.e., the field must be well lit. Thirdly, there must be gentle opening of the plane by continuous traction and counter traction, but not so much that the tissue tears or rips.

In his discussion, Heald describes what is encircled within the "Holy Plane" and what is outside the "Holy Plane." Within the plane one finds the rectum and its circumferential mesentery, the mesorectum. He described the rectum and the mesorectum as one distinct lymphovascular entity and noted "the tumor is more apt to spread initially along the field of active lymphatic and venous flow." If one accepts that the vast majority of rectal cancers and their lymphatic metastases are confined to this envelope of tissue, one can understand how removing it intact might lead to very low rates of local failure.

Outside the "Holy Plane," one finds those structures that should be preserved: the sympathetic and parasympathetic pelvic nerves and the major vessels (of primary concern are the veins) of the pelvis. He notes that there are two bloodless planes of dissection in the pelvis: one just inside the inferior hypogastric nerves, which is the proper plane, and one just outside the inferior hypogastric nerves, the wrong plane.

With regard to the ultra-low anastomosis that results after TME, Heald points out that the rectum and mesorectum are attached to the pelvic floor by a clean "tube" of anorectal muscle. The mesorectum has a very definite end, lying 1–2 cm above the anorectal angle. Beyond this point, there is no mesentery, just a muscular tube of bowel (Fig. 2). During TME, it is in this area caudal to the mesorectum where the distal division of the bowel and construction of the "ultra-low stapled anastomosis" occur. A stapled anastomosis in this location will place the circular staple line approximately 1.5–2 cm above the dentate line. If one were to dissect this muscular tube more distally into the anus, it would be found to be continuous with the intersphincteric space. Carried more distally, the line of dissection would exit at the anal verge in the intersphincteric groove. This anatomic understanding is critically important in conceptualizing and conducting an intersphincteric LAR, which is discussed below.

TOWARD USE OF SPHINCTER SPARING RESECTIONS

The abdominal perineal resection has fallen out of favor in the last two decades as the result of a number of factors. Not only has recognition of the proper surgical technique and requirement for TME of mid- and low-rectal cancers contributed to this trend, but technical advances and redefinition of the relative importance of circumferential and longitudinal margins along with better understanding of acceptable margin distances have also been significant influences. The technique of rectal reconstruction has changed such that patients also have a better functional result. Additionally, there is also better appreciation of the contribution that appropriately utilized multimodality chemoradiation therapy makes, both as an adjunct to achieve sphincter preservation, and to improve oncologic outcomes.

Technical Advances

Improvement in surgical instrumentation has dramatically impacted the surgical treatment of rectal cancer. Heald's imperatives for oncologic proctectomy included operating under direct vision in a well-lighted field. Several manufacturers responded to this need and now produce and market specially designed pelvic retractors that have a fiber-optic cord mounted on the retractor so that the depths of the pelvis can be illuminated (Fig. 1). This means that fascial planes, nerves, and other pertinent anatomy that were once poorly visualized in the depths of the dark pelvis are now seen more clearly.

Advances in stapling instruments that both secure and transect the rectum have made it possible to perform ultra-low anastomoses. Narrow, low profile staplers allow the surgeon to place a staple line across the rectum in the narrowest portion of the pelvis at the level of the anorectal ring or below. This, used in combination with a circular stapler, allows the surgeon to construct a quick and reliable "double-stapled" anastomosis, even at the level of the anal canal. These instruments have revolutionized low pelvic surgery.

Margins

In contradiction to longstanding dogma, it is now clear that 5 cm distal margins are not needed to achieve good local control for rectal cancers. A 2 cm margin is quite adequate, based on the fact that distal intramural spread and/or retrograde lymphatic extension are rare, and when they do occur, the prognosis is poor despite the surgery. Similarly, the distal resection margin does not appear to predict local recurrence. Williams et al *(26)* showed that in a group of 50 rectal cancer specimens, there was no intramural spread distal to the tumor 75% of the time; in 14% of the specimens, there was distal spread less than a centimeter; and in just five cases, there was distal spread >1 cm. All five of these patients had poorly differentiated, stage III tumors and developed distant metastatic disease within 3 years. Pollett and Nichols *(27)* showed in a series of over 300 rectal cancer specimens that length of the distal margin did not correlate with risk of local failure. Data from the Large Bowel Cancer Group Project corroborated these findings *(28)*. More recent data suggest that even narrower distal margins may be adequate for the very lowest of tumors, especially when resection follows neoadjuvant chemoradiation therapy. Distal margins of 1 cm or less may be sufficient in radical attempts at sphincter preservation *(29,30)*.

It now appears that the circumferential resection margin (CRM) – previously referred to as the deep, lateral, or radial margin – is more critical to oncologic outcome than length of distal margin. The CRM is often measured in millimeters, and a positive CRM places the patient at great risk for local failure. This has been demonstrated by Quirke et al *(31)* who looked carefully at a group of 26 APR specimens and 26 LAR specimens. The CRM was positive in ten specimens from each group, and 75% of these margin-positive patients developed a local recurrence. Only one patient with a negative deep margin developed local failure. Surprisingly, the lateral margin, (measured microscopically from the deep edge of the tumor) was no different in LAR vs. APR specimens.

CRM involvement has also been shown to predict distant recurrence and overall survival. *(32)* A CRM of <1 mm, whether as direct tumor extension, lymph node metastasis, or intravascular growth, should be considered positive. In a report by Adam et al the local failure was observed in 74% of patients with a margin of <1 mm compared to 10% for a margin >1 mm *(33)*. Data from the North Central Cancer Treatment Group showed that if the CRM was 0–1 mm, the local failure rate was 25%, compared to only 3% if the CRM was >1 cm *(34)*. Birbeck et al described a local failure rate of 58% when CRM was positive, 28% if CRM was <1 mm, and 10% when CRM was 1 mm or more *(35)*.

Several authors have concluded that CRM is an acceptable rectal cancer oncologic endpoint that predicts both local recurrence and disease-free survival *(31,33,35–38)*. A negative CRM is critical in achieving good oncologic outcomes. Precise consideration of the anatomy of proper rectal cancer resection leads one to the conclusion that the deep margin, for all but the lowest and most advanced rectal tumor, is not maximized by performing an abdominal perineal resection. Unless a tumor has invaded the sphincter complex, one can legitimately ask, why should this complex and the anus be removed? This concept is developed in more detail, below.

CHANGING CONCEPTS IN SPHINCTER-PRESERVING RECTAL CANCER RESECTION

From a historical standpoint, the critical issue in rectal cancer surgery has been the distal margin. The classic question has been at what level in the rectum does a patient go from being a candidate for sphincter preservation to APR, i.e., "how low can you go?" If one accepts the historic 5 cm rule, then most patients with a low-rectal tumor will require APR. If one accepts the 2 cm rule as an adequate distal margin, then more patients will be treated with an LAR; however, most patients with tumors near the anorectal ring would not be treated with sphincter-preserving resection.

A more modern concept focuses on the deep (radial) margin more than the distal margin. The critical issue, then, for tumors in the lower rectum, even those within the anal canal itself, is whether the tumor has invaded the external sphincter muscle (Fig. 3). If the muscles

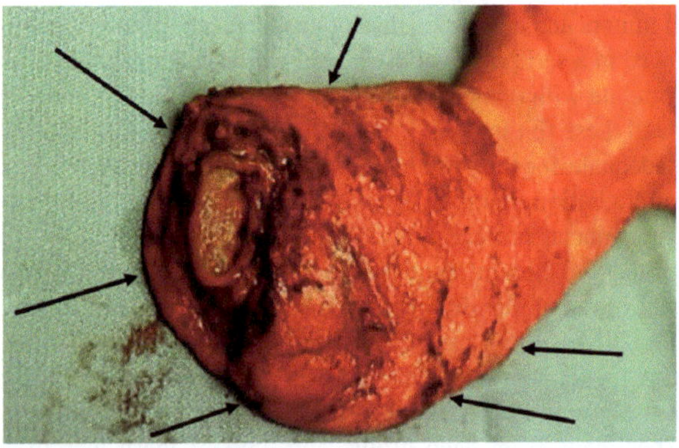

Fig. 3. Total mesorectal excision: the Fascia Propria. The arrows point out the smooth edge of the mesorectum, the fascia propria, after a TME. If there has not been extension of tumor through this fascial envelope, the sphincters should, from technical standpoint, be spared.

of the pelvic floor/external sphincter are not involved with the tumor, why remove them? Compared to historical dogma, contemporary surgical resection focuses more on deep (radial) margins vs. the distal margin. Surgical techniques are available that can preserve the anus and sphincters, even for very low tumors. The surgeon relies on meticulous technique and the use of neoadjuvant chemoradiation therapy to assure a negative deep margin. This approach should ensure a low rate of local recurrence.

SPHINCTER SPARING RESECTIONS

Basic Technical Concepts

Despite the level of the tumor in the rectum, any sphincter sparing resection (SSR) will start with a complete mobilization of the left colon to provide appropriate length of bowel for an anastomosis in the depths of the pelvis. There should be absolutely no tension on the anastomosis, whether it is constructed in the mid-rectum after resection of an upper rectal cancer, or at the dentate line after an intersphincteric LAR for a tumor at the upper aspect of the anal canal. For distal tumors, when reconstruction is performed with either a colonic J-pouch or a transverse coloplasty pouch, complete mobilization is of particular importance. The following are the steps to achieve this necessary length.

First the left colon is mobilized along its lateral peritoneal and retroperitoneal attachments over to the midline (the aorta). The omentum is removed from the distal transverse colon and the splenic flexure is taken down along the inferior edge of the pancreas, at the base of the transverse mesocolon, over to the middle colic vessels. The peritoneum to the right of the inferior mesenteric artery (IMA) is incised and the IMA is taken at its origin off of the aorta. The left colic artery is taken at its origin off of the IMA and the inferior mesenteric vein (IMV) is taken at the inferior edge of the pancreas. Taking the IMV is the final step in "straightening-out" the left colon so it will easily reach the pelvis. The marginal vessel at the sigmoid-descending colon is then isolated and clamped distally. It is divided proximally, good pulsatile flow is confirmed, and it is ligated. The bowel is divided at this point with a linear cutting stapler. At this point the left colon has been freed from its mesenteric attachments at the midline, which assures complete mobility, and its blood supply is the middle colic artery carried through the marginal vessel high in the mesentery. This type of complete mobilization is generally not required when performing an abdominal perineal resection. The extensive mesenteric mobilization is performed not necessarily for oncologic reasons, but for length reasons.

Low Anterior Resection

STANDARD LAR FOR UPPER RECTAL CANCER

For tumors in the upper rectum, surgery involves anterior resection (dissection and/or anastomosis does not go beneath the anterior peritoneal reflection) or LAR (anastomosis occurs beneath the anterior peritoneal reflection). These operations result in a colorectal anastomosis. This is typically a straight, double-stapled anastomosis with the distal bowel divided with a TA or PI type stapler, and the anastomosis constructed with a circular stapler. These operations should be performed according to the principles of TME. Mobilization should take place in defined anatomic planes, under direct vision using sharp dissection. The mesorectum is divided at a point approximately 5 cm below the distal edge of the tumor. It is at this point that the bowel is also divided.

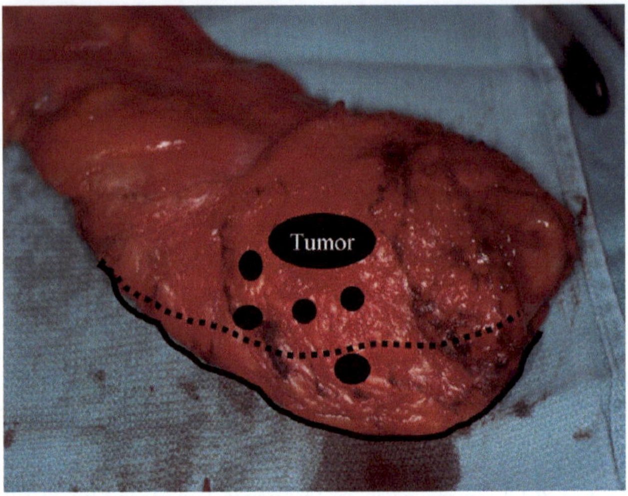

Fig. 4. Illustration of complete vs. incomplete total mesorectal excision. In this TME specimen, the dissection has taken place on the smooth surface of the mesorectum (*the solid line*). An incomplete mesorectal excision (*the dotted line*) may potentially leave tumor deposits intact, resulting in local recurrence.

Two concepts are important with this operation. The first is that the mesorectum and the bowel are divided at the same point. This is a critical concept. Many local, so-called mesorectal recurrences, occur because the surgeon "cones-in" on the rectum by coming through the mesorectum starting at a point too close to the tumor. The surgeon is happy that a 5 cm distal margin is obtained at the level of the bowel wall, but the real issue is the margin on the mesentery. Tumor outside the bowel wall (in the mesorectum, deep to the tumor) may be left intact if the surgeon does not take the mesorectal dissection just behind the fascia propria of the mesorectum, down to the point of the distal resection margin. The mesorectum is divided perpendicular to the distal rectal margin (Fig. 4).

The second important concept is that of distal rectal washout performed just before the bowel is divided distally *(39)*. There is good evidence that tumor cells are shed into the lumen of the bowel. This may be obvious on proctoscopy where portions of tumor are frequently (and easily) separated from the primary mass. The concept of the distal rectal washout is that these cells must not be incorporated in the distal staple line placed on the rectum when performing a double-stapled type of anastomosis. Once the mesorectum is divided distally, a right angle bowel clamp is placed just distal to the tumor and a cytotoxic solution (dilute alcohol, iodine solution) or sterile water is flooded into the distal rectum through a rectal tube or a bulb-type syringe. Once the distal bowel has been "washed-out," the distal staple line is placed. Again, the goal is to minimize the chance of incorporating tumor cells into the distal staple lines.

LAR for Mid- and Low-Rectal Cancer

For tumors in the mid-rectum, the left colon is mobilized as described above and the distal dissection is carried out according to the principles of TME. For mid-rectal tumors, the bowel is divided distally, just past the lower edge of the mesorectum, at the upper aspect of the anal canal. At this point the bowel is simply a muscular tube. Also at this point, the rectal diameter tapers down significantly as it transitions into the anal canal and it can be taken distally, for a double-stapled anastomosis, with a 30-mm stapler. There is no need for a larger stapler, as the bowel can almost always fit into this type of stapler. In fact, if it does not, then one is probably not at the proper level in the rectum. This is very consistent. Distal rectal washout is conducted as described above, and the anastomosis is carried out with a circular stapler. At this level, reconstruction is almost always carried out using a colonic J-pouch. The anastomosis following a TME with stapled colonic J-pouch to anal anastomosis will be situated about 1.5–2.0 cm above the dentate line, in very close proximity to the anorectal ring. This anastomosis is nearly always diverted temporarily with a loop ileostomy. For patients who have been treated with neoadjuvant chemoradiation therapy, this operation will typically be followed by a course of adjuvant chemotherapy. The loop ileostomy is generally closed when this course is completed.

For some tumors in the low-rectum, the resection and the reconstruction can be managed as described above for mid-rectal tumors. For the very low lesions, there are two techniques that allow for sphincter preservation. The first option is a hand-sewn coloanal anastomosis (simply a reconstructive option), and the second is a resection and reconstruction technique known as an intersphincteric proctectomy with coloanal anastomosis.

Hand-Sewn LAR with Colonic Pouch to Anal Anastomosis

The hand-sewn coloanal anastomosis is simply a technique used for reconstruction when there is not enough room in the pelvis to place the PI-30 stapler at the upper aspect of the anal canal (generally in a deep and very narrow male pelvis) or in the situation where an adequate margin can be obtained from the abdominal approach, but not enough margin for placing a distal staple line. The TME is conducted in the standard fashion down to the anal canal. However, instead of placing a staple gun distally, as would be performed for a double-stapled anastomosis, the bowel is occluded just distal to the tumor, and then it is simply divided with electrocautery from above, within the anal canal, usually about 0.5–1.0 cm above the dentate line. The specimen is passed off the table, and the patient is placed in a more exaggerated lithotomy position to expose the anus and perineum. The surgeon then works from between the legs and the anus is then effaced with a number of heavy sutures to better expose/efface the anal canal. Eight, 3-0 absorbable sutures are then placed at the cut edge of the distal bowel and these are tacked to the drapes. An assistant then passes the proximal bowel (almost always fashioned into a colonic J-pouch) into the pelvis. Different colored sutures placed at the apical colotomy on the pouch, used to mark right, left, anterior, and posterior, are then grasped with a clamp passed through the anus by the perineal operator. The pouch is then pulled down into the anal canal. Starting with the anterior, posterior, left, and right anal sutures, the hand-sewn colonic J-pouch to anal anastomosis is performed. The remaining four preplaced sutures are then placed using a small lighted Hill-Ferguson retractor for exposure in the anal canal. Additional sutures, usually eight to ten more, are placed, as needed. Unless the patient has a very long anal canal, there is usually no need to perform a mucosectomy of the anal canal. Rather, based on being in the right plane during the dissection, the bowel has been divided only 5–10 mm above the dentate line, and this is where the anastomosis is fashioned. Performing the anastomosis as such preserves the tissues of the anal canal. The colonic J-pouch to anal anastomosis is constructed within the anal canal, if possible.

Intersphincteric Proctectomy with Colonic Pouch to Anal Anastomosis

For the lowest of rectal cancers, the final technique for sphincter-preserving resection is an intersphincteric proctectomy with colonic pouch to anal anastomosis. This operation is

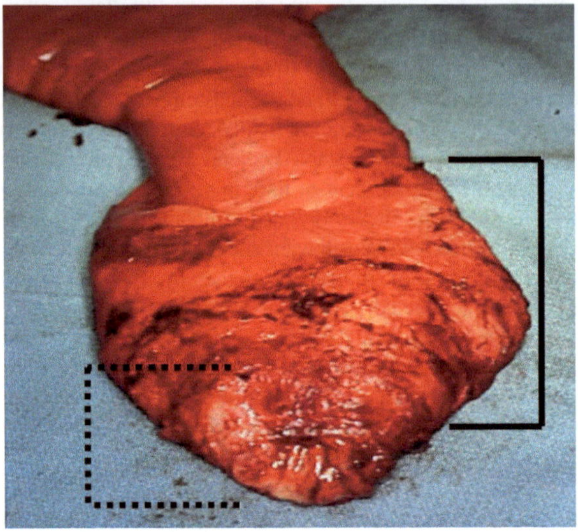

Fig. 5. An intersphincteric resection specimen. The *solid line* marks the mesorectum. The *dotted line* marks the anal canal above the *dentate line* which includes the mucosa, the submucosa and full thickness upper portion of the internal sphincter muscle.

chosen for patients with tumors that are located either just above or just below the anorectal ring but have not invaded the external sphincter muscle or pelvic floor. These operations leave very little margin for error in terms of the deep and distal margins. Most tumors treated with this technique are managed with neoadjuvant chemoradiation therapy to maximize these narrow margins and to decrease the volume of intraluminal tumor so as to avoid intraoperative tumor seeding. The validity of this operation is based on the concept that it is the deep tumor margin that is most critical. If the deep margin does not involve the skeletal muscle, then there is no reason to remove it. The intersphincteric resection is based anatomically on the concept (put forth by Heald in his writings on the TME) that if one follows the muscular tube of anorectum distally, one eventually exits on the anoderm in the intersphincteric groove at the anal verge (Fig. 5). This operation removes the upper aspect of the internal sphincter muscle (sometimes more), and as such, there will be functional changes. Patients chosen for this type of operation must be motivated, have a well-functioning sphincter mechanism and have normal premorbid continence.

The senior author performs this operation in two phases. The first part of the operation is conducted with the patient in the prone-jack-knife position. This is the most critical part of the operation and this position provides the best exposure to the anal canal and the most comfortable position for the surgeon. The anus is effaced with either a Lone Star retractor or heavy sutures. The anal canal is visualized using a lighted Hill-Ferguson or Sawyer retractor, and the anal canal mucosa is incised at the dentate line. The incision is circumferential and it extends through the mucosa, the submucosa, and directly through the internal sphincter muscle into the intersphincteric groove onto the external sphincter muscle. The dissection should begin away from the tumor so that the proper plane can be identified as an initial step and the area involved by the cancer can be approached last. The surgeon will know he is in the correct plane when he sees the anal canal tissue start to retract upwards as all of its attachments at the anus are disconnected. The most difficult part of the dissection is anterior.

The plane here is frequently not as clear. There are fibers of the internal sphincter and the external sphincter that interdigitate. In the male, it is important not to proceed too deep, as it is possible to actually dissect deep to the lower edge of the prostate, putting the urethra at great risk. Again, where possible, it is best to perform the posterior and lateral portions of the dissection prior to the anterior component. Finding the proper plane laterally and then dissecting toward the prostate from the side facilitates this process. The dissection proceeds proximally, staying just on the external sphincter muscle. The critical issue with this part of the dissection is whether the external sphincter muscle is free of tumor. If the surgeon has judged incorrectly, and this plane on the external sphincter muscle is not clean, attempts at sphincter preservation should be aborted, and the involved muscle will need to be resected. If not, dissection proceeds to a point well above the tumor. Often this plane can be followed up into the pelvis to a point just beneath the seminal vesicles in the male or the cervix in the female. When this proximal point is reached, the distal aspect of the "tube" of rectum is oversewn with a running suture, the pelvis is irrigated, the anal effacement sutures are removed, and the patient is turned and placed into the modified lithotomy position for the second phase of the operation.

The abdominal part of the operation is conducted and then the pelvic dissection proceeds in the usual fashion until it meets with the plane that has been developed from below. Once the specimen has been removed and the colonic pouch has been fashioned, the patient is placed in an exaggerated lithotomy position, the anus is effaced again and a hand-sewn colonic pouch to anal anastomosis is conducted as described above. This anastomosis is constructed at the dentate line and there is no real need to work up in the anal canal. The anastomotic sutures are placed deep to include anoderm and internal sphincter muscle. The effacement sutures are removed, the anastomosis retracts into the anal canal, and the anastomosis is diverted with a loop ileostomy.

Results with LAR and Intersphincteric Proctectomy

The issue of APR vs. LAR will likely never be resolved by a prospective, randomized trial, but there is abundant data indicating that local recurrence rates and survival figures are not adversely affected by aggressive attempts at sphincter preservation. Multiple reports have detailed good oncologic and functional results with LAR. Other reports have detailed experiences with intersphincteric proctectomy with reconstruction *(40–50)*. Local recurrence figures have been acceptably low, typically <10–12%. In a series of 92 patients reported by Rullier using the intersphincteric resection technique for tumors situated 1.5–4.5 cm from the anal verge, the rate of complete microscopic resection (R0) was 89%, with a 98% negative distal margin rate and 89% negative circumferential margin rate. In 58 patients with a follow-up of >24 months, the rate of local recurrence was 2% and the 5-year overall and disease-free survivals were 81 and 70%, respectively. Seventy-two of these patients had T3 disease and 81 patients were treated with preoperative chemoradiotherapy *(47)*. In another series of 121 patients undergoing intersphincteric resection and coloanal anastomosis, the median distance of the inferior margin of the tumor to the anal margin was 3 cm (range, 1–5 cm). One-hundred and seventeen of these patients had rectal cancer and 113 patients underwent curative resection. With a median follow-up time of 93 (range, 24–185) months, the local recurrence rate was 5.3% and most of these recurrences developed in the first 2 years *(49)*. The largest series of intersphincteric resections comes from Japan, where Saito reported on 228 patients undergoing intersphincteric proctectomy at seven Japanese institutions. One-hundred and three patients had T3 tumors and 78 had T2 disease. While not standardly performed in Japan, 57 patients with T3 tumors were treated with neoadjuvant chemoradiation therapy.

Complete microscopic curative surgery was achieved in 225 of the 228 patients. During the median observation time of 41 months, the rate of local recurrence was 5.8% at 3 years and 5-year overall and disease-free survival rates were 91.9 and 83.2%, respectively *(50)*.

Functional disturbances following almost any rectal cancer surgery are common, but a good quality of life can be achieved, even after intersphincteric proctectomy with coloanal anastomosis *(51–58)*. Comparing 37 patients undergoing conventional coloanal anastomosis to 40 patients undergoing intersphincteric resection and coloanal anastomosis, Bretagnol et al found that there was no difference in stool frequency, fragmentation, urgency, dyschezia, and alimentary restriction between the two groups. However, patients undergoing intersphincteric resection had worse continence and needed more antidiarrheal drugs. Quality of life after intersphincteric resection was altered based on the subscale of embarrassment in the Fecal Incontinence Quality of Life score, but not as measured by the SF-36, a second quality of life questionnaire *(54)*.

Reconstruction with a colonic J-pouch or a transverse coloplasty pouch (discussed below) can help minimize functional disturbances. In a report from Willis et al looking specifically at the issue of the colonic pouch vs. straight coloanal anastomosis after intersphincteric resection, patients undergoing pouch construction had significantly better outcomes in terms of stool frequency and urgency. On physiologic testing, these patients fared better in terms of maximum tolerated volume, threshold volume, and compliance. Interestingly, continence was not different between groups *(52)*. In addition, medical treatment with antidiarrheal agents, low residue diets, antispasmodic agents, enemas, and biofeedback can all help with regards to functional disturbances. Obviously, the intersphincteric operation removes (at least) the upper aspect of the internal sphincter and this will lower the resting tone of the anus *(59)*. The patient chosen for this type of operation must have a normal external sphincter and must understand that achieving normal continence may be a challenge. The authors' experience has been that in properly chosen and motivated patients, conversion to a permanent colostomy is rarely requested. The patient is given at least a year (or more) to adapt to the new anatomy before this type of conversion is even considered.

Reconstruction After LAR and Coloanal Anastomosis

As LAR replaced APR, and as the level of the anastomosis moved down to the anal canal, the bowel dysfunction that followed was appreciated and came to be known as the LAR syndrome. It can be reasonably stated that almost every patient treated with LAR (especially those who undergo a TME with an anastomosis constructed at the anorectal ring or below) will have some degree of functional difficulty. The symptoms of LAR syndrome include fecal urgency, frequency, tenesmus, a feeling of incomplete evacuation, clustering of bowel movements (multiple small volume stools over a period of time, as if one bowel movement empties itself in "clusters" instead of all at once), and sometimes incontinence. The symptoms generally improve over a period of 1–2 years. The etiology of this syndrome is not well understood. Possible explanations include impairment of internal anal sphincter function, decrease in anal canal sensation, disappearance of the recto-anal inhibitory reflex, and/or a disruption of local reflexes and communication between the rectum and the anus. The data supporting any of these concepts is inconsistent. The only consistent theme is that the neorectal reservoir lacks the type of compliance found in the native rectum. There is now data that would suggest that the cause of the syndrome is extrinsic denervation of the neorectum that takes place during the extensive efforts made to mobilize the left colon so that it will reach, without tension, to the anus *(60)*.

Recognizing the syndrome, in 1986, Lazorthes *(61)* and Parcs, *(62)* in the same volume of the British Journal of Surgery, described in separate studies their experience with reconstruction using, instead of a straight coloanal anastomosis, a colonic J-pouch to anal anastomosis. Both reported improved function after a low colorectal or coloanal anastomosis using this approach. Over the next decade, a number of studies clarified issues surrounding colonic J-pouch reconstruction. Initially, pouches were made too large and did not empty appropriately *(62–64)*. The proper size has now been determined to be in the range of 5–7 cm *(65–67)* Pouches that were anastomosed to the rectum, too far from the anus, were also found to be problematic. It became clear that a pouch should be used only for reconstruction at the lowest levels, within about 2 cm of the dentate line or 3–4 cm of the anal verge *(52,68,69)* Above this, and the pouch may not empty well. A number of prospective randomized trials concluded that reconstruction using a colonic J-pouch to anal anastomosis was superior to a straight coloanal anastomosis *(70,71)*. It was widely felt that the pouch reconstruction was primarily helpful in the first year or two following surgery. Thereafter, it was felt that even after a straight anastomosis, the neorectal compliance improved and the functional differences resolved. However, two long-term studies suggest that the functional superiority of pouch reconstruction is durable. Dehni et al compared 47 pouch patients to 34 straight patients, with a mean follow-up of 5 years, and found that for every variable measured (frequency, clustering, use of antidiarrheals, need to restrict diet, and overall disruption of social or professional life as a result of bowel function), the pouch patients fared better *(72)*. Hida et al evaluated 5 year follow-up of 46 pouch patients vs. 48 straight patients, and again, for every variable measured (number of bowel movements per day or night, urgency and soilage), the pouch patients did better *(73)*. A meta-analysis of multiple studies published on colonic J-pouch formation support the functional superiority of this reconstruction over the straight coloanal anastomosis *(74)*.

For a variety of reasons, including perceived evacuation problems in some patients with colonic J-pouches and the technical difficulties associated with placing a bulky pouch into the depths of a narrow male pelvis (particularly when the anastomosis is at the dentate line), a different type of pouch, the transverse coloplasty pouch, was described, first by Z'graggen in 1999, *(75,76)* then by Fazio in 2000 *(77)*. The concept was to duplicate J-pouch function without creating a pouch. From a technical standpoint, an 8–10 cm long longitudinal colotomy is made starting about 4–5 cm from the end of the colon. The colotomy is then closed transversely, similar to the closure of a strictureplasty. Since a "straight" anastomosis is constructed with the coloplasty pouch, the problems with placement of a bulky pouch to or down into the anal canal in a narrow, deep pelvis are obviated. A large, multicenter, international trial was conducted to answer the question of whether this type of pouch works as well as a colonic J-pouch *(78)*. Patients who could not undergo colonic J-pouch placement were randomized to straight coloanal vs. transverse coloplasty pouch placement. Patients in whom a colonic J-pouch was feasible were randomized to J-pouch vs. transverse pouch placement. With 364 patients randomized, the authors found that the J-pouch was functionally superior to the transverse coloplasty pouch and that the transverse pouch was superior to a straight anastomosis (Fig. 6).

Temporary Diversion After Coloanal Anastomosis

An anastomosis at or beneath the anorectal ring, as one constructs following TME or intersphincteric proctectomy with coloanal anastomosis, is considered a high-risk anastomosis. This is based on a significant rate of anastomotic leak and the morbid consequences of a leak

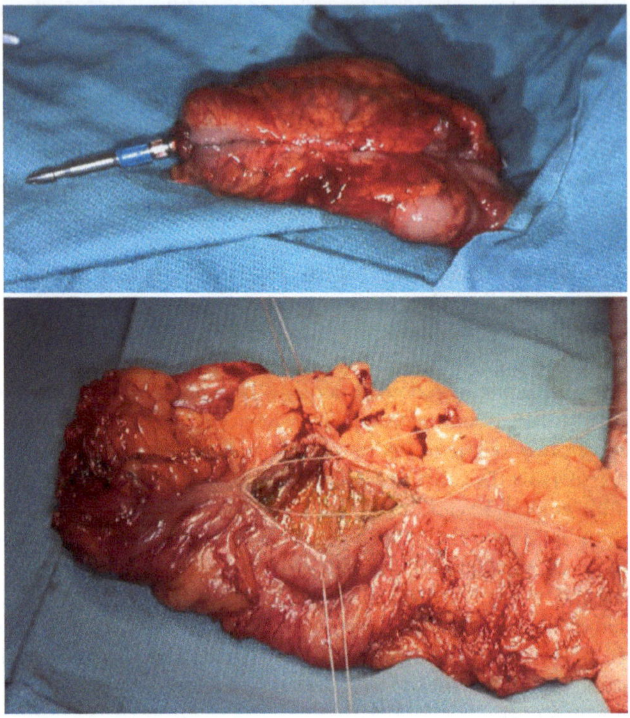

Fig. 6. Two types of colonic pouches. The upper photo is a 7 cm colonic J-pouch ready to be approximated to the anus for a double-stapled anastomosis. The lower photo is a transverse coloplasty pouch being prepared. There is an 8–10 cm longitudinal colotomy being closed transversely about 4 cm from the end of the colon.

at this level. As such, these patients frequently undergo temporary enteral diversion with a loop ileostomy. Leak rates as high as 40% have been reported when routine radiographic evaluation is performed. The "true" leak rate is probably somewhere in the 1–15% range, and appears to be lower among patients undergoing diverting stoma *(79–81)*. In an early study by Heald's group, *(81)* clinically significant anastomotic complications were seen in 15% of 75 patients without an ostomy, and in only 0.8% of 125 diverted patients. This is in the setting of diversion being used selectively for patients thought by the surgeon to be at high risk of anastomotic leak. Based on these results, Heald recommends temporary diversion for all patients undergoing TME. In the Dutch TME Trail, TME was associated with an anastomotic leak rate of 12%, with absence of a protective stoma associated with an increased risk of anastomotic breakdown and a greater need for surgical intervention following leak diagnosis. The authors concluded that every patient undergoing TME should have a protective stoma *(82,83)*. Eriksen evaluated leak rates in a prospective study of 1958 patients undergoing anterior resection for rectal cancer with TME from 1993–1998. The overall leak rate was 11.6% and multivariate analysis showed that the risk of leakage was significantly higher in men, patients treated with neoadjuvant radiation therapy, and when the anastomosis was <6 cm from the anal verge. The authors concluded that a low anastomosis after TME should be protected through placement of a diverting stoma. Prospective and randomized trials support the concept that temporary diversion should accompany reconstruction with a low anastomosis after TME *(84,85)*.

The consequences of a leak at this level in the pelvis can be very significant *(86)*. While some would argue that a diverting stoma does not reduce the anastomotic leak rate, few would disagree with the concept that the consequences of anastomotic leak are significantly reduced when a stoma is in place *(79,87)*. In the diverted patient, pelvic sepsis can almost always be treated by simply placing a drain. In the nondiverted patient, drains may suffice, but a return to the operating room to construct a diversion may be in order. The consequences of a leak include formation of significant fibrosis in and around the neorectum which can adversely affect bowel function. In addition, pelvic sepsis can lead to a hard, static, and fibrotic pelvic floor that simply does not function properly. Combining these potential problems with the already problematic bowel function that can accompany these operations and the value in trying to avoid pelvic sepsis become clear. In addition, an uneventful postoperative recovery allows patients to receive adjuvant chemotherapy in a timely fashion. There is data to suggest that pelvic sepsis following rectal cancer resection places patients at an increased risk of worsened oncologic outcome *(88,89)*. All told, temporary diversion after TME with reconstruction seems prudent *(90)*.

ABDOMINOPERINEAL RESECTION

For the vast majority of tumors in the upper-, mid-, and low-rectum, as long as baseline bowel and sphincter function is satisfactory, a SSR is indicated. For tumors in the distal rectum, the current indication for APR is tumor fixation to the pelvic floor or external sphincter muscle. In this setting, curative tumor resection requires resection of the continence mechanism and, short of creating a colo-perineal anastomosis and surrounding it with either a gracillis neosphincter *(91)* or an artificial bowel sphincter, *(92)* a permanent colostomy will be the end result. As stated previously, while APR was once considered the "gold standard" operation for patients with rectal cancer, it can now be fairly stated that the LAR, conducted according to the principles of TME, has supplanted the APR. With regard to the APR, the following issues should be considered: (1) an APR may actually be inferior to LAR as an oncologic procedure, and a multidisciplinary approach and extraordinary operative approaches may be needed to optimize oncologic outcomes, and (2) poor perineal wound healing is frequently encountered following APR, especially in patients who have been treated with neoadjuvant chemoradiation therapy, and flap closure may be indicated.

Oncologic Adequacy of the Standard APR

For decades, the APR was the standard radical operation for rectal cancer against which all other operations were compared. Its place as an effective cancer operation was unquestioned. Despite this, there is now considerable data suggesting that there may be significant oncologic drawbacks surrounding the use of APR for rectal cancer. In a population-based observational study from Leeds in the UK, Haward et al were able to show that in over 3,500 rectal cancer patients treated in the Yorkshire Regional Health Authority, there was a statistically significant survival advantage for those patients treated with anterior resection as compared to these treated with an APR *(93)*. The analysis also indicated that colorectal specialist and high-volume colorectal cancer surgeons were more likely to offer SSR. Based on analysis of a smaller set of data, the authors concluded that the differences seen were not a function of significant differences in stage distribution between those treated with LAR vs. APR. Law and Chu, from Hong Kong, reported that in a series of 504 patients with rectal cancer treated surgically with TME-type resections, for the 69 patients treated with APR, as compared to the 435 treated with LAR, the local recurrence rate was higher (23% vs. 10.2%) and the cancer-specific survival rate was lower (60% vs. 74%). On subgroup analysis of patients with tumors <6 cm from the anal verge, patients treated with LAR had local recurrence rates less than those treated with APR. There was no difference in the rate of distant metastatic disease development between these groups, suggesting that the difference in survival was based on the difference in the rate of local recurrence *(22)*. Marr and colleagues reported local recurrence and survival figures for 608 patients operated for rectal cancer in Leeds between 1986 and 1997 *(94)*. Compared to LAR patients, APR patients had a higher local recurrence rate (22.3% vs. 13.5%, $p<0.002$) and a lower survival rate (52.3% vs. 65.8%, $p<0.003$). Based on careful pathologic measurements of the volume of tissue removed outside of the muscularis propria of the rectum (less for APR specimens than for LAR specimens) and linear dimensions of transverse slices of tissue containing tumor, median posterior and lateral margins were smaller for APR specimens relative to LAR specimens. Corresponding to this, the rate of CRM positivity was higher in the APR group than in the LAR group (36% vs. 22%, $p<0.002$). They conclude that the oncologic drawback with APR is that poor results are a reflection of a high rate of CRM involvement in APR specimens. Based on careful pathologic specimen evaluation and the fact that the stage distribution between APR and LAR patients was similar, and the depth of tumor infiltration only slightly greater in the APR group, the authors conclude that the poor results after APR are a result of the removal of less tissue at the level of the tumor in an APR. This problem has not been diminished by TME and they suggest that a change to a more radical approach for APR be considered. Data from the Dutch TME Trial *(95)* suggests that part of the problem with APR may be the high rate of incomplete TME in patients undergoing APR compared to those undergoing an LAR (66% vs. 27%). This is notable when considering the fact that when local recurrence rates in patients with a negative CRM were analyzed, the overall recurrence rate was increased in the group undergoing incomplete mesorectal excision (28.6% vs. 14.9%, $p<0.03$) *(95)*. den Dulk et al using data from APR patients participating in the Dutch TME Trial reported that the involved CRM rate for APR patients was 29.6% overall with an astonishingly high rate of 44% for anteriorly situated tumors. Anterior tumor location, advanced T-stage, and higher N-stage were independent risk factors for an involved CRM. Similarly, positive CRM, advanced T-stage and high N-stage were risk factors for local recurrence *(96)*. Nagtegaal et al again using data from the Dutch TME Trial, reported that patients treated with APR, as compared to those treated with LAR, had a higher rate of CRM involvement (30.4% vs. 10.7%, $p<0.002$), a higher rate of specimen perforation (13.7% vs. 2.5%, $p<0.001$) and, surprisingly, by careful pathologic specimen examination, the plane of dissection around the tumor was within the sphincter muscles, the submucosa or the rectal lumen in more than one-third of APR specimens *(97)*. Not surprisingly, the survival for patients undergoing APR, as opposed to LAR, was worse (38.5% vs. 57.6%, $p<0.008$). The authors concluded that the disappointing results for this operation might be greatly improved by adoption of different surgical techniques (that result in wider margins and less frequent CRM involvement) and/or the more frequent use of neoadjuvant chemoradiation therapy for this group of patients.

In contrast to the above, there is data suggesting APR results in equivalent oncologic outcomes relative to LAR. Data from the Norwegian Rectal Cancer Project looked at over 2,100 patients with rectal cancer treated at 47 centers and found that on multivariate analysis, tumor distance from the anal verge, but not the operative technique (APR vs. LAR), influenced the risk of local recurrence *(98)*. Chuwa and Seow-Choen from Singapore evaluated oncologic outcomes of 791 patients undergoing curative resections for rectal cancer, 12.1% of whom underwent APR. They found no difference in local recurrence rates or 5-year survival between those treated with APR vs. sphincter-preserving resections *(99)*.

The issue with much of the literature regarding the disappointing results of APR for the treatment of low-rectal cancers is that patients either did not receive preoperative chemoradiotherapy or they were treated with short course radiation therapy (five times 5 Gy over 5 days with surgery to follow within a week). This short course approach does not allow sufficient time for tumor downstaging, *(100)* so it is unlikely that it will in any way alter the high rate of CRM involvement for the bulky, very low-rectal cancer that typically is treated with an APR. Additionally, there is little doubt that the anatomy in the depths of the pelvis in the funnel of the levators and external sphincters makes dissection difficult and this can result in CRM compromise. Similarly, anterior tumors are problematic. The mesorectum is thin anteriorly in men and particularly so in women. There is not a clear anatomic plane outside the sphincters and pelvic floor that allows the surgeon to very precisely separate the specimen from adjacent organs such as the vagina, the urinary sphincter, and the postprostatic urethra in men. Simply put, in many (if not most) cases, there just is not much room for error in the anterior dissection (Fig. 7). The difference between a negative CRM and a multivisceral resection may only be a few millimeters. Even for lateral or posterior tumors, when studying the anatomy of the rectum and the mesorectum, one appreciates that below a point, the rectum is no longer surrounded by the mesorectum. There is simply a muscular tube as the rectum transitions into the anus. Tumors with extension outside the bowel wall in this location are problematic and margins can be very slight.

To manage these problems, a multidisciplinary approach makes the most sense, with operation preceded by a long course of neoadjuvant chemoradiation therapy, which has been consistently shown to downstage rectal cancers *(6,7)*. This downstaging effect may help reduce the incidence of an involved CRM for these low tumors. It is also reasonable for the surgeon to constantly bear in mind the importance of obtaining a wide margin of normal tissue at the level of the tumor. During APR, the levators are taken at their attachments on the pelvic sidewall, and the anococcygeal ligament is taken just over the coccyx. In women, the anterior margin is taken just on the posterior vaginal wall, or includes the posterior vaginal wall if necessary,

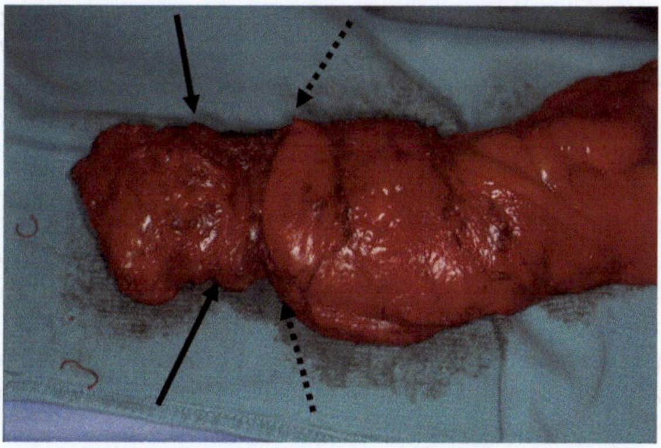

Fig. 7. An abdominoperineal resection specimen. The *dotted arrows* mark the end of the mesorectum. The *solid arrows* mark the lower edge of the pelvic floor just above the perineal portion of the specimen. It is in this zone that the CRM is at risk.

and then anteriorly through the transverse perineal muscles. In men, the dissection is performed just on the posterior aspect of the prostate, it is carried down the posterior aspect of the rectourethralis muscles and just over the urethra before coming down through the perineal body.

One can argue that the optimal exposure for the perineal portion of an APR is with the patient in a prone jack-knife position. This is the senior author's preferred approach. The abdominal dissection is taken down past the coccyx posteriorly, onto the pelvic floor laterally, and then anteriorly down to the distal aspect of the prostate in males or the mid-vagina in females. The rectum is pushed into the pelvis, the abdomen is closed, the colostomy is matured, and the patient is repositioned on the operative table. The perineal incision is made out over the ischiorectal fat pads and extends from the tip of the coccyx to the perineal body. The dissection is taken down through the subcutaneous fat, into the ischiorectal fossae, and down to the anococcygeal ligament posteriorly. The pelvis is entered sharply just over the tip of the coccyx, and the pelvic floor muscles are "hooked" with the index finger and are taken widely on the pelvic sidewall bilaterally. Typically, the rectal specimen is then delivered through the wound giving optimal exposure for the anterior dissection, which is generally the most technically demanding portion of the operation. The prone position optimizes this anterior exposure. There are potential downsides to this repositioning, including anesthesia concerns in turning the patient, the difficulty in using a rectus myocutaneous muscle flap for perineal reconstruction or vaginal wall reconstruction (if needed), and the possibility of having to perform an additional position change should it become clear during the perineal phase that a multivisceral resection will be required to achieve negative margins. The tremendous exposure, in most cases, compensates for these downsides.

Perineal Wound Healing After APR

Aside from the potential oncologic issues detailed above, another potential drawback of the APR is the tendency for delayed perineal wound healing, particularly when preceded by the neoadjuvant use of chemoradiation therapy. In this setting, the rate of perineal wound morbidity has been reported to be from 10 to 40%. In the Swedish Rectal Cancer Trial, patients in the irradiated group had a twofold increase in perineal wound infection from 10 to 20% *(101)*. In the Dutch TME Trial, APR patients treated with short course radiotherapy had a perineal wound complication rate of 31% *(102)*. In a Polish trial evaluating short vs. long course radiation, the short course patients had a 29% incidence of perineal wound complications vs. 21% for those treated with the long course regimen *(103)*. In a study of patients undergoing APR at Memorial Sloan-Kettering Cancer Center, 30% of patients who had been previously treated with preoperative chemoradiation therapy experienced a perineal wound infection compared to 13% who had not been irradiated. In patients treated with both preoperative and intraoperative radiation therapy, the rate of infection was 61%. Thirty days after surgery, the perineal wound was still open in 19% of the surgery-alone patients, 51% of the preoperative radiation group and in 83% of the patients who had pre- and intraoperative radiation *(104)*. Delayed perineal wound healing can present a significant obstacle for patients in whom a course of adjuvant chemotherapy is planned.

In the past, perineal wounds were often left open to heal by second intention. Today, they are usually closed primarily. There is some data that suggests that using antibiotic impregnated fleece in the pelvis and the perineum can reduce the incidence of perineal wound infection *(105)*. Successful use of various myocutaneous flaps has also been reported. The rectus myocutaneous flap, based on the inferior epigastric pedicle, is a useful flap for closing a difficult perineum, particularly following posterior vaginectomy *(106–111)*. However, when a pelvic exenteration is performed and dual stomas are required, the placement of the second stoma on the side from which the flap was harvested can be problematic. Also, if the perineal portion of the operation is to be performed with the patient in the prone jack-knife position, using this flap may be problematic and may require the help of a cooperative and creative plastic surgeon. Shibat et al reported on their experience using unilateral or bilateral gracillis muscle flaps for perineal wound closure after radiation therapy and APR for primary or recurrent rectal cancer *(112)*. Flap closure resulted in a lower incidence of perineal wound infection than seen in a comparable group of patients who had primary closure. Successful use of gluteal flaps and posterior thigh flaps have also been described *(113,114)*.

Frequency of APR Utilization

While the issue of restricting the treatment of rectal cancer to surgeons with special training and sufficient volume to maintain skills has gained support in some parts of the world, in the United States, where there are no restrictions, the issues surrounding APR are particularly critical as a large number of these operations continue to be performed. Recent data from Ricciardi et al based on a review of a large national database, showed that while the rate of SSR improved from 27% in 1988 to 48% in 2003, the majority of rectal cancer patients still undergo an APR for treatment of their disease *(115)*. This is viewed as problematic *(116)*. Ultimately, while the choice of operation for any one patient with rectal cancer depends on multiple tumor and patient characteristics, there is data to suggest that higher surgeon or hospital caseload is associated with an increased utilization of SSRs. Using the same large national database referenced above, Purves and colleagues were able to show that rectal cancer patients treated by high-volume surgeons, defined as surgeons doing more that ten rectal cancer resections a year, were five times more likely to be treated with a sphincter sparing procedure than those treated by low volume rectal cancer surgeons (defined as surgeons doing one to three rectal cancer operations a year) *(117)*. Data from a national audit in the Netherlands showed that the APR vs. LAR ratio dropped by 32% comparing sequential time periods in the mid- to late-1990s *(118)*. The authors of this study attributed this increased use of SSRs to a change in surgical attitude that accompanied the teaching of proper technique and the control of operation at the time of the Dutch TME trial. A Swedish study also showed that APR rates may decline in a region when rectal cancer operations are performed by fewer, better trained surgeons *(24)*.

Quality of Life After APR

The secondary goal in treating patients with rectal cancer is optimizing quality of life, and for most patients, it has generally been assumed that this translates into a SSR. As detailed above, much effort has been extended toward sparing sphincter function with the thought that this would provide, for properly selected patients, the best quality of life. While there are obvious body image issues that may come with permanent colostomy placement, there is a "price to be paid" in terms of abnormal bowel function when a low anastomosis is constructed. Recent studies, using various instruments for measuring quality of life, suggest that the differences experienced by patients having an APR vs. an LAR are not as significant as one might predict. In a prospective study of 249 patients treated for rectal cancer (46 APR and 203 LAR) using validated quality of life instruments, Schmidt and colleagues found that quality of life for patients undergoing an LAR was not different than that of patients undergoing APR *(119)*. APR patients experienced more sexual dysfunction while LAR patients suffered more bowel dysfunction. Using data from the Norwegian Rectal Cancer

Database, Guren et al found that in 319 rectal cancer patients (229 LAR and 90 APR), LAR patients had better body image and better preserved male sexual function compared to APR patients; however, there were no differences in overall quality of life *(120)*. Patients with a very low anastomosis (<3 cm from the anal verge) had worse bowel function than those with a higher anastomosis but still had a better overall quality of life than patients treated with an APR. This led the authors to conclude that impairment in functional outcome does not necessarily have a major impact on quality of life. They also found that radiation had an overall negative impact on quality of life. Using treatment trade-off (where the certainty of a stoma was hypothetically weighed against the risk of incontinence) and time trade-off (where the remaining life expectancy was traded off to avoid a permanent stoma or fecal incontinence) methods, Bossema et al, using patients participating in the Dutch TME trial, found that most patients preferred LAR over APR even if LAR involved a risk of fecal incontinence *(121)*. Seventy-one percent of LAR patients would chose LAR even if they would suffer monthly incontinence, and 32% would chose LAR even if the incontinence episodes were daily. However, APR patients would give up less remaining years of life to be without a stoma than LAR patients to be without monthly incontinence.

Patients treated by either operation can have a good quality of life, and preoperatively, they should be counseled as such. The decision as to whether a rectal cancer is better treated with a SSR or an APR is a complex one based on the exact location of the tumor, the stage of the tumor, the patient's baseline bowel and anal function, overall health status, and perhaps most importantly, their personal desires in terms of how they would rather be treated once they have had appropriate counseling.

BEYOND: LAPAROSCOPIC RECTAL CANCER RESECTION

Four prospective randomized controlled trials have evaluated the oncologic adequacy of laparoscopic colectomy, *(122–125)* proving it to be at least equivalent to open surgery in experienced hands. Only one of these trials included comparison of laparoscopic and open radical proctectomy, and when early outcomes were published, there was a nonsignificant trend toward margin positivity in the laparoscopic group *(123)*. However, a follow-up study by the same group demonstrated no difference in local recurrence rates *(126)*.

That laparoscopic colon resections are technically challenging is widely appreciated by colorectal and laparoscopic surgeons *(127,128)*. These challenges intensify in deep pelvic surgery, and recognition of these differences lends some degree of uncertainty to extrapolation of results from the colectomy experience to radical proctectomy. From a technical standpoint, whether performing open and laparoscopic proctectomy, limited exposure is the primary obstacle to performing TME. The bony confines of the pelvis impede visualization and hinder distraction of tissue necessary for identification of tissue planes. In some respects, the laparoscopic approach provides superior visualization by placing the video lens in the pelvis and by replacing the surgeon's hand with narrow instruments. Even so, dissection is arduous. Loss of tactile sensory input and mechanical limitations of laparoscopic stapling devices demand careful planning of rectal transection to avoid compromising the distal margin or even worse, incorporating the tumor bed in the staple line. Surgeons who contributed laparoscopic colectomy data to the COSTG (Clinical Outcomes of Surgical Therapy Study Group) trial had to first prove technical proficiency *(122)*. The number of surgeons performing laparoscopic proctectomies is small but growing, and many surgeons have tried to address the technical challenges of the pure laparoscopic approach by developing hand assisted and hybrid approaches.

Pending completion of larger, prospective randomized controlled trials comparing laparoscopic and open radical proctectomy, surrogate markers of oncologic adequacy have been used in retrospective or nonrandomized prospective studies to assess early outcomes. A meta-analysis of 2,071 patients showed no difference in lymph node harvest or radial margin positivity between laparoscopic and open procedures *(129)*. Another study utilizing the grading system for mesorectal fascial integrity defined by the Dutch TME trial found no difference between operative approaches in a nonrandomized series of 25 patients *(130)*.

Differences in functional outcomes and economic implications of laparoscopic vs. open approaches have also been evaluated. Retrospective review of bladder and sexual dysfunction among patients enrolled in a randomized, controlled trial comparing laparoscopic and open resection found an increased incidence of male sexual dysfunction in laparoscopically resected rectal cancer patients. It was noted, however, that the preponderance of patients in the laparoscopic group with erectile and ejaculatory problems had either locally advanced or very low tumors *(131)*. This trend was also reported in a follow-up of the CLASICC (Medical Research Council Conventional vs. Laparoscopic-Assisted Surgery In Colorectal Cancer) trial. Male patients undergoing laparoscopic proctectomy had an excess incidence of sexual and bladder dysfunction compared to laparoscopic colectomy and open proctectomy patients. Interestingly, the TME rate in the laparoscopic proctectomy group was higher than in the open group despite the fact that the groups were well matched with regard to tumor level and T-stage. In the CLASICC trial, tumor fixity and uncertainty about margin clearance were the most common reasons for conversion from laparoscopic to open proctectomy. The authors speculated that difficulty in assessing tumor location may have led laparoscopic surgeons to dissect more widely. Additionally, wider resection margin is associated with increased risk of encroachment on pelvic nerves *(132)*. Two more recent trials suggest that bladder and sexual dysfunction rates are the same or better following laparoscopic compared to open TME *(133,134)*. Although none of these studies constitute level I data, it is possible that refinement of laparoscopic TME skills enhances surgeons' ability to identify and preserve pelvic nerves by capitalizing on the superior pelvic visualization made possible by laparoscopic instrumentation.

It has been shown that reconstruction with a colonic J-pouch rather than straight colorectal or coloanal anastomosis following open LAR results in superior bowel function. Laparoscopic colonic J-pouch reconstruction is technically feasible, but it was uncertain whether this approach would confer the same advantages to laparoscopically resected patients that it does to open. A study that randomized patients undergoing laparoscopic proctectomy to either straight anastomosis or colonic J-pouch formation found that J-pouch patients had decreased stool frequency, improved perineal irritation, and less use of diarrheal medications than those with straight anastomoses. J-pouch patients also returned to work and full activities sooner *(135)*.

Efforts to discern the financial impact of performing an operation laparoscopically or open have been confounded by numerous issues such as selection bias (i.e., allocation of technically challenging patients to conventional surgery), cultural factors (length of stay and reliance on intermediate care after hospital discharge), complication profiles (i.e., potential influence of the procedural learning curve), difficulty assessing indirect costs (nursing care intensity), and valuation of quality of life. It appears that higher operative costs of laparoscopic colectomy are offset by lower utilization of services after leaving the operating room *(136,137)*. With regard to proctectomy specifically, a cost–benefit analysis of laparoscopic vs. open radical proctectomy evaluated clinical outcomes and expense in 168 rectal adenocarcinoma patients randomized to either approach. The laparoscopic patients experienced shorter postoperative recovery, improved 1-year quality of life, and no compromise of oncologic outcome at early follow-up, but at increased cost ($351/patient) *(138)*.

Table 1
Laparoscopic vs. open proctectomy oncologic outcomes meta-analysis (Anderson et al.) *(139)*

Outcome measure	*No. of articles*	*N*	*Lap (mean)*	*Open (mean)*	*p Value*
Positive radial margin (%)	10	1,504	5	8	ns
Distance radial margin (%)	5	642	0.5 cm	0.6 cm	ns
Lymph node harvest (*n*)	17	2,442	10[a]	11[a]	0.001
Local recurrence (%)[b]	16	2,277	7	8	ns
Distant failure (%)[b]	10	1,408	13	14	ns
Overall survival (%)[c]	11	1,995	72	65	ns

[a]Median number of lymph nodes
[b]Mean follow-up 33 months
[c]At average 4.4 years

Longer-term oncologic outcomes with laparoscopic proctectomy are now being reported. A meta-analysis of 24 comparative rectal cancer publications included data on 1,403 laparoscopic and 1,755 open proctectomies (Table 1). There was no difference between the groups with regard to mean radial margin positivity (5% laparoscopic vs. 8% open, p=n.s.) or mean radial margin distance (0.5 cm laparoscopic vs. 0.6 cm open, p=n.s.). A small difference in median lymph node harvest was noted despite comparable neoadjuvant radiation therapy rates in the laparoscopic and open groups (10 laparoscopic vs. 11 open, $p=0.001$). This difference may be attributable to three studies whose open lymph node harvest rate was substantially greater than the laparoscopic rate *(139)*.

In this meta-analysis, 16 of the 24 publications analyzed included sufficient data to compare local recurrence (LR) rates at a mean follow-up of 33 months and found no difference. The mean LR rate was 7% in the laparoscopic group and 8% in the open group (p=n.s.). Of the ten studies with sufficient distant failure data, there was likewise no difference (12% lap, 14% open, p=n.s.). Survival rates established from 11 studies also showed no difference at an average 4.4 year follow-up (72% laparoscopic vs. 65% open, p=n.s.).

The consistency of the results among these preliminary studies is encouraging and suggests that laparoscopic proctectomy may be comparable to an open approach. In lieu of having results from large, randomized controlled trials with long-term follow-up, laparoscopic colorectal surgeons are proceeding cautiously. Despite apparent perioperative quality of life advantages enjoyed by patients undergoing laparoscopic resections, surgeons and patients alike must remain cognizant of the primary goal of treatment: curative extirpation of rectal cancer. Every effort must be made to avoid compromising this goal.

REFERENCES

1. Miles W. The radical abdomino-perineal operation for cancer of the pelvic colon. *BMJ*. 1910;941–943.
2. Miles W. *Cancer of the Rectum*. London: Harrison; 1926.
3. Dixon CF. Anterior resection for malignant lesions of the upper part of the rectum and lower part of the sigmoid. *Ann Surg*. 1948;128:425–442.
4. Williams NS. The rationale for preservation of the anal sphincter in patients with low rectal cancer. *Br J Surg*. 1984;71:575–581.

5. Sauer R, Becker H, Hohenberger W, et al. Preoperative versus postoperative chemoradiotherapy for rectal cancer. *N Engl J Med*. 2004;351:1731–1740.
6. Crane CH, Skibber JM, Birnbaum EH, et al. The addition of continuous infusion 5-FU to preoperative radiation therapy increases tumor response, leading to increased sphincter preservation in locally advanced rectal cancer. *Int J Radiat Oncol Biol Phys*. 2003;57:84–89.
7. Onaitis MW, Noone RB, Fields R, et al. Complete response to neoadjuvant chemoradiation for rectal cancer does not influence survival. *Ann Surg Oncol*. 2001;8:801–806.
8. Habr-Gama A, Perez RO, Proscurshim I, et al. Patterns of failure and survival for nonoperative treatment of stage c0 distal rectal cancer following neoadjuvant chemoradiation therapy. *J Gastrointest Surg*. 2006;10:1319–1328. discussion 28–29.
9. Wibe A, Eriksen MT, Syse A, Myrvold HE, Soreide O. Total mesorectal excision for rectal cancer – what can be achieved by a national audit? *Colorectal Dis*. 2003;5:471–477.
10. Raub WF. From the National Institutes of Health. *JAMA*. 1991;265:2173.
11. Heald RJ, Husband EM, Ryall RD. The mesorectum in rectal cancer surgery – the clue to pelvic recurrence? *Br J Surg*. 1982;69:613–616.
12. Heald RJ. The 'Holy Plane' of rectal surgery. *J R Soc Med*. 1988;81:503–508.
13. Colorectal Cancer Collaborative Group. Adjuvant radiotherapy for rectal cancer: a systematic overview of 8,507 patients from 22 randomised trials. *Lancet*. 2001;358:1291–1304.
14. Heald RJ, Moran BJ, Ryall RD, Sexton R, MacFarlane JK. Rectal cancer: the Basingstoke experience of total mesorectal excision, 1978–1997. *Arch Surg*. 1998;133:894–899.
15. Kapiteijn E, Marijnen CA, Nagtegaal ID, et al. Preoperative radiotherapy combined with total mesorectal excision for resectable rectal cancer. *N Engl J Med*. 2001;345:638–646.
16. Cawthorn SJ, Parums DV, Gibbs NM, et al. Extent of mesorectal spread and involvement of lateral resection margin as prognostic factors after surgery for rectal cancer. *Lancet*. 1990;335: 1055–1059.
17. Arbman G, Nilsson E, Hallbook O, Sjodahl R. Local recurrence following total mesorectal excision for rectal cancer. *Br J Surg*. 1996;83:375–379.
18. Enker WE, Thaler HT, Cranor ML, Polyak T. Total mesorectal excision in the operative treatment of carcinoma of the rectum. *J Am Coll Surg*. 1995;181:335–346.
19. Arenas RB, Fichera A, Mhoon D, Michelassi F. Total mesenteric excision in the surgical treatment of rectal cancer: a prospective study. *Arch Surg*. 1998;133:608–611. discussion 11–12.
20. Fernandez-Represa JA, Mayol JM, Garcia-Aguilar J. Total mesorectal excision for rectal cancer: the truth lies underneath. *World J Surg*. 2004;28:113–116.
21. Heald RJ, Smedh RK, Kald A, Sexton R, Moran BJ. Abdominoperineal excision of the rectum – an endangered operation. Norman Nigro Lectureship. *Dis Colon Rectum*. 1997;40:747–751.
22. Law WL, Chu KW. Abdominoperineal resection is associated with poor oncological outcome. *Br J Surg*. 2004;91:1493–1499.
23. Heald RJ. Rectal cancer: the surgical options. *Eur J Cancer*. 1995;31A:1189–1192.
24. Martling AL, Holm T, Rutqvist LE, Moran BJ, Heald RJ, Cedemark B. Effect of a surgical training programme on outcome of rectal cancer in the County of Stockholm. Stockholm Colorectal Cancer Study Group, Basingstoke Bowel Cancer Research Project. *Lancet*. 2000;356:93–96.
25. Ruo L, Pfitzenmaier J, Guillem JG. Autonomic nerve preservation during pelvic dissection for rectal cancer. *Clin Colon Rectal Surg*. 2002;15:35–41.
26. Williams NS, Dixon MF, Johnston D. Reappraisal of the 5 centimetre rule of distal excision for carcinoma of the rectum: a study of distal intramural spread and of patients' survival. *Br J Surg*. 1983;70:150–154.
27. Pollett WG, Nicholls RJ. The relationship between the extent of distal clearance and survival and local recurrence rates after curative anterior resection for carcinoma of the rectum. *Ann Surg*. 1983;198:159–163.
28. Phillips RK, Hittinger R, Blesovsky L, Fry JS, Fielding LP. Local recurrence following 'curative' surgery for large bowel cancer: I. The overall picture. *Br J Surg*. 1984;71:12–16.
29. Ueno H, Mochizuki H, Hashguchi Y, et al. Preoperative parameters expanding the indication of sphincter preserving surgery in patients with advanced low rectal cancer. *Ann Surg*. 2004; 239:34–42.

30. Karanjia ND, Schache DJ, North WR, Heald RJ. 'Close shave' in anterior resection. *Br J Surg*. 1990;77:510–512.
31. Quirke P, Durdey P, Dixon MF, Williams NS. Local recurrence of rectal adenocarcinoma due to inadequate surgical resection. Histopathological study of lateral tumour spread and surgical excision. *Lancet*. 1986;2:996–999.
32. Hall NR, Finan PJ, al-Jaberi T, et al. Circumferential margin involvement after mesorectal excision of rectal cancer with curative intent. Predictor of survival but not local recurrence? *Dis Colon Rectum*. 1998;41:979–983.
33. Adam IJ, Mohamdee MO, Martin IG, et al. Role of circumferential margin involvement in the local recurrence of rectal cancer. *Lancet*. 1994;344:707–711.
34. Stocchi L, Nelson H, Sargent DJ, et al. Impact of surgical and pathologic variables in rectal cancer: a United States community and cooperative group report. *J Clin Oncol*. 2001;19:3895–3902.
35. Birbeck KF, Macklin CP, Tiffin NJ, et al. Rates of circumferential resection margin involvement vary between surgeons and predict outcomes in rectal cancer surgery. *Ann Surg*. 2002;235:449–457.
36. de Haas-Kock DF, Baeten CG, Jager JJ, et al. Prognostic significance of radial margins of clearance in rectal cancer. *Br J Surg*. 1996;83:781–785.
37. Ng IO, Luk IS, Yuen ST, et al. Surgical lateral clearance in resected rectal carcinomas. A multivariate analysis of clinicopathologic features. *Cancer*. 1993;71:1972–1976.
38. Glynne-Jones R, Mawdsley S, Pearce T, Buyse M. Alternative clinical end points in rectal cancer – are we getting closer? *Ann Oncol*. 2006;17:1239–1248.
39. Sayfan J, Averbuch F, Koltun L, Benyamin N. Effect of rectal stump washout on the presence of free malignant cells in the rectum during anterior resection for rectal cancer. *Dis Colon Rectum*. 2000;43:1710–1712.
40. Teramoto T, Watanabe M, Kitajima M. Per anum intersphincteric rectal dissection with direct coloanal anastomosis for lower rectal cancer: the ultimate sphincter-preserving operation. *Dis Colon Rectum*. 1997;40:S43-S47.
41. Rullier E, Zerbib F, Laurent C, et al. Intersphincteric resection with excision of internal anal sphincter for conservative treatment of very low rectal cancer. *Dis Colon Rectum*. 1999;42: 1168–1175.
42. Kohler A, Athanasiadis S, Ommer A, Psarakis E. Long-term results of low anterior resection with intersphincteric anastomosis in carcinoma of the lower one-third of the rectum: analysis of 31 patients. *Dis Colon Rectum*. 2000;43:843–850.
43. Marks G, Mohiuddin M, Masoni L, Montoro A. High-dose preoperative radiation therapy as the key to extending sphincter-preservation surgery for cancer of the distal rectum. *Surg Oncol Clin N Am*. 1992;1:71–86.
44. Tiret E, Poupardin B, McNamara D, Dehni N, Parc R. Ultralow anterior resection with intersphincteric dissection – what is the limit of safe sphincter preservation? *Colorectal Dis*. 2003;5:454–457.
45. Saito N, Ono M, Sugito M, et al. Early results of intersphincteric resection for patients with very low rectal cancer: an active approach to avoid a permanent colostomy. *Dis Colon Rectum*. 2004;47:459–466.
46. Hohenberger W, Merkel S, Matzel K, Bittorf B, Papadopoulos T, Gohl J. The influence of abdomino-peranal (intersphincteric) resection of lower third rectal carcinoma on the rates of sphincter preservation and locoregional recurrence. *Colorectal Dis*. 2006;8:23–33.
47. Rullier E, Laurent C, Bretagnol F, Rullier A, Vendrely V, Zerbib F. Sphincter-saving resection for all rectal carcinomas: the end of the 2-cm distal rule. *Ann Surg*. 2005;241:465–469.
48. Chin CC, Yeh CY, Huang WS, Wang JY. Clinical outcome of intersphincteric resection for ultra-low rectal cancer. *World J Gastroenterol*. 2006;12:640–643.
49. Schiessel R, Novi G, Holzer B, et al. Technique and long-term results of intersphincteric resection for low rectal cancer. *Dis Colon Rectum*. 2005;48:1858–1865. discussion 65–67.
50. Saito N, Moriya Y, Shirouzu K, et al. Intersphincteric resection in patients with very low rectal cancer: a review of the Japanese experience. *Dis Colon Rectum*. 2006;49:S13-S22.
51. Renner K, Rosen HR, Novi G, Holbling N, Schiessel R. Quality of life after surgery for rectal cancer: do we still need a permanent colostomy? *Dis Colon Rectum*. 1999;42:1160–1167.

52. Willis S, Kasperk R, Braun J, Schumpelick V. Comparison of colonic J-pouch reconstruction and straight coloanal anastomosis after intersphincteric rectal resection. *Langenbecks Arch Surg.* 2001;386:193–199.
53. Bittorf B, Stadelmaier U, Gohl J, Hohenberger W, Matzel KE. Functional outcome after intersphincteric resection of the rectum with coloanal anastomosis in low rectal cancer. *Eur J Surg Oncol.* 2004;30:260–265.
54. Bretagnol F, Rullier E, Laurent C, Zerbib F, Gontier R, Saric J. Comparison of functional results and quality of life between intersphincteric resection and conventional coloanal anastomosis for low rectal cancer. *Dis Colon Rectum.* 2004;47:832–838.
55. Vorobiev GI, Odaryuk TS, Tsarkov PV, Talalakin AI, Rybakov EG. Resection of the rectum and total excision of the internal anal sphincter with smooth muscle plasty and colonic pouch for treatment of ultralow rectal carcinoma. *Br J Surg.* 2004;91:1506–1512.
56. Takase Y, Oya M, Komatsu J. Clinical and functional comparison between stapled colonic J-pouch low rectal anastomosis and hand-sewn colonic J-pouch anal anastomosis for very low rectal cancer. *Surg Today.* 2002;32:315–321.
57. Park JG, Lee MR, Lim SB, et al. Colonic J-pouch anal anastomosis after ultralow anterior resection with upper sphincter excision for low-lying rectal cancer. *World J Gastroenterol.* 2005;11:2570–2573.
58. Pocard M, Sideris L, Zenasni F, et al. Functional results and quality of life for patients with very low rectal cancer undergoing coloanal anastomosis or perineal colostomy with colonic muscular graft. *Eur J Surg Oncol.* 2007;33:459–462.
59. Schiessel R, Karner-Hanusch J, Herbst F, Teleky B, Wunderlich M. Intersphincteric resection for low rectal tumours. *Br J Surg.* 1994;81:1376–1378.
60. Lee WY, Takahashi T, Pappas T, Mantyh CR, Ludwig KA. Surgical autonomic denervation results in altered colonic motility: an explanation for low anterior resection syndrome? *Surgery.* 2008;143:778–783.
61. Lazorthes F, Fages P, Chiotasso P, Lemozy J, Bloom E. Resection of the rectum with construction of a colonic reservoir and colo-anal anastomosis for carcinoma of the rectum. *Br J Surg.* 1986;73:136–138.
62. Parc R, Tiret E, Frileux P, Moszkowski E, Loygue J. Resection and colo-anal anastomosis with colonic reservoir for rectal carcinoma. *Br J Surg.* 1986;73:139–141.
63. Mortensen NJ, Ramirez JM, Takeuchi N, Humphreys MM. Colonic J pouch-anal anastomosis after rectal excision for carcinoma: functional outcome. *Br J Surg.* 1995;82:611–613.
64. Nicholls RJ, Lubowski DZ, Donaldson DR. Comparison of colonic reservoir and straight colo-anal reconstruction after rectal excision. *Br J Surg.* 1988;75:318–320.
65. Hida J, Yasutomi M, Fujimoto K, et al. Functional outcome after low anterior resection with low anastomosis for rectal cancer using the colonic J-pouch. Prospective randomized study for determination of optimum pouch size. *Dis Colon Rectum.* 1996;39:986–991.
66. Hida J, Yasutomi M, Maruyama T, Tokoro T, Wakano T, Uchida T. Enlargement of colonic pouch after proctectomy and coloanal anastomosis: potential cause for evacuation difficulty. *Dis Colon Rectum.* 1999;42:1181–1188.
67. Banerjee AK, Parc R. Prediction of optimum dimensions of colonic pouch reservoir. *Dis Colon Rectum.* 1996;39:1293–1295.
68. Ikeuchi H, Kusunoki M, Shoji Y, Yamamura T, Utsunomiya J. Functional results after "high" coloanal anastomosis and "low" coloanal anastomosis with a colonic J-pouch for rectal carcinoma. *Surg Today.* 1997;27:702–705.
69. Hida J, Yasutomi M, Maruyama T, et al. Indications for colonic J-pouch reconstruction after anterior resection for rectal cancer: determining the optimum level of anastomosis. *Dis Colon Rectum.* 1998;41:558–563.
70. Seow-Choen F, Goh HS. Prospective randomized trial comparing J colonic pouch-anal anastomosis and straight coloanal reconstruction. *Br J Surg.* 1995;82:608–610.
71. Hallbook O, Pahlman L, Krog M, Wexner SD, Sjodahl R. Randomized comparison of straight and colonic J pouch anastomosis after low anterior resection. *Ann Surg.* 1996;224:58–65.

72. Dehni N, Tiret E, Singland JD, et al. Long-term functional outcome after low anterior resection: comparison of low colorectal anastomosis and colonic J-pouch-anal anastomosis. *Dis Colon Rectum*. 1998;41:817–822. discussion 22–23.
73. Hida J, Yoshifuji T, Tokoro T, et al. Comparison of long-term functional results of colonic J-pouch and straight anastomosis after low anterior resection for rectal cancer: a five-year follow-up. *Dis Colon Rectum*. 2004;47:1578–1585.
74. Heriot AG, Tekkis PP, Constantinides V, et al. Meta-analysis of colonic reservoirs versus straight coloanal anastomosis after anterior resection. *Br J Surg*. 2006;93:19–32.
75. Z'Graggen K, Maurer CA, Mettler D, Stoupis C, Wildi S, Buchler MW. A novel colon pouch and its comparison with a straight coloanal and colon J-pouch – anal anastomosis: preliminary results in pigs. *Surgery*. 1999;125:105–112.
76. Z'Graggen K, Maurer CA, Birrer S, Giachino D, Kern B, Buchler MW. A new surgical concept for rectal replacement after low anterior resection: the transverse coloplasty pouch. *Ann Surg*. 2001;234:780–785. discussion 5–7.
77. Fazio VW, Mantyh CR, Hull TL. Colonic "coloplasty": novel technique to enhance low colorectal or coloanal anastomosis. *Dis Colon Rectum*. 2000;43:1448–1450.
78. Fazio VW, Zutshi M, Remzi FH, et al. A randomized multicenter trial to compare long-term functional outcome, quality of life, and complications of surgical procedures for low rectal cancers. *Ann Surg*. 2007;246:481–488. discussion 8–90.
79. Dehni N, Schlegel RD, Cunningham C, Guiguet M, Tiret E, Parc R. Influence of a defunctioning stoma on leakage rates after low colorectal anastomosis and colonic J pouch-anal anastomosis. *Br J Surg*. 1998;85:1114–1117.
80. Ho YH, Brown S, Heah SM, et al. Comparison of J-pouch and coloplasty pouch for low rectal cancers: a randomized, controlled trial investigating functional results and comparative anastomotic leak rates. *Ann Surg*. 2002;236:49–55.
81. Karanjia ND, Corder AP, Holdsworth PJ, Heald RJ. Risk of peritonitis and fatal septicaemia and the need to defunction the low anastomosis. *Br J Surg*. 1991;78:196–198.
82. Peeters KC, Tollenaar RA, Marijnen CA, et al. Risk factors for anastomotic failure after total mesorectal excision of rectal cancer. *Br J Surg*. 2005;92:211–216.
83. Eriksen MT, Wibe A, Norstein J, Haffner J, Wiig JN. Anastomotic leakage following routine mesorectal excision for rectal cancer in a national cohort of patients. *Colorectal Dis*. 2005; 7:51–57.
84. Matthiessen P, Hallbook O, Rutegard J, Simert G, Sjodahl R. Defunctioning stoma reduces symptomatic anastomotic leakage after low anterior resection of the rectum for cancer: a randomized multicenter trial. *Ann Surg*. 2007;246:207–214.
85. Poon RT, Chu KW, Ho JW, Chan CW, Law WL, Wong J. Prospective evaluation of selective defunctioning stoma for low anterior resection with total mesorectal excision. *World J Surg*. 1999;23:463–467. discussion 7–8.
86. Pata G, D'Hoore A, Fieuws S, Penninckx F. Mortality risk analysis following routine versus selective defunctioning stoma formation after total mesorectal excision for rectal cancer. *Colorectal Dis*. 2009;11(8):797–805.
87. Wong NY, Eu KW. A defunctioning ileostomy does not prevent clinical anastomotic leak after a low anterior resection: a prospective, comparative study. *Dis Colon Rectum*. 2005;48: 2076–2079.
88. Law WL, Choi HK, Lee YM, Ho JW, Seto CL. Anastomotic leakage is associated with poor long-term outcome in patients after curative colorectal resection for malignancy. *J Gastrointest Surg*. 2007;11:8–15.
89. McArdle CS, McMillan DC, Hole DJ. Impact of anastomotic leakage on long-term survival of patients undergoing curative resection for colorectal cancer. *Br J Surg*. 2005;92:1150–1154.
90. Huser N, Michalski CW, Erkan M, et al. Systematic review and meta-analysis of the role of defunctioning stoma in low rectal cancer surgery. *Ann Surg*. 2008;248:52–60.
91. Sato T, Konishi F, Endoh N, Uda H, Sugawara Y, Nagai H. Long-term outcomes of a neo-anus with a pudendal nerve anastomosis contemporaneously reconstructed with an abdominoperineal excision of the rectum. *Surgery*. 2005;137:8–15.

92. Romano G, La Torre F, Cutini G, Bianco F, Esposito P. Total anorectal reconstruction with an artificial bowel sphincter: report of five cases with a minimum follow-up of 6 months. *Colorectal Dis*. 2002;4:339–344.
93. Haward RA, Morris E, Monson JR, Johnston C, Forman D. The long term survival of rectal cancer patients following abdominoperineal and anterior resection: results of a population-based observational study. *Eur J Surg Oncol*. 2005;31:22–28.
94. Marr R, Birbeck K, Garvican J, et al. The modern abdominoperineal excision: the next challenge after total mesorectal excision. *Ann Surg*. 2005;242:74–82.
95. Nagtegaal ID, van de Velde CJ, van der Worp E, Kapiteijn E, Quirke P, van Krieken JH. Macroscopic evaluation of rectal cancer resection specimen: clinical significance of the pathologist in quality control. *J Clin Oncol*. 2002;20:1729–1734.
96. den Dulk M, Marijnen CA, Putter H, et al. Risk factors for adverse outcome in patients with rectal cancer treated with an abdominoperineal resection in the total mesorectal excision trial. *Ann Surg*. 2007;246:83–90.
97. Nagtegaal ID, van de Velde CJ, Marijnen CA, van Krieken JH, Quirke P. Low rectal cancer: a call for a change of approach in abdominoperineal resection. *J Clin Oncol*. 2005;23:9257–9264.
98. Wibe A, Syse A, Andersen E, Tretli S, Myrvold HE, Soreide O. Oncological outcomes after total mesorectal excision for cure for cancer of the lower rectum: anterior vs. abdominoperineal resection. *Dis Colon Rectum*. 2004;47:48–58.
99. Chuwa EW, Seow-Choen F. Outcomes for abdominoperineal resections are not worse than those of anterior resections. *Dis Colon Rectum*. 2006;49:41–49.
100. Marijnen CA, Nagtegaal ID, Klein Kranenbarg E. No downstaging after short-term preoperative radiotherapy in rectal cancer patients. *J Clin Oncol*. 2001;19:1976–1984.
101. Swedish Rectal Cancer Trial. Initial report from a Swedish multicentre study examining the role of preoperative irradiation in the treatment of patients with resectable rectal carcinoma. *Br J Surg*. 1993;80:1333–1336.
102. Marijnen CA, Kapiteijn E, van de Velde CJ, et al. Acute side effects and complications after short-term preoperative radiotherapy combined with total mesorectal excision in primary rectal cancer: report of a multicenter randomized trial. *J Clin Oncol*. 2002;20:817–825.
103. Bujko K, Nowacki MP, Kepka L, Oledzki J, Bebenek M, Kryj M. Postoperative complications in patients irradiated pre-operatively for rectal cancer: report of a randomised trial comparing short-term radiotherapy vs chemoradiation. *Colorectal Dis*. 2005;7:410–416.
104. Nissan A, Guillem JG, Paty PB, et al. Abdominoperineal resection for rectal cancer at a specialty center. *Dis Colon Rectum*. 2001;44:27–35. discussion 6.
105. Gruessner U, Clemens M, Pahlplatz PV, Sperling P, Witte J, Rosen HR. Improvement of perineal wound healing by local administration of gentamicin-impregnated collagen fleeces after abdominoperineal excision of rectal cancer. *Am J Surg*. 2001;182:502–509.
106. Khoo AK, Skibber JM, Nabawi AS, et al. Indications for immediate tissue transfer for soft tissue reconstruction in visceral pelvic surgery. *Surgery*. 2001;130:463–469.
107. de Haas WG, Miller MJ, Temple WJ, et al. Perineal wound closure with the rectus abdominis musculocutaneous flap after tumor ablation. *Ann Surg Oncol*. 1995;2:400–406.
108. Bell SW, Dehni N, Chaouat M, Lifante JC, Parc R, Tiret E. Primary rectus abdominis myocutaneous flap for repair of perineal and vaginal defects after extended abdominoperineal resection. *Br J Surg*. 2005;92:482–486.
109. McAllister E, Wells K, Chaet M, Norman J, Cruse W. Perineal reconstruction after surgical extirpation of pelvic malignancies using the transpelvic transverse rectus abdominal myocutaneous flap. *Ann Surg Oncol*. 1994;1:164–168.
110. Tei TM, Stolzenburg T, Buntzen S, Laurberg S, Kjeldsen H. Use of transpelvic rectus abdominis musculocutaneous flap for anal cancer salvage surgery. *Br J Surg*. 2003;90:575–580.
111. D'Souza DN, Pera M, Nelson H, Finical SJ, Tran NV. Vaginal reconstruction following resection of primary locally advanced and recurrent colorectal malignancies. *Arch Surg*. 2003;138:1340–1343.
112. Shibata D, Hyland W, Busse P, et al. Immediate reconstruction of the perineal wound with gracilis muscle flaps following abdominoperineal resection and intraoperative radiation therapy for recurrent carcinoma of the rectum. *Ann Surg Oncol*. 1999;6:33–37.

113. Hurwitz DJ, Swartz WM, Mathes SJ. The gluteal thigh flap: a reliable, sensate flap for the closure of buttock and perineal wounds. *Plast Reconstr Surg*. 1981;68:521–532.
114. Judge BA, Garcia-Aguilar J, Landis GH. Modification of the gluteal perforator-based flap for reconstruction of the posterior vagina. *Dis Colon Rectum*. 2000;43:1020–1022.
115. Ricciardi R, Virnig BA, Madoff RD, Rothenberger DA, Baxter NN. The status of radical proctectomy and sphincter-sparing surgery in the United States. *Dis Colon Rectum*. 2007;50:1119–27. discussion 26–27.
116. Ludwig KA, Mantyh CM. The status of radical proctectomy and sphincter-sparing surgery in the United States. Invited commentary. *Dis Colon Rectum*. 2007;50:1126–1127.
117. Purves H, Pietrobon R, Hervey S, Guller U, Miller W, Ludwig K. Relationship between surgeon caseload and sphincter preservation in patients with rectal cancer. *Dis Colon Rectum*. 2005;48: 195–202. discussion 4.
118. Engel AF, Oomen JL, Eijsbouts QA, Cuesta MA, van de Velde CJ. Nationwide decline in annual numbers of abdomino-perineal resections: effect of a successful national trial? *Colorectal Dis*. 2003;5:180–184.
119. Schmidt CE, Bestmann B, Kuchler T, Longo WE, Kremer B. Prospective evaluation of quality of life of patients receiving either abdominoperineal resection or sphincter-preserving procedure for rectal cancer. *Ann Surg Oncol*. 2005;12:117–123.
120. Guren MG, Eriksen MT, Wiig JN, et al. Quality of life and functional outcome following anterior or abdominoperineal resection for rectal cancer. *Eur J Surg Oncol*. 2005;31:735–742.
121. Bossema E, Stiggelbout A, Baas-Thijssen M, van de Velde C, Marijnen C. Patients' preferences for low rectal cancer surgery. *Eur J Surg Oncol*. 2008;34:42–48.
122. Clinical Outcomes of Surgical Therapy Study Group. A comparison of laparoscopically assisted and open colectomy for colon cancer. *N Engl J Med*. 2004;350:2050–2059.
123. Guillou PJ, Quirke P, Thorpe H, et al. Short-term endpoints of conventional versus laparoscopic-assisted surgery in patients with colorectal cancer (MRC CLASICC trial): multicentre, randomised controlled trial. *Lancet*. 2005;365:1718–1726.
124. Lacy AM, Delgado S, Castells A, et al. The long-term results of a randomized clinical trial of laparoscopy-assisted versus open surgery for colon cancer. *Ann Surg*. 2008;248:1–7.
125. Buunen M, Veldkamp R, Hop WC, et al. Survival after laparoscopic surgery versus open surgery for colon cancer: long-term outcome of a randomised clinical trial. *Lancet Oncol*. 2009;10:44–52.
126. Jayne DG, Guillou PJ, Thorpe H, et al. Randomized trial of laparoscopic-assisted resection of colorectal carcinoma: 3-year results of the UK MRC CLASICC Trial Group. *J Clin Oncol*. 2007;25:3061–3068.
127. Veenhof AA, Engel AF, van der Peet DL, et al. Technical difficulty grade score for the laparoscopic approach of rectal cancer: a single institution pilot study. *Int J Colorectal Dis*. 2008;23:469–475.
128. Park JS, Kang SB, Kim SW, Cheon GN. Economics and the laparoscopic surgery learning curve: comparison with open surgery for rectosigmoid cancer. *World J Surg*. 2007;31:1827–1834.
129. Aziz O, Constantinides V, Tekkis PP, et al. Laparoscopic versus open surgery for rectal cancer: a meta-analysis. *Ann Surg Oncol*. 2006;13:413–424.
130. Breukink SO, Grond AJ, Pierie JP, Hoff C, Wiggers T, Meijerink WJ. Laparoscopic vs open total mesorectal excision for rectal cancer: an evaluation of the mesorectum's macroscopic quality. *Surg Endosc*. 2005;19:307–310.
131. Quah HM, Jayne DG, Eu KW, Seow-Choen F. Bladder and sexual dysfunction following laparoscopically assisted and conventional open mesorectal resection for cancer. *Br J Surg*. 2002;89: 1551–1556.
132. Jayne DG, Brown JM, Thorpe H, Walker J, Quirke P, Guillou PJ. Bladder and sexual function following resection for rectal cancer in a randomized clinical trial of laparoscopic versus open technique. *Br J Surg*. 2005;92:1124–1132.
133. Tsang WW, Chung CC, Kwok SY, Li MK. Laparoscopic sphincter-preserving total mesorectal excision with colonic J-pouch reconstruction: five-year results. *Ann Surg*. 2006;243:353–358.
134. Yang L, Yu YY, Zhou ZG, et al. Quality of life outcomes following laparoscopic total mesorectal excision for low rectal cancers: a clinical control study. *Eur J Surg Oncol*. 2007;33:575–579.

135. Liang JT, Lai HS, Lee PH, Huang KC. Comparison of functional and surgical outcomes of laparoscopic-assisted colonic J-pouch versus straight reconstruction after total mesorectal excision for lower rectal cancer. *Ann Surg Oncol*. 2007;14:1972–1979.
136. Delaney CP, Kiran RP, Senagore AJ, Brady K, Fazio VW. Case-matched comparison of clinical and financial outcome after laparoscopic or open colorectal surgery. *Ann Surg*. 2003;238:67–72.
137. Ridgway PF, Boyle E, Keane FB, Neary P. Laparoscopic colectomy is cheaper than conventional open resection. *Colorectal Dis*. 2007;9:819–824.
138. Braga M, Frasson M, Vignali A, Zuliani W, Capretti G, Di Carlo V. Laparoscopic resection in rectal cancer patients: outcome and cost-benefit analysis. *Dis Colon Rectum*. 2007;50:464–471.
139. Anderson C, Uman G, Pigazzi A. Oncologic outcomes of laparoscopic surgery for rectal cancer: a systematic review and meta-analysis of the literature. *Eur J Surg Oncol*. 2008;34:1135–1142.

6 T4 and Recurrent Rectal Cancer

Jason Park and Jose Guillem

INTRODUCTION

More than 41,000 cases of rectal cancer are diagnosed annually in the United States *(1)*. Most patients present with primary tumor (T-stage) limited to the rectal wall or perirectal fat, although 6–13% of patients present with locally advanced T4 disease *(2–4)*. In addition, 5–30% of rectal cancer patients undergoing surgical resection will go on to develop a locoregional recurrence *(5)*. Locally invasive T4 and recurrent rectal cancer have similarities: (1) both entities often involve other structures or organs, (2) accurate preoperative evaluation with modern imaging techniques is critical for planning therapy, (3) multimodality therapy has a prominent role in treating both diseases, and (4) in cases selected for surgery, en bloc resection to include contiguously involved structures and negative resection margins are associated with superior disease-free and overall survival in both patient populations. In the following chapter, we will review definitions and classifications of both locally advanced T4 and recurrent rectal cancer, briefly describe their clinical and radiographic evaluation, and then focus on issues pertaining to the surgical management and outcomes of both diseases.

CLASSIFICATION AND NOMENCLATURE

T4 Rectal Cancer

T4 rectal cancer is defined by the American Joint Committee on Cancer (AJCC) TNM staging system as a primary tumor that directly invades other organs or structures, and/or perforates visceral peritoneum *(6)*. A tumor that is adherent to other organs or structures is also classified as a T4 lesion. However, if there is no tumor present in the adhesion on microscopic examination, the classification should be pT3 according to the AJCC staging system.

The frequency with which specific organs are involved in T4 rectal cancer varies with series. The sites most commonly involved include the pelvic sidewall, posterior vaginal wall,

From: *Current Clinical Oncology: Rectal Cancer*,
Edited by: B.G. Czito and C.G. Willett, DOI: 10.1007/978-1-60761-567-5_6,

uterus, or adnexa in women, and the pelvic sidewall, bladder, prostate, or seminal vesicles in men. Multiples organs are involved in 25% of T4 rectal cancer cases *(2–4)*.

Locally Recurrent Rectal Cancer

Although there is no standard classification system for recurrent rectal cancer, we previously described a system that classifies pelvic recurrences based on anatomic region(s) of the pelvis involved with disease (Fig. 1) *(7)*. This system facilitates a more standardized treatment approach and allows for a better comparison of outcomes in this heterogeneous population.

Pelvic recurrence can be classified as involving the axial, anterior, posterior, or lateral regions:

1. Axial region recurrences include both mucosal and soft tissue recurrences. This category includes local recurrence following a transanal excision, anastomotic recurrence following a low anterior resection (LAR) with primary reconstruction, recurrence in

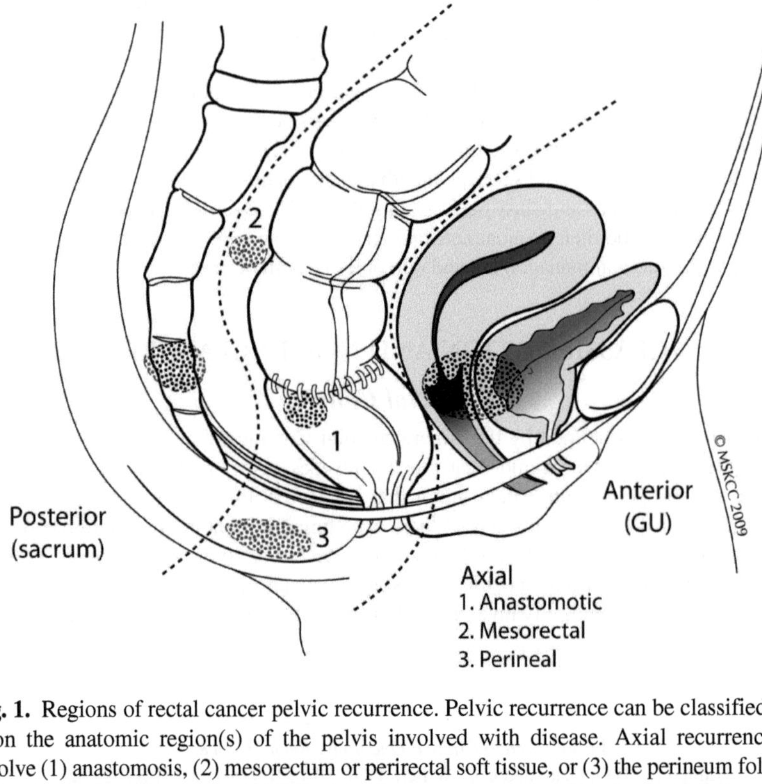

Fig. 1. Regions of rectal cancer pelvic recurrence. Pelvic recurrence can be classified based upon the anatomic region(s) of the pelvis involved with disease. Axial recurrences can involve (1) anastomosis, (2) mesorectum or perirectal soft tissue, or (3) the perineum following abdominal perineal resection (APR). Anterior recurrences involve the genitourinary (GU) tract including the bladder, vagina, uterus, seminal vesicles, and prostate. Posterior recurrences involve the sacrum and presacral fascia. Lateral recurrences (not shown) involve the soft tissue of the pelvic sidewall and lateral bony pelvis.

the mesorectum, as well as the relatively uncommon perineal recurrence following an abdominal perineal resection (APR).

2. Anterior region recurrences involve the genitourinary (GU) tract. In women, this includes the vagina, uterus, urinary bladder and distal ureters. In men, this includes the prostate, seminal vesicles, bladder, and distal ureters.
3. Posterior region recurrences involve the sacrum and coccyx.
4. Lateral region recurrences involve the soft tissue and structures of the pelvic sidewall (iliac vessels, lateral pelvic lymph nodes, pelvic ureters, pelvic nerves, sidewall musculature), and lateral bony pelvis.

Recurrences often involve more than one anatomic region. In a review of 101 patients with a pelvic recurrence of colorectal cancer at Memorial Sloan-Kettering Cancer Center, we found the axial region to be involved in 38 patients, the anterior region in 47 patients, the posterior region in 42 patients, and the lateral region in 47 patients *(7)*.

EVALUATION

Clinical Evaluation

Although no specific gastrointestinal (GI) symptoms can distinguish T4 rectal cancers from less advanced lesions, symptoms such as changes in bowel habits, obstipation, blood per rectum, tenesmus, and pelvic or perianal pain should be elicited in any patient being assessed for a primary rectal cancer. Patients being followed after restorative proctocolectomy or any local procedure for rectal cancer should be assessed for similar complaints. Tumor involvement of the GU tract may present as vaginal bleeding or urinary symptoms, such as pneumaturia, hematuria, and frequent urinary tract infections. Involvement of the pelvic sidewall may present with neurogenic pain in a sciatic distribution.

Digital rectal examination (DRE) and rigid sigmoidoscopy are also essential for evaluating patients suspected of having primary rectal cancer or recurrent pelvic disease. The DRE enables assessment of (1) size, (2) degree of fixation, and (3) location of disease relative to the upper part of the anorectal ring. Fixed lesions suggest involvement of the surrounding pelvic structures. In patients with status post-radical resection or a local procedure for rectal cancer in whom a digital examination is possible (i.e., restorative resections, nonrestorative resections with Hartmann's pouch, any local procedure), a careful DRE can pick up subtle changes in the pelvis such as increasing fullness or firmness. In general, with time the initial postsurgical fibrosis should abate and the tissue should become supple. Rigid proctoscopy is usually performed in conjunction with the DRE. This allows delineation of tumor orientation (anterior, lateral, or posterior) and circumferential involvement (evaluated as a percentage of the entire bowel wall circumference), and allows the most precise measurement of tumor distance from the anal verge. On follow-up of patients who have undergone a previous APR, the perineal area should also be assessed for tenderness, mass lesions, or persistent fistula, which may reflect recurrence.

The physical examination should include an examination of surrounding structures that may be involved by tumor. In females, a bimanual pelvic examination may reveal involvement of the rectovaginal septum, vagina or uterus, and adnexa. Neuromuscular examination of the lower extremities may identify findings that reflect sciatic nerve involvement. The inguinal regions should also be examined to assess for nonregional adenopathy. A full colonoscopy should be performed to exclude synchronous lesions that may alter treatment plans.

Imaging

Accurate pretreatment evaluation and staging is needed to (1) delineate the extent of locoregional involvement and (2) ascertain the presence or absence of metastatic disease. This information is of critical importance in determining the optimal approach and sequence of treatment modalities, and in selecting patients for potential surgical resection. The most common imaging studies currently used to acquire this information are endorectal ultrasound (ERUS), computed tomography (CT), magnetic resonance imaging (MRI), and positron emission tomography (PET) scan.

Given the multitude of imaging modalities from which to choose, it is important to understand the type of information that each provides and to have specific reasons for ordering each test. In the setting of primary disease, our practice is to include, as part of the initial evaluation: (1) locoregional staging with ERUS and (2) an assessment of distant metastasis with contrast-enhanced CT scan of the chest, abdomen, and pelvis. We selectively obtain PET–CT scans in patients when further characterization of indeterminate distant lesions found on CT scan is required.

In the setting of locally recurrent disease, all patients undergo extensive evaluation in order to rule out extrapelvic disease. The metastatic workup consists of a dedicated CT scan of the chest, abdomen and pelvis and, more recently, a PET–CT scan to rule out distant metastatic disease. PET–CT can also be used in cases of equivocal recurrence to assess for uptake in areas of concern.

Finally, all patients with suspected locally advanced or recurrent rectal cancer in the pelvis who are being considered for possible resection of local disease undergo a phased array MRI with focus on the specific area identified on ERUS, CT, or PET–CT, in order to obtain detailed information regarding pelvic anatomy and possible involvement of pelvic structures. In our opinion, MRI is currently the imaging modality of choice for assessing the resectability of locally advanced and recurrent lesions, given its excellent delineation of soft tissue structures. It is anticipated that ongoing efforts aimed at improving the ability of MRI to distinguish postoperative/postradiation fibrosis from cancer will further enhance the ability of the surgeon to identify those patients most likely to successfully undergo curative resection.

MANAGEMENT OF T4 OR PELVIC RECURRENCE OF RECTAL CANCER

Following the diagnosis and evaluation of disease extent for T4 or recurrent rectal cancer, it is necessary to establish a plan with regard to: (1) multimodality treatment and (2) the selection of patients for surgical resection. Patients will fall into one of four categories based on: the resectability of local disease; the presence of extrapelvic disease; and the presence of symptoms. A management algorithm based on these categories is presented in Figs. 2 and 3. Other important considerations with regard to treatment include patient age and the presence of comorbid conditions.

Category I: Resectable, Isolated Pelvic Disease

The determination of resectability of locally advanced and recurrent rectal cancer remains a challenge and the criteria for resectability vary considerably amongst centers. We define a resectable case as one in which we anticipate achieving a negative (R0) microscopic resection margin with acceptable risk and morbidity to the patient. Tumors that are fixed to critical

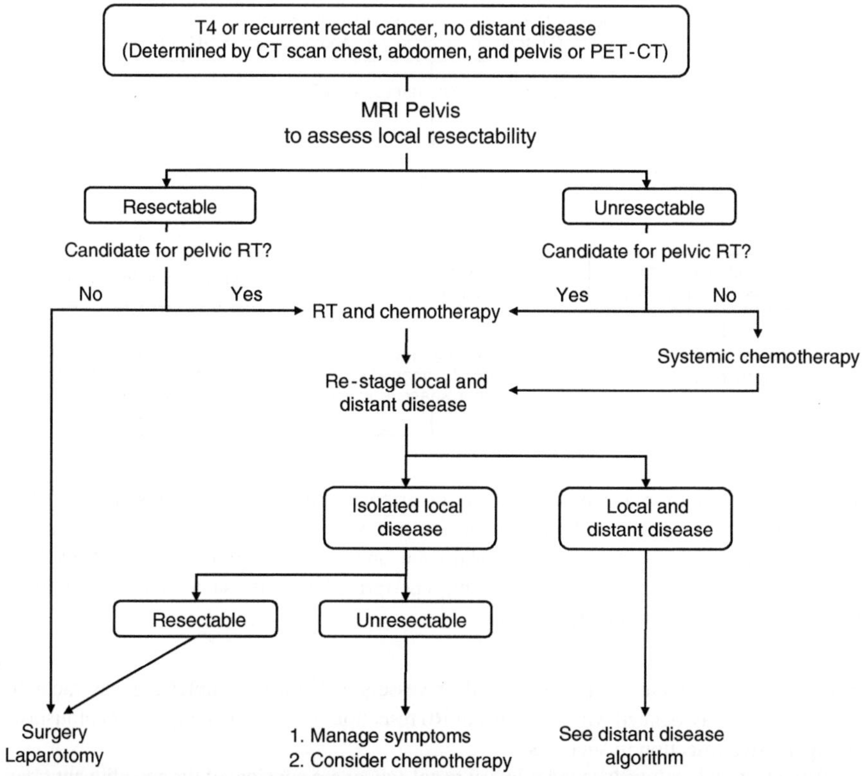

Fig. 2. Algorithm for management of T4 or recurrent rectal cancer in the absence of distant metastasis. The presence or absence of distant metastasis is determined by an intravenous contrast-enhanced computed tomography (CT) scan of the chest, abdomen, and pelvis or a positron emission tomography (PET)–CT scan. Pelvic magnetic resonance imaging (MRI) is used to assess local resectability. In patients who have not previously received a full course of pelvic radiation, radiation therapy (RT) may be given with a radiosensitizing dose of chemotherapy. Restaging is performed using the same imaging modalities that were used for the initial evaluation.

structures or organs that are neither amenable to nor appropriate for radical en bloc resection would be considered unresectable.

At our institution, we review all patients with complex locally advanced and recurrent rectal cancers with a multidisciplinary team consisting of members from the departments of surgery (which can include colorectal, hepatobiliary, plastic, orthopedic, and urologic surgeons), radiation oncology, medical oncology, gastroenterology, radiology, and pathology. During these conferences, the likelihood of obtaining an R0 resection, the need for neoadjuvant therapies, and the appropriateness of approach are thoroughly discussed on a case-by-case basis. In our opinion, broad, diffuse involvement of the proximal sacrum (S1 or higher), diffuse circumferential pelvic sidewall involvement, extension through the sciatic foramina, or encasement of the sciatic nerve usually render patients technically unresectable due to the low likelihood of being able to achieve an R0 resection and the extremely high rate of associated

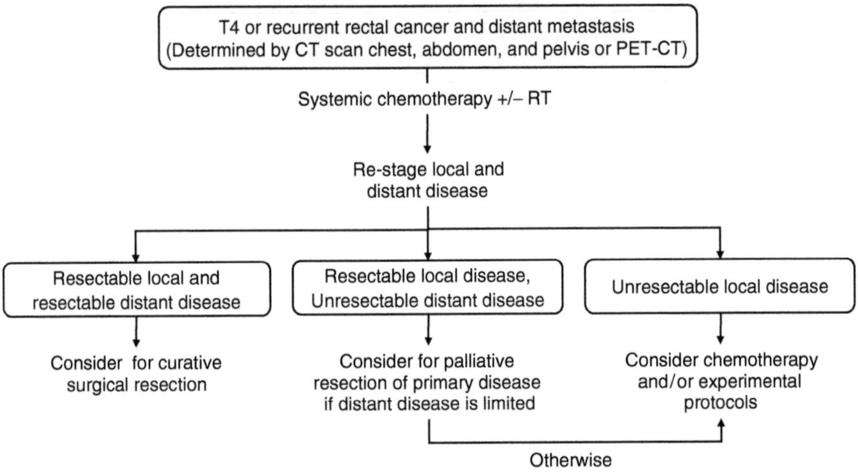

Fig. 3. Algorithm for management of T4 or recurrent rectal cancer in the presence of distant metastasis. The presence or absence of distant metastasis is determined by an intravenous contrast-enhanced CT scan of the chest, abdomen, and pelvis or a PET–CT scan. Pelvic MRI is used to assess local resectability. Restaging is performed using the same imaging modalities that were used for the initial evaluation.

morbidity. Involvement of the external iliac vessels and bilateral ureteric encasement by disease are also associated with low rates of R0 resection, which may temper our enthusiasm for aggressive resection in such cases.

Patients with locally advanced primary rectal cancer are considered for neoadjuvant treatments prior to surgical resection. At our institution, we administer long course external beam radiation therapy (RT), usually in combination with chemotherapy, to patients with T4 rectal cancer who are to undergo resection. Patients with recurrent rectal cancer limited to the pelvis are also considered for preoperative chemoradiation if they have not previously received RT. We then wait approximately 6 weeks following completion of preoperative chemoradiation to maximize tumor response before proceeding to surgery.

The goal of surgical resection of T4 and recurrent rectal cancer limited to the pelvis is complete extirpation of tumor and involved viscera with R0 margins. This may include partial resections of involved hollow viscera such as bladder or vagina, or more radical procedures involving entire and sometimes multiple organs. The reported R0 resection rates in patients who undergo surgical exploration and attempted resection with curative intent ranges from 48 to 79% for T4 and recurrent disease despite careful patient selection *(4,5,8-11)*. In bulky tumors, a positive margin may reflect advanced disease rather than inadequate surgery.

The ability to achieve an R0 resection margin has significant prognostic value for both primary T4 and recurrent rectal cancers. For patients with primary T4 rectal cancer who are selected for surgery, retrospective studies have shown that an R0 resection margin status is associated with improved local control and overall survival. A review of patients with locally advanced colon and rectal cancer who were selected for surgery at M.D. Anderson Cancer Center found a median survival of 34 months and 5-year overall survival of 52% in patients who underwent R0 resections compared to a median survival of 11 months and 5-year overall survival of 0% in those who underwent non-R0 resections *(12)*. When R0 margins can be obtained in patients with locally invasive T4 cancer, survival rates appear comparable to those of patients with tumors that do not involve adjacent organs *(13)*.

For patients with a pelvic recurrence of rectal cancer who are selected for surgery, resection margin status has been shown to be the most consistent predictor of outcome in multiple retrospective reviews. A review of patients with recurrent rectal cancer who were selected for surgical resection and intraoperative radiation therapy (IORT) at our institution found that patients who underwent R0 resections had a 5-year disease-free survival (DFS) of 30% and a 5-year disease-specific survival (DSS) of 51%, compared to a 5-year DFS and DSS of 9 and 14%, respectively, for those undergoing non-R0 resections *(5)*. R0 resection margin status was found to be associated with DFS and DSS on multivariate analysis. Failures occurred following re-resection in 60% of cases overall, with only 33% of these developing isolated local re-recurrence, 45% experiencing distant failure, and 22% experiencing combined local and distant failures.

Extended resections for locally advanced and recurrent rectal cancer can be associated with significant morbidity and occasional mortality, which underscores the need to carefully balance the risks and benefits of resection. The precise type and incidence of complication varies with procedure, but commonly reported postoperative complications include pelvic sepsis, perineal wound problems, fistula, and bowel obstruction *(8-10)*.

Category II: Unresectable, Isolated Pelvic Disease

Patients with unresectable, locally advanced rectal cancer should be treated with neoadjuvant therapy. Our current treatment of choice is long course external beam RT in combination with chemotherapy. Following chemoradiation therapy, patients are reassessed radiographically for tumor response. Selected patients are considered for surgery after neoadjuvant treatment if: (1) the lesion has responded sufficiently to convert it to one that is technically resectable with R0 margins and (2) no evidence of distant disease is found. If the disease remains unresectable or there is evidence of progression, patients are considered for further chemotherapy.

Treatment options for patients with isolated, unresectable pelvic recurrence are similar to those with T4 primary disease, and include combined modality therapy. If the patient has not received prior radiation, external beam RT in combination with chemotherapy may result in sufficient response to convert a previously unresectable lesion to one that is resectable. Entrapment of small bowel in the pelvis following prior pelvic surgery sometimes limits the ability to deliver external beam RT.

For patients with an impending obstruction who are being considered for neoadjuvant treatment with chemoradiation, an open or laparoscopic end-loop colostomy can be performed to divert patients while they are being treated *(14)*. Patients with a near obstruction are at risk of progression to complete obstruction from edema from RT, and it is important to ensure that at least a 1-cm lumen is maintained in these cases.

Category III: Asymptomatic Local Disease in the Setting of Distant Metastasis

Patients with locally advanced primary or recurrent disease and distant metastasis present a challenging situation. These patients represent a heterogenous population and it is difficult to define an all-encompassing strategy. Options vary depending on extent of primary and metastatic disease, presence of symptoms, and patient age and comorbidities. Overall, the prognosis for patients with T4 rectal cancer or pelvic recurrence in the setting of synchronous distant metastasis is poor. Retrospective data from the University of Minnesota found that patients with T4 rectal cancer and synchronous distant metastasis had a median survival of 7 months and no patients in their series underwent curative resection *(4)*. They also found no difference in survival when either a palliative resection or colostomy was performed in these patients.

For patients with primary T4 rectal cancer and isolated distant metastasis, a strategy aimed at cure can be adopted if both lesions appear resectable. Neoadjuvant therapy can be initiated in these cases with more intensive systemic chemotherapy regimens to decrease the likelihood of progression of metastasis, followed by chemoradiation therapy should further preoperative shrinkage of the tumor be deemed necessary. After neoadjuvant treatment, patients are restaged and considered for resection of their primary and metastatic disease.

For patients presenting with locally recurrent and isolated distant disease, surgery can be considered in highly selected patients with resectable lesions. However, there is only limited data supporting this approach. In a small series of 42 patients from our institution with locally recurrent colorectal cancer and synchronous resectable distant (M1) disease who were selected for surgery, an R0 resection was achieved in 22 (52%) patients with either synchronous or staged resection of their locally recurrent and M1 disease *(15)*. The ability to achieve an R0 resection was associated with survival on multivariate analysis, with a median survival of 23 months in the R0 group compared to 7 months in the non-R0 group. It is, however, important to understand that this study was a retrospective review of a group of highly selected patients and therefore cannot make any claims on the benefit of intervention over case selection alone.

For unresectable local or distant disease from either primary or recurrent disease, treatment should be aimed at best palliation, which can include external beam RT and chemotherapy in selected patients.

Category IV: Symptomatic Local Disease in the Setting of Distant Metastasis

Patients with local symptoms and distant metastasis are treated with the same neoadjuvant principles as those without symptoms, but the management of symptoms becomes a priority in this group of patients. The main symptoms that require intervention are obstruction, bleeding, pain, and chronic pelvic sepsis. Patients with bowel obstruction can be managed with a diverting colostomy or palliative resection in very selected cases with limited hepatic involvement and adequate hepatic function to withstand pelvic surgery. We prefer to perform a diverting colostomy in order to minimize recovery time and shorten the time interval to initiation of systemic treatment. However, in patients with a short life expectancy and in whom surgical therapy is prohibitive, bowel obstruction can be palliated using endoscopic stenting. Patients presenting with bleeding per rectum or tumor-related pain can be managed with external beam RT or, in some cases, palliative resection.

SURGICAL CONSIDERATIONS

Preoperative Preparation

Extended resections of primary and recurrent rectal cancers are best undertaken by individuals with training and experience with these procedures. Pelvic resections that involve adjacent structures are not standard operations. The primary surgeon must have experience working in anatomic plans outside of those required for conventional resection in order to perform a complete resection in a safe manner. In addition, extended resections often require the active participation of other specialists who have interest and experience with these cancers: radiation oncologists, urologists, and plastic and orthopedic surgeons. The institution must also be capable of providing adequate intraoperative support and perioperative care to optimize outcomes.

Special consideration should be given to women with recurrent disease who have undergone a previous hysterectomy since the recurrence will often involve the base of the bladder or be surgically inseparable from it. Similarly, men who are status post-APR often have a posteriorly retroflexed bladder that may be involved or inseparable from recurrent tumor. Prior irradiation, particularly if delivered in the distant past, should be taken into consideration as the dissection may be difficult in fibrotic tissue. Lastly, close proximity or involvement of major pelvic vessels should prompt a preoperative consultation with a vascular surgeon.

An often neglected aspect of preparation for surgery is the amount of education and counseling required to prepare patients and their family for surgery. Extended pelvic surgery for rectal cancer is associated with major complications, prolonged hospitalization, and a significant risk of local and distant recurrence. In addition, patients' long-term quality of life may be affected by a nonhealing perineal wound, bowel, urinary, or sexual dysfunction, or the need for a colostomy or ileal conduit. These issues must be discussed with patients and their family preoperatively, in order to set appropriate expectations and inform the consent process.

Conduct of Operation

The conduct of radical surgery requires: (1) a thorough exploration of the abdominopelvic cavity, (2) en bloc resection of tumor and involved structures, and (3) reconstruction of the GI and GU tracts, as well as the perineum as indicated.

Cystoscopy and bilateral ureteric stent placement is recommended for all patients with suspected locally advanced T4 disease and patients with a pelvic recurrence, especially when bladder and/or pelvic sidewall involvement is suspected. The standard operative approach is a laparotomy and exploration to exclude the presence of metastatic disease in peritoneum, periaortic lymph nodes or liver. Alternatively, a diagnostic laparoscopy can be considered in patients with T4 rectal cancer and selected patients with recurrent disease in order to assess for metastatic disease. If unresectable extrapelvic or locally recurrent disease is found and confirmed on frozen section, an end-loop or double barreled colostomy are options in cases of impending obstruction.

Tumors may be adherent to adjacent organs or structures by direct tumor invasion and/or inflammatory adhesions. Twenty-two percent of adherent primary rectal cancers that are resected have malignant invasion on subsequent histologic analysis, but the distinction between adherence from inflammation and malignant invasion is impossible to make intraoperatively, particularly in the setting of prior pelvic irradiation or surgery *(16)*. Consequently, locally invasive primary rectal cancers with adjacent organ involvement should be treated by en bloc resection to include any adherent tissues when technically feasible. Procedures in which tumors are transected at the site of local adherence are considered incomplete resections and are associated with a higher incidence of treatment failure. Authors from the University of Sydney reviewed 126 patients with primary rectal cancer found to have an adherent tumor on exploration. Patients who underwent en bloc resection had a lower pelvic recurrence rate than those who had separation of the tumor (17% vs. 39%) *(16)*.

Surgical Management Based on Location of Disease

Anterior Disease

T4 and recurrent rectal cancer involving the GU tract require en bloc resection of involved pelvic viscera to achieve R0 resection margins. Limited involvement of structures such as dome of bladder and posterior vagina can be treated adequately with partial resection, provided wide negative margins are achieved. In female patients, the rectum and vagina are in close proximity and share a communicating lymphatic system; therefore, recurrences can be seen in the posterior vaginal wall following rectal cancer resection. A review of patients who underwent a partial vaginectomy during resection for primary rectal cancer at our institution found a local failure rate of 16% and a 5-year overall survival of 46% *(17)*. Local recurrence was more commonly found in patients with positive margins. These results support en bloc resection for locally advanced rectal cancers involving the vagina with the aim of achieving negative margins, which is associated with decreased recurrence and increased survival.

Tumors involving the bladder trigone or cervix usually require a pelvic exenteration. Total pelvic exenteration (TPE) involves en bloc removal of the rectum, internal genitalia structures, bladder and distal ureters. Posterior pelvic exenteration entails en bloc resection of the rectum and internal genitalia structure, but leaves the bladder and distal ureters intact. Pelvic exenteration is a formidable procedure requiring thorough preoperative evaluation and accurate intraoperative assessment for metastatic disease. It is associated with a high risk of morbidity and therefore should not be attempted unless the surgeon anticipates an R0 resection margin. Operating room times can range from 3 to 10 h for these procedures, with a median reported blood loss of 3,800 mL *(18)* .When total cystectomy is indicated, options for urinary diversion include ileal conduit and continent reservoirs. Urinary complications contribute significantly to postoperative morbidity after TPE. Early complications of urinary diversion in patients undergoing TPE include anastomotic leak, while late complications include ureteric strictures.

In a review of patients from our institution with advanced primary or locally recurrent rectal cancer undergoing TPE, we found that an R0 resection was achieved in 73% of cases *(19)*. Median DSS for all patients was 49 months. Five-year survival rates of 23–28% have been reported for patients with locally recurrent rectal cancer requiring pelvic exenteration *(11)*. Reported postoperative complication rates for TPE range from 22% to 78% and in-house hospital mortality rates range from 0 to 10% *(19,20)*. The most commonly reported complications include iatrogenic bladder or ureter injury, wound infection (abdominal or perineal), or fecal or urinary fistula.

Posterior Disease

Tumors can be tethered posteriorly to the sacrum. In carefully selected patients, en bloc resection of the bony pelvis can be performed with acceptable morbidity and adequate oncologic outcomes. When sacral involvement is limited to the sacral fascia or superficial periosteum, an en bloc resection with periosteal elevation may achieve negative margins, but this can result in significant hemorrhage. When bony invasion of the sacrum is present, R0 resection may still be achieved in select patients using a combined abdominosacral approach. A sacrectomy may be performed in combination with an APR or pelvic exenteration, depending on the extent of pelvic disease. These are formidable and technically demanding operations, which entail long operating room times and may involve significant blood loss.

Major complications associated with this procedure include intestinal and urinary fistula, wound complications, pulmonary embolus, and bladder dysfunction. Bladder dysfunction is related to the level of sacral transection, and sacral transection below S3 will usually not affect urinary continence. Mild urinary dysfunction may occur with unilateral division of S2 or S1 nerve roots. Resection of both S2 nerve roots leads to bladder dysfunction, whereas bilateral S1 nerve root resection results in complete bladder denervation. The reported operative mortality rates range from 0 to 9% in series from specialized centers *(2,21)*.

LATERAL DISEASE

Lateral disease along the pelvic sidewall is the least likely to be salvaged with surgical resection *(7)*. These tumors often adhere to the bony pelvis or invade the sciatic nerve or ureter – all of which are associated with a low likelihood of R0 resection. This operation may entail partial ureterectomy as well as partial resection of major arteries and veins, including the iliac vessels, in select patients.

AXIAL DISEASE

Recurrent disease limited to the axial anatomic region most likely represents tumor implantation into the mesorectum during local excision, failure to obtain an adequate distal margin during LAR, or perineal implantation of tumor during APR. For high axial anastomotic recurrences, sphincter preservation may be an option. However, significant lateral extension often requires a combined abdominoperineal approach to ensure negative circumferential margins. For perineal soft tissue recurrences following APR, wide local excision may render the patient free of disease. However, perineal disease is often a sign of disease deeper in the pelvis, thereby necessitating a combined abdominoperineal approach.

RADIATION AND CHEMOTHERAPY

Although a comprehensive discussion of chemoradiation therapy in the treatment of rectal cancer is beyond the scope of this chapter, it is important to recognize the role of preoperative chemoradiation therapy in treating patients with locally advanced rectal cancer as well as some patients with recurrent disease. The improvement in locoregional control in patients with locally advanced rectal cancer undergoing preoperative external beam RT was demonstrated in a recent randomized trial *(22)*. For advanced primary disease, RT may facilitate resection by downsizing disease and possibly induce a sufficient response to convert a previously unresectable lesion to a resectable one *(23,24)*.

For recurrent disease, the role of external beam RT may be limited by previous pelvic radiation. However, recent advances in conformal radiotherapy techniques, including the use of intensity-modulated radiotherapy (IMRT), has allowed reradiation of select patients with local recurrence with an additional dose of 30–40 Gy. Whether preoperative reirradiation with chemosensitization in locally recurrent disease will successfully downsize a significant proportion of patients to allow for R0 resection (with corresponding improvement in survival) remains to be seen.

Intraoperative Radiation Therapy

IORT allows the delivery of an increased dose of radiation to a specific target field while concurrently limiting the exposure of normal surrounding tissue. It can be applied to areas of close or questionable resection margins. A previous study of patients with locally recurrent rectal cancer demonstrated that surgical resection plus IORT achieved a high rate of local control (67%) and 5-year DFS and DSS of 22 and 39%, respectively, although the selection bias inherent in retrospective studies precludes the ability to draw definitive conclusions about the independent contribution of the IORT treatment effects *(5)*. To date, no studies have been performed in a randomized, controlled manner to document a survival advantage for patients treated with IORT.

RECONSTRUCTION FOR PERINEAL DEFECTS

Perineal wound complications are a major cause of morbidity after APR for locally advanced or recurrent rectal cancer, particularly in patients who have received preoperative RT. In selected patients, the incidence of wound complications may be decreased with use of a myocutaneous flap to reconstruct the perineum. The use of myocutaneous flaps can achieve perineal closure and reduce pelvic dead space using a pedicle of well-vascularized, nonirradiated tissue, which in theory can improve healing and decrease the risk of infection.

Options for perineal reconstruction include rectus abdominus myocutaneous (RAM), gracilis muscle (unilateral or bilateral), and gluteal muscle flaps. A study from our institution found that patients with RAM reconstruction following RT and APR had significantly lower perineal wound complication rates compared to matched controls (16% vs. 44%), despite increased rates of vaginectomy and IORT use in the RAM group *(25)*. The wound complication rate after RAM reconstruction in our series was also lower than the rates reported in the literature following gracilis or gluteal muscle flap reconstruction. However, the use of the rectus abdominus muscle limits potential colostomy sites, which must be taken into account when planning procedures. The long-term effect of the RAM technique on the development of abdominal wall hernias has yet to be determined.

SUMMARY

The management of patients with T4 and recurrent rectal cancer remains a challenge. Accurate preoperative imaging is required to determine the extent of local disease and exclude the presence of distant metastases. This information is absolutely essential in directing management decisions regarding multimodality therapy and selecting patients for potentially curative surgery.

Surgical resection for T4 and recurrent rectal cancer involves complete extirpation of the tumor and involved viscera with R0 resection margins. These extended resections are a major undertaking and are associated with high rates of morbidity and potentially devastating effects on function and quality of life. However, careful patient selection may result in prolonged survival when disease can be completely resected with negative margins. This therapy should be carefully planned and carried out within the context of a multidisciplinary team and undertaken in specialized centers that have experience with this approach. Future strategies should be aimed at improving preoperative imaging in order to better select those patients most likely to be amenable to an R0 resection and perhaps to help define the operative plane best suited for achieving an R0 resection. In addition, given the rates of distant failures seen in these patients, further developments leading to improved, novel systemic therapies are needed.

REFERENCES

1. American Cancer Society. *Cancer Facts & Figures 2008*. Atlanta: American Cancer Society; 2008.
2. Moriya Y, Akasu T, Fujita S, Yamamoto S. Aggressive surgical treatment for patients with T4 rectal cancer. *Colorectal Dis*. 2003;5:427–431.

3. Sanfilippo NJ, Crane CH, Skibber J, et al. T4 rectal cancer treated with preoperative chemoradiation to the posterior pelvis followed by multivisceral resection: patterns of failure and limitations of treatment. *Int J Radiat Oncol Biol Phys.* 2001;51:176–183.
4. Yiu R, Wong SK, Cromwell J, Madoff RD, Rothenberger DA, Garcia-Aguilar J. Pelvic wall involvement denotes a poor prognosis in T4 rectal cancer. *Dis Colon Rectum.* 2001;44:1676–1681.
5. Shoup M, Guillem JG, Alektiar KM, et al. Predictors of survival in recurrent rectal cancer after resection and intraoperative radiotherapy. *Dis Colon Rectum.* 2002;45:585–592.
6. American Joint Committee on Cancer. *Cancer Staging Manual.* Chicago: American Joint Committee on Cancer; 2002.
7. Moore HG, Shoup M, Riedel E, et al. Colorectal cancer pelvic recurrences: determinants of resectability. *Dis Colon Rectum.* 2004;47:1599–1606.
8. Heriot AG, Byrne CM, Lee P, et al. Extended radical resection: the choice for locally recurrent rectal cancer. *Dis Colon Rectum.* 2008;51:284–291.
9. Hahnloser D, Nelson H, Gunderson LL, et al. Curative potential of multimodality therapy for locally recurrent rectal cancer. *Ann Surg.* 2003;237:502–508.
10. Garcia-Aguilar J, Cromwell JW, Marra C, Lee SH, Madoff RD, Rothenberger DA. Treatment of locally recurrent rectal cancer. *Dis Colon Rectum.* 2001;44:1743–1748.
11. Salo JC, Paty PB, Guillem J, Minsky BD, Harrison LB, Cohen AM. Surgical salvage of recurrent rectal carcinoma after curative resection: a 10-year experience. *Ann Surg Oncol.* 1999;6:171–177.
12. Talamonti MS, Shumate CR, Carlson GW, Curley SA. Locally advanced carcinoma of the colon and rectum involving the urinary bladder. *Surg Gynecol Obstet.* 1993;177:481–487.
13. Tjandra JJ, Kilkenny JW, Buie WD, et al. Practice parameters for the management of rectal cancer (revised). *Dis Colon Rectum.* 2005;48:411–423.
14. Koea JB, Guillem JG, Conlon KC, Minsky B, Saltz L, Cohen A. Role of laparoscopy in the initial multimodality management of patients with near-obstructing rectal cancer. *J Gastrointest Surg.* 2000;4:105–108.
15. Hartley JE, Lopez RA, Paty PB, Wong WD, Cohen AM, Guillem JG. Resection of locally recurrent colorectal cancer in the presence of distant metastases: can it be justified? *Ann Surg Oncol.* 2003;10:227–233.
16. Darakhshan A, Lin BP, Chan C, Chapuis PH, Dent OF, Bokey L. Correlates and outcomes of tumor adherence in resected colonic and rectal cancers. *Ann Surg.* 2008;247:650–658.
17. Ruo L, Paty PB, Minsky BD, Wong WD, Cohen AM, Guillem JG. Results after rectal cancer resection with in-continuity partial vaginectomy and total mesorectal excision. *Ann Surg Oncol.* 2003;10:664–668.
18. Yeung RS, Moffat FL, Falk RE. Pelvic exenteration for recurrent and extensive primary colorectal adenocarcinoma. *Cancer.* 1993;72:1853–1858.
19. Jimenez RE, Shoup M, Cohen AM, Paty PB, Guillem J, Wong WD. Contemporary outcomes of total pelvic exenteration in the treatment of colorectal cancer. *Dis Colon Rectum.* 2003;46:1619–1625.
20. Ike H, Shimada H, Yamaguchi S, Ichikawa Y, Fujii S, Ohki S. Outcome of total pelvic exenteration for primary rectal cancer. *Dis Colon Rectum.* 2003;46:474–480.
21. Wells BJ, Stotland P, Ko MA, et al. Results of an aggressive approach to resection of locally recurrent rectal cancer. *Ann Surg Oncol.* 2007;14:390–395.
22. Sauer R, Becker H, Hohenberger W, et al. Preoperative versus postoperative chemoradiotherapy for rectal cancer. *N Engl J Med.* 2004;351:1731–1740.
23. Braendengen M, Tveit KM, Berglund A, et al. Randomized phase III study comparing preoperative radiotherapy with chemoradiotherapy in nonresectable rectal cancer. *J Clin Oncol.* 2008;26:3687–3694.
24. Mathis KL, Nelson H, Pemberton JH, Haddock MG, Gunderson LL. Unresectable colorectal cancer can be cured with multimodality therapy. *Ann Surg.* 2008;248:592–598.
25. Chessin DB, Hartley J, Cohen AM, et al. Rectus flap reconstruction decreases perineal wound complications after pelvic chemoradiation and surgery: a cohort study. *Ann Surg Oncol.* 2005;12:104–110.

7 Surgical Management of Pulmonary Metastases

Loretta Erhunmwunsee and Thomas A. D'Amico

INTRODUCTION

Approximately 10–20% of patients with colorectal cancer will develop metastases to the lungs, the second most common site of systemic disease (*1*). The 5-year survival of these patients is less than 5% without treatment. Most stage IV colorectal cancer patients are treated palliatively with chemotherapeutic regimens that have been shown to prolong survival in patients with unresectable disease (*2*). Although chemotherapeutic regimens do offer significant improvements in overall survival, the combination of surgery and systemic therapy offers the best option for cure in selected patients with pulmonary colorectal metastases.

PATIENT EVALUATION

Because up to 40% of rectal cancer patients will develop distant spread, there must be close follow-up after curative resection to rule out locally recurrent or metastatic disease. Few patients with spread to the lung will develop symptoms that prompt metastatic work-up (*3,4*). Instead, the majority of pulmonary metastases will be detected via surveillance CT scans or rising carcinoembryonic antigen (CEA) levels, which are usually obtained at least twice annually during the first several years after resection (*5*). On CT, pulmonary metastases are typically smooth, well-circumscribed, peripheral and frequently numerous. CEA is involved in intercellular recognition and attachment and may promote the adhesion of tumor cells to each other or to host cells (*6*). The marker is elevated in the presence of colorectal cancer but should normalize after resection if all disease has been removed. Interval elevation of CEA is strongly associated with recurrent disease, in either the liver or the lung. Eight percent of patients with a history of colorectal cancer and a rising CEA were found to have a pulmonary nodule in a study by Irshad and associates (*7*). Because of the high detection

From: *Current Clinical Oncology: Rectal Cancer*,
Edited by: B.G. Czito and C.G. Willett, DOI: 10.1007/978-1-60761-567-5_7,

rates of pulmonary metastases via CT and CEA, their use in regular surveillance is associated with early detection.

Pulmonary nodules in patients with current or prior history of colorectal cancer cannot be assumed to be metastatic. In patients with only one pulmonary nodule, approximately half will be colorectal metastases. Primary lung cancer will make up most of the other half, and some lesions are not malignant *(4)*. Biopsy or tissue diagnosis from isolated nodules is not necessary prior to surgery because resection is indicated whether the lesion is a primary lung tumor or a metastatic lesion. Bronchoscopy, however, may be warranted, if a lesion is centrally located on radiographic imaging. This procedure would be important to rule out endobronchial involvement, which has been reported in up to 28% of patients *(4)*.

Nevertheless, once a nodule is found, it is imperative that extrapulmonary disease is excluded. Abdominal CT, PET scan and colonoscopy are typically performed to assess for the presence of metastatic disease at other sites. Patients with neurologic symptoms or acute bony pain undergo head CT and bone scan, respectively. Typically, the presence of extrapulmonary colorectal metastases suggests disease that will not benefit from resection and palliation is frequently recommended. Metastasis to the liver is the only exception, as there may be a survival benefit to resection of both *(8)*.

OUTCOMES

Although there are no prospective, randomized trials evaluating the benefit of pulmonary metastasectomy in patients with colorectal carcinoma metastatic to the lungs, there are many reports demonstrating outcomes following resection. Rotolo et al examined outcomes of 23 patients after pulmonary resection of single metastasis from colorectal cancer. In this series, patients experienced a 5-year survival of 56% and median survival of 74 months *(9)*. In a study by Welter et al, the outcomes of 175 patients with pulmonary metastases secondary to colorectal cancer were analyzed, many of whom had more than one metastasis. They observed a 5-year survival of 39% and median survival of 47 months *(10)*. Casali et al studied 142 patients also with colorectal cancer metastatic to the lungs. They found similar results: an overall 5-year survival of 36% and median survival of 47 months *(11)*. Lo and colleagues retrospectively evaluated 80 patients who had pulmonary metastatic colorectal carcinoma, with 5-year survival of 42.5% *(12)*. These results (see Table 1) are impressive given patients with untreated metastatic disease from colorectal cancer typically have a median survival of less than 10 months and a 5-year survival rate of less than 5% *(13)*.

Unfortunately, most patients who undergo pulmonary metastasectomy will develop pulmonary recurrence. Many studies have shown the utility of re-resection of recurrent pulmonary metastases *(10,14)* and there is evidence that repeat pulmonary resection for locally recurrent disease is not an ominous prognostic factor *(15)*. There is ample evidence that lung metastasectomy is associated with improved outcomes. For this reason, pulmonary metastasectomy and re-resection, when indicated, are now performed routinely in selected patients with metastatic colorectal cancer.

PROGNOSTIC FACTORS

In spite of the improved outcomes from pulmonary metastasectomy, the survival of most patients with pulmonary colorectal metastases will not be improved by pulmonary resection. Thus, much focus has gone into determining which patients with pulmonary colorectal metastases should in fact undergo surgery and which patients should not be offered futile resection.

Table 1
Survival following pulmonary resection for metastatic colorectal carcinoma

	No. of patients	*Median survival (months)*	*5-Year overall survival*	*10-Year overall survival*
Rotolo *(9)*	23	74	56%	~
Welter *(10)*	175	47.2	39.1%	20%
Lo *(12)*	80	46.6	42.5%	35.5%
Casali *(11)*	142	47	36%	~

~ not reported

In the 1960s, Thomford et al *(16)* recommended that patients proceed to pulmonary metastasectomy only if the following indications were met: (1) control of the primary site, (2) lack of other distant metastatic disease including the liver, (3) a technically feasible operation was possible, and (4) adequate cardiopulmonary reserve was present. Since then others have worked to refine the operative indications by discovering variables that are associated with poor outcomes. In the 1980s, Mansel et al recommended that patients with more than one lung metastasis not undergo metastasectomy because of decreased benefit *(17)*. In 1997, the International Registry of Lung Metastases*(18)* reported the outcome of 5,206 patients with pulmonary metastases from various tumor types, including epithelial cancers, sarcomas, germ cell tumors and melanomas. This registry proposed a prognostic stratification based on three variables that independently influenced outcomes: resectability, disease-free interval (DFI) and number of pulmonary metastases. This study suggested that patients with greater than one nodule and a DFI<3 years had worse outcomes.

Lo and colleagues suggested that high preoperative CEA level (>20 mg/ml) and short DFI (<12 months) were negative predictive factors for survival following metastasectomy, whereas the number of pulmonary metastases did not have an effect on outcomes. Lo et al recommend that tumors with high serum CEA levels and short DFI have an aggressive behavior and that patients with these tumors are less likely to benefit from pulmonary metastasectomy *(12)*. In another study, Irshad and colleagues found that more than one pulmonary lesion, a DFI<2 years, and moderately or poorly differentiated colorectal cancer carried a poor prognosis *(7)*.

Casali and colleagues detected a survival difference based on the presence of metastases in mediastinal nodes and suggest that nodal status should be considered in the selection of patients for lung metastasectomy *(11)*. Saito et al also reported worse outcomes with patients who had hilar or mediastinal lymph node metastases. They also suggest that an elevated prethoracotomy CEA level (>10 ng/ml) was associated with lower survival *(14)*. Onaitis and colleagues evaluated 377 patients and discovered that DFI<1 year and numerous metastases (>3) were independent predictors of recurrence, recommending that these patients be treated nonoperatively *(19)*.

Review of these studies (Table 2) demonstrates that there is not yet a consensus about which variables should be used to determine operability. In studies that reported on its importance, elevated CEA levels have generally shown prognostic importance *(12,14,20,21)*. Although studies have not agreed on what value is important, most use a CEA value in the 5–20 ng/ml range. The majority of studies also suggest that the DFI between resection of the primary tumor and pulmonary metastasectomy is an important prognostic factor *(7,11,12,18,19)*. The definition of a short DFI, however, has not been specified, as it ranges from 1 to 3 years depending on the study. Well-designed clinical trials must be performed to determine exactly

Table 2
Prognostic factors associated with survival following pulmonary metastasectomy for colorectal cancer (by multivariate analysis)

	No. of patients	*No. of mets*	*DFI*	*CEA level*	*Nodal disease*	*Incomplete resection*	*Bilaterality*
Onaitis *(19)*	377	SS (>3)	SS (<1 year)	~	~	~	~
Welter *(10)*	175	SS (>1)	ns	ns	ns	~	~
Lo *(12)*	80	ns	SS (<1 year)	SS (>20 μg/dl)	~	SS	~
Casali *(11)*	142	ns	ns	~	SS	~	~
Saito *(14)*	165	ns	ns	SS (>10 μg/dl)	SS	~	ns
Irshad *(7)*	49	SS (>1)	SS (<2 years)	~	~	~	SS
Pastorino *(18)*	5,206	SS (>1)	SS (<3 years)	~	~	~	~
Girard *(21)*	86	ns	ns	SS (>5 ng/ml)	~	SS	~

ns not significant; *SS* statistically significant; ~ not reported; *DFI* disease-free interval which variables should be prioritized in consideration of resection. In the meantime, thoracic surgeons and oncologists should work together in deciding which patients are surgical candidates, using the NCCN recommendations as guidelines *(5)*. According to NCCN guidelines, the current criteria for resectability of colorectal metastases to the lungs are: (1) the primary tumor must have been resected for cure; (2) complete resection of pulmonary metastases with maintenance of adequate function must be feasible; (3) resectable extrapulmonary metastases do not preclude resection; and (4) re-resection can be considered in selected patients.

Most pulmonary metastases are located peripherally (in the outer one-third of the lung) and are frequently subpleural*(22)* and thus amenable to wedge resection. For lesions that are more centrally located, segmentectomy, lobectomy, and (rarely) pneumonectomy are required for complete resection. Among the 5,206 patients that were analyzed in the International Registry of Lung Metastases, 67% underwent a wedge resection, 9% segmentectomy, 21% lobectomy or bilobectomy, and 3% pneumonectomy *(18)*. Pfannschmidt et al performed a systematic review of 20 studies that focused on the outcomes of pulmonary metastasectomy of colon cancer origin. In this review, 13 of the studies concluded that the extent of lung resection was not prognostic for survival, whereas one study suggested that the type of resection influenced outcomes *(15)*. These results have led thoracic surgeons to favor performing smaller procedures to preserve as much normal lung as possible while achieving negative operative margins.

Many surgical approaches have been used throughout the years in the resection of lung metastasis, namely median sternotomy, the clamshell incision, and posterolateral thoracotomy. The median sternotomy and clamshell incisions are still favored by a few surgeons because of their exposure of both lung fields and because of the ability to palpate both lungs for lesions undetected by CT; however, studies have not shown increased survival with the increased detection of these lesions *(23)*. Presently, the majority of surgeons perform either posterolateral thoracotomy or video-assisted thoracoscopic surgery (VATS). VATS resection is favored by most surgeons who are experienced with the technique because of its association with smaller incisions, less pain, a reduction in hospital-stay and because VATS survival outcomes are similar to those from thoracotomy in the resection of pulmonary metastases *(24-28)*.

CONTROVERSIAL ISSUES

Numerous studies support the use of surgery in selected patients with colorectal cancer and pulmonary metastases, yet several issues remain unresolved. The number of nodules is an important prognostic factor, yet there is no consensus on the upper limit which would make a patient oncologically inoperable. The timing of surgical resection is also unsettled. For patients with bilateral nodules, the use of systemic and biologic therapy may be offered preoperatively, postoperatively, or between staged procedures. Additionally, there is a lack of agreement on the optimal surgical approach. Proponents of thoracotomy insist that the ability to palpate the lung is essential, yet there is no evidence of improved survival, and the use of the thoracoscopic approach is increasing.

CONCLUSION

Pulmonary metastases develop in 10–20% of patients with colorectal cancer and are usually detected via surveillance CT scans and elevated serum CEA levels. After careful evaluation, patients who meet established criteria may be offered pulmonary metastasectomy.

Communication between oncologists and thoracic surgeons is required to determine the timing of surgery and systemic therapy. Resection, either by thoracotomy or VATS approaches, may be performed in selected patients, with improvement in survival and minimal complications. In patients with resectable pulmonary recurrence following pulmonary metastasectomy, re-resection should be considered.

REFERENCES

1. Saclarides TJ, Krueger BL, Szeluga DJ, Warren WH, Faber LP, Economou SG. Thoracotomy for colon and rectal cancer metastases. *Dis Colon Rectum*. 1993;36:425–429.
2. Ruers TJ, Josten JJ, Wiering B, et al. Comparison between local ablative therapy and chemotherapy for non-resectable colorectal liver metastases: a prospective study. *Ann Surg Oncol*. 2007;14:1161–1169.
3. Weyant MJ, Rusch VW. Lung metastases. In: Abeloff M, ed. *Abeloff's Clinical Oncology*. 3rd ed. Philadelphia: Churchill Livingstone; 2004.
4. Rusch VW. Pulmonary metastasectomy: current indications. *Chest*. 1995;107:322–331.
5. Last accessed on National Comprehensive Cancer Network: Clinical Practice Guidelines in Oncology. Rectal Cancer. Available at http://www.nccn.org/professionals/physician_gls/PDF/rectal.pdf. November 30, 2008.
6. Gutman M, Fidler IJ. Biology of human colon cancer metastasis. *World J Surg*. 1995;19:226–234.
7. Irshad K, Ahmad F, Morin JE, Mulder DS. Pulmonary metastases from colorectal cancer: 25 years of experience. *Can J Surg*. 2001;44:217–221.
8. Joosten J, Bertholet J, Keemers-Gels M, Barendregt W, Ruers T. Pulmonary resection of colorectal metastases in patients with or without history of hepatic metastases. *J Cancer Surg*. 2008;34:895–899.
9. Rotolo N, De Monte L, Imperatori A, Dominioni L. Pulmonary resections of single metastases from colorectal cancer. *Surg Oncol*. 2007;16:5141–5144.
10. Welter S, Jacobs J, Krbek T, Krebs B, Stamatis G. Long-term survival after repeated resection of pulmonary metastases from colorectal cancer. *Ann Thorac Surg*. 2007;84:203–210.
11. Casali C, Stefani A, Stornelli E, Moranti U. Prognostic factors and survival after resection of lung metastases from epithelial tumors. *Interact Cardiovasc Thorac Surg*. 2006;5:317–321.
12. Lo C, Chu C, Zhu T, Ma C, Ko K, Ho K. Pulmonary resection for metastases from colorectal cancer. *Surg Pract*. 2007;11:147–153.
13. Simmonds PC. Palliative chemotherapy for advanced colorectal cancer: systematic review and meta-analysis. *Br Med J*. 2000;321:531–535.
14. Saito Y, Omiya H, Kohno K, et al. Pulmonary metastasectomy for 165 patients with colorectal carcinoma: a prognostic assessment. *J Thorac Cardiovasc Surg*. 2002;124:1007–1013.
15. Pfannschmidt J, Dienemann H, Hoffsmann H. Surgical resection of pulmonary metastases from colorectal cancer: a systematic review of published series. *Ann Thorac Surg*. 2007;84:324–338.
16. Thomford NR, Woolner LB, Clagett OT. The surgical treatment of metastatic tumor in the lung. *J Thorac Cardiovasc Surg*. 1965;49:357–363.
17. Mansel JK, Zinsmeister AR, Pairolero PC, Jett JR. Pulmonary resection of metastatic colorectal adenocarcinoma: ten year experience. *Chest*. 1986;89:109–112.
18. Pastorino U, Buyse M, Friedel G, et al. Long-term results of lung metastasectomy: prognostic analyses based on 5206 cases. *J Thorac Cardiovasc Surg*. 1997;113:37–49.
19. Onaitis MW, Haney J, Petersen R, et al. Factors influencing outcome after pulmonary resection for colorectal cancer metastases in the current era. *J Clin Oncol*. 2008;26:4024 [abstract].
20. Girard P, Grunenwald D, Baldeyrou P, Spaggiari L, Regnard J, Levasseur P. Resectable lung metastases from colorectal cancer: look at the serum CEA level! *Ann Thorac Surg*. 1996;62:1888–1889.
21. Girard P, Ducreux M, Baldeyrou P, et al. Surgery for lung metastases from colorectal cancer: analysis of prognostic factors. *J Clin Oncol*. 1996;14:2047–2053.

22. Crow J, Slavin G, Kreel L. Pulmonary metastasis: a pathologic and radiologic study. *Cancer*. 1981; 47:2595–2602.
23. Roth JA, Pass HI, Wesley MN, White D, Putnam JB, Seipp C. Comparison of median sternotomy and thoracotomy for resection of pulmonary metastases in patients with adult soft-tissue sarcomas. *Ann Thorac Surg*. 1986;42:134–138.
24. Dowling RD, Landreneau RJ, Miller DL. Video-assisted thoracoscopic surgery for resection of lung metastases. *Chest*. 1998;113:2–5.
25. Liu H, Lin PJ, Hsieh M, Chang J, Chang C. Application of thoracoscopy for lung metastases. *Chest*. 1995;107:266–268.
26. Ninomiya M, Nakajima J, Tanaka M, et al. Effects of lung metastasectomy on respiratory function. *Jpn J Thorac Cardiovasc Surg*. 2001;49:17–20.
27. Nakajima J, Murakawa T, Fukami T, Takamoto S. Is thoracoscopic surgery justified to treat pulmonary metastasis from colorectal cancer? *Interact Cardiovasc Thorac Surg*. 2007;7:212–217.
28. Mutsaerts EL, Zoetmulder FA, Meijer S, Bass P, Hart AA, Rutgers EJ. Long term survival of thoracoscopic metastasectomy vs metastasectomy by thoracotomy in patients with a solitary pulmonary lesion. *Eur J Surg Oncol*. 2002;28:864–868.

8 Surgical and Ablative Management of Liver Metastases

Srinevas K. Reddy and Bryan M. Clary

INTRODUCTION

Colorectal liver metastases (CRLM) will develop in up to 50% of patients within 5 years of primary tumor diagnosis *(1)* and are discovered on preoperative imaging or at primary tumor resection in 15–25% of patients *(2–6)*. However, only 15–30% of patients with CRLM are eligible for surgical extirpation *(7–13)*. Due in part to traditional nihilistic views concerning the prognosis of metastatic disease, population cohort studies reveal that only 4–6% of patients with CRLM undergo partial hepatectomy *(14)*. Enhancements in surgical technique, preoperative imaging, critical care, understanding of hepatic anatomy, and systemic chemotherapeutics have dramatically altered the prognosis of resectable CRLM. Numerous prospective clinical trials and large case series have demonstrated long-term survival after surgical extirpation of CRLM is achievable. The objectives of this chapter are to (1) outline the modern criteria for resectability of CRLM, (2) delineate recent developments that have both expanded and narrowed the criteria for resectability, and (3) describe the long-term outcomes and the variables associated with survival after resection of CRLM. For the purposes of this review, no distinction will be made between liver metastases from colon and rectal cancer as most studies do not show a difference in survival by primary disease site (Table 1).

RESECTABILITY OF COLORECTAL LIVER METASTASES

Criteria for Resectability

While there are no universal standards, the criteria for resectable CRLM at most large volume centers have evolved over the past 20 years. Older studies established certain clinicopathologic factors as negative predictors of survival after surgical extirpation that became contraindications for resection, including the presence of more than three liver lesions, hilar adenopathy, extrahepatic metastatic disease (EHD), or the inability to achieve at least 1-cm resection margins *(12,15)*. However, most of these earlier studies, which included small

From: *Current Clinical Oncology: Rectal Cancer*,
Edited by: B.G. Czito and C.G. Willett, DOI: 10.1007/978-1-60761-567-5_8,

Table 1
Factors associated with overall survival from large retrospective series of hepatic resection for colorectal metastases (listed chronologically)

Author	*n*	*Chemo*	*Median OS*	*3 Year OS (%)*	*5 Year OS (%)*	*Gender*	*Age*	*Primary node*	*Rectal tumor*	*Primary T stage*	*Primary stage group*	*CEA*	*DFI*	*EHD*	*CLM volume*	*No.*	*Bilobar*	*Size*	*Satellitosis*	*Portal nodes*	*Grade*	*DOS*	*Blood tx*	*Anatomic*	*Margin*	*Postop chemo*	*Hospital volume*
Hughes et al *(100,101)*,[a]	800[b]	NR			32			•				•	•	•		•									•		
Doci et al *(102)*	100	NR	28		30						•				•												
Ooijen et al *(103)*	118[b]	NR	26		21																						
Donato et al *(106)*	102[b]	39% postop	29	36		•							•														
Hohenberger et al *(104)*	141	NR	34			•						•	•		•												
Nordlinger et al *(90)*	1,568[b]	35% postop		44	28		•	•		•		•	•			•		•							•		
Jamison et al *(105)*	280	33% postop	32	46	27									•					•								
Jenkins et al *(107)*,[a]	149	NR		42	25									•											•		
Ohlsson et al *(108)*	111	18% postop	25	37	25							•		•							•	•	•				
Cady et al *(109)*	244	NR										•				•									•		
Bakalakos et al *(110)*	238	100% postop	23														•								•		
Kokudo et al *(111)*	132	57% postop		57	42								•					•		•						•	
Harms et al *(112)*	245	65% postop	35										•							•					•		
Fong et al *(91)*	1,001	NR	42	57	37			•				•	•	•		•		•							•		
Ambiru et al *(113)*	168	62% postop	23	42	26			•								•									•	•	
Iwatsuki et al *(92)*	305	67% postop			32								•	•		•	•			•					•		
Harmon et al *(114)*,[a]	121	NR	42		46								•					•									
Bradley et al *(115)*,[a]	134	50% postop		50	36											•											
Seifert et al *(116)*	120	NR	30		31													•							•		
Choti et al *(117)*	226	52% preop	46	57	40							•										•			•		
Ercolani et al *(118)*	245	41% postop		53	34										•												
Mala et al *(119)*	146	0 postop	37		29			•				•													•		
Kato et al *(120)*	585[b]	55% postop		53	39							•	•	•											•		

Hofmann et al *(121,122)*	597	NR			33		•						•				•	•		•			•			
Laurent et al *(123)*	311	44% postop		53	36	•	•	•							•											
Nagashima et al *(124)*	151[b]	NR		56[c]	49[c]								•		•		•									
Nicoli et al *(125)*	228	42% postop			16																					
Schindl et al *(126)*	307[b]	0		52[c]	36[c]					•	•		•		•											
Pawlik et al *(33)*	557[b]	60% postop	74	74	58										•		•									
Wei et al *(127)*	423	32% postop	53		47	•									•		•							•		
Tanaka et al *(128)*	156	Most postop		54	43												•			•						
Tsai et al *(129)*	145	100% postop			41																					
Figueras et al *(130)*	545	65% postop[d]	44	60	42								•		•										•	
Jonas et al *(131)*	685	35%[e]			37										•				•		•			•		
Minagawa et al *(132,133)*	598[b]	NR		52[c]	38[c]		•				•				•				•							
Niu et al *(134)*	415	45% postop	32	45	29						•		•				•			•						
Parks et al *(135)*	792[b]	46% postop	41	55	33											•								•	•	
Shah et al *(136)*	841[b]	NR	48	59	43										•						•					•
Malik et al *(93)*,[f]	687	10% preop- Most postop	50	62	45										•											
Zakaria et al *(94)*	662	33% postop	–	NR	37							•					•		•			•				
Rees et al *(137)*	929	NR	43	NR	36		•				•		•		•		•			•				•		
Reddy et al *(138)*	230	50%[g]	42	55	38		•				•														•	

[a]Multivariate analysis not performed[b]Multiinstitutional study

[c]Reported for test cohorts

[d]19% received multiagent posthepatectomy chemotherapy and 18% received prehepatectomy chemotherapy

[e]35% received pre or posthepatectomy chemotherapy; 12% received multiagent chemotherapy

[f]Inflammatory response to tumor also independently associated with overall and disease-free survival

[g]50% each received pre and posthepatectomy chemotherapy; 35 and 32% received multiagent chemotherapy

OS overall survival after hepatic resection, *Median* median overall survival after hepatic resection reported in months, *Chemo* percentage of patients treated with prehepatectomy or posthepatectomy chemotherapy, *CEA* carcino-embryonic antigen, *NR* not reported, *No.* number of liver metastases, *Size* size of largest liver metastases, *DFI* disease-free interval from primary tumor resection to discovery or resection of liver metastases, *Primary node* node positive primary disease, *EHD* extrahepatic metastatic disease, *Bilobar* bilobar distribution of CLM, *Margin* positive/negative or width of hepatic resection margin, *Grade* grade of primary tumor or liver metastases, *Blood tx* intraoperative blood product transfusion, *Portal nodes* nodes in the hepatoduodenal ligament, *Anatomic* anatomic hepatic resection, *CLM volume* hepatic tumor volume, *DOS* date of hepatic resection, *Satellitosis* satellite lesions around main CLM, *Postop chemo* posthepatectomy chemotherapy number of patients who met "exclusion" criteria for resection, were from an era in which the mortality of major (three or more segments) hepatectomy exceeded 20%, and did not include adjunctive, contemporary chemotherapeutics *(16,17)*. Moreover, most of these studies used only univariate statistical analyses and did not account for competing risk factors that may have affected survival *(17)*. For example, microscopically positive margins or negative margins of less than 1 cm are frequently associated with multifocal disease, large tumor size, bilateral distribution of disease, and EHD *(17,19,20)*. New resectability criteria deemphasize old standards of disease burden but instead focus on what remains after potential extirpation *(12)*. This new paradigm includes the ability to achieve (1) a negative hepatic resection margin; (2) a residual liver remnant of at least two contiguous segments with intact biliary drainage, vascular inflow/outflow, and adequate size to provide sufficient hepatic function after resection; and (3) the ability to completely remove and/or ablate EHD *(16,17)*. The volume threshold of liver remnant required is not well established and is dependent on the extent of disease and/or existing injury in the nontumor bearing liver. One proposal calls for consideration of resection when the future liver remnant is at least 30% of the total liver volume in setting of a normal liver to as high as 50% when fibrosis, macrosteatosis, or cirrhosis is present *(17)*. However, there is no consensus method for determining synthetic function of a future liver remnant before partial hepatectomy.

Resection Margin

While the traditional goal of surgical extirpation of CRLM has been a 1 cm margin of uninvolved liver, more recent studies suggest that the width of microscopically negative resection margin is less relevant than achieving a negative surgical margin (R_0) with regard to long-term survival. In a large retrospective study comprising 557 patients who underwent resection of CRLM, Pawlik et al *(21)* found that patients with a positive microscopic surgical margin (R_1) had higher overall recurrence (51% vs. 39%, $p=0.04$) and a worse 5-year actuarial survival (17% vs. 64%, $p=0.01$) compared to patients who underwent R_0 resection. In contrast, the width of negative surgical margin did not affect overall survival or surgical margin site recurrence. In a large study comprising 663 liver resections by Figueras et al, *(18)* a negative resection margin less than 1 cm was associated with hepatic recurrence on univariate ($p=0.0123$) but not multivariate analysis. A multicenter retrospective analysis of 333 patients found no difference in local or overall recurrence-free survival among patients with resection margins ≥10 vs. 3–5 mm. Patients with 1–2 mm margins or positive resection margins experienced shorter overall ($p=0.003$) and intrahepatic ($p<0.0005$) recurrence-free survival compared to patients with resection margins ≥3 mm. However, extent of negative margin did not impact overall survival *(22)*. From these data, Konopke et al *(22)* conclude that the indications for resection can be extended to cases in which a 1-cm margin cannot be obtained and suggest that the use of modern resection techniques (cavi-pulse ultrasound aspirator, harmonic scalpel, and/or water-jet dissector) may eradicate disease in adjacent, nonresected parenchyma, thereby leading to underestimation of negative resection margin width. In a study comprising 176 patients *(20)*, positive resection margins, surgical margin ≤9 mm and >9 mm resection margin were present in 43, 110, and 23 patients, respectively. Five patients developed surgical margin recurrence, which was not associated with the resection margin width. Similarly, margin status was not associated with recurrence-free ($p=0.343$) or overall ($p=0.364$) survival. While Are et al *(19)* note that a margin width of >1 cm ($p<0.01$) and margin width treated as a continuous variable were both associated with prolonged survival after hepatic resection among a cohort of 1,019 patients, these investigators note that a subcentimeter resection margin is associated with a longer median survival compared to patients not undergoing resection and treated with conventional chemotherapeutics (median 42 vs. 20–24 months). Thus, these investigators argue that while a resection margin >1 cm is associated with superior outcomes, the inability to achieve ≥1 cm margin should not preclude attempts at hepatic resection as long as negative resection margins are deemed achievable. In contrast, a study by de Haas et al *(23)* described 436 patients (74 and 83% of which were treated with pre and posthepatectomy chemotherapy, respectively) who underwent an R_1 resection (44%) or R_0 resection (54%). No difference in overall survival was seen in R_0 vs. R_1 resection patients (5-year 61% vs. 57%, $p=0.27$). Despite a difference in intrahepatic recurrence (17% vs. 28%, $p=0.004$), there was no difference in recurrence at the surgical margin (15% vs. 12%). In addition to the above data, other investigators cite several reasons why a 1 cm surgical margin is not always necessary. First, Kokudo et al *(24)* report the detection of micrometastases (via K-ras and p53 genetic mutations) in only 2% of all CRLM and that all micrometastases were within 4 mm of the visible hepatic lesion. Moreover, Ng et al *(25)* compared 25 untreated CRLM to 26 CRLM treated with chemotherapy (25/26 treated with irinotecan, leucovorin, and 5-fluorouracil) before hepatic resection and found that chemotherapy treated tumors regressed concentrically in most cases with central necrosis and viable peripheral cells "drawn in" to the center. Discrete islands of tumor cells were observed in only four patients and all were within 4 mm of the main lesion. These two observations suggest that an anticipated resection margin of <1 cm can still result in R_0 resection in most cases. Additionally, while a positive or "close" margin on initial resection may increase the chance of local recurrence, repeat hepatectomy can still result in long-term survival *(26–32)*. Pawlik and Vauthey *(33)* make similar arguments, citing the fact that most CRLM are well circumscribed with relatively few cases of satellitosis, extension into Glisson's sheath, and/or micrometastases. Thus, the inability to obtain a 1 cm surgical margin is no longer a contraindication for resection of CRLM.

Extrahepatic Metastatic Disease

Despite inferior survival outcomes when compared to patients without EHD (Table 1), recent studies have shown that long-term survival is possible after resection of CRLM in the setting of resectable EHD. Many older studies demonstrating dismal survival after surgical extirpation of CRLM in the presence of EHD were from an era where contemporary chemotherapeutics were not used and were comprised of relatively few patients who underwent concomitant or staged resection of EHD *(17,34)*. Elias et al *(34)* report long-term outcomes of 75 patients who underwent R_0 resection of CRLM and EHD in which the most common sites were peritoneal carcinomatosis (25%), local primary recurrence (16%), and hilar lymph nodes (13%). Three- and 5-year overall survival were 45 and 28% after a median follow-up of 4.9 years and was not different compared to 219 patients without EHD (56 and 33%, respectively, $p=0.15$). On multivariate analysis, more than five CRLM ($p=0.02$) and multiple sites of EHD ($p=0.04$) were associated with survival although not the particular site of EHD ($p=0.17$). Further analysis suggested that it is the overall number of metastases (potentially reflecting a more aggressive tumor biology) and not the presence of EHD that was associated with survival *(35)*. In a study comprising 47 patients treated with chemotherapy before hepatic resection and with regional nodal disease, Adam et al *(36)* noted that patients who underwent resection of CRLM and regional nodal disease had worse overall survival compared to 710 patients without regional nodal disease (3- and 5-year overall survival 38% and 18% vs. 68% and 53%, respectively, $p<0.001$). Location of regional lymph node metastases influenced overall survival as pedicular nodal disease has favorable survival (5-year 25%) compared to celiac (0%) and para-aortic (0%) disease. Celiac location of nodal disease retained significance in association with overall survival on multivariate analysis (HR 4.7, $p<0.001$). Several centers have recently reported long-term outcomes after combined resections of liver and lung colorectal metastases – either presenting synchronously or metachronously. Of 131 patients who underwent resection of hepatic and pulmonary CRLM, Miller et al *(37)* described 32 patients with synchronous colorectal and pulmonary metastases. While the survival of these patients was shorter when compared to patients with metachronous lesions (median 3.5 vs. median 5.5 years, $p=0.0003$), long-term survival in patients with synchronous disease was longer than that demonstrated with treatment with contemporary chemotherapeutics alone. Other smaller series have indicated similar long-term outcomes for synchronous liver and lung metastases *(38,39)*. We agree with Pawlik et al *(17)* and Adam et al *(36)* that patients with resectable CRLM and EHD should initially be treated with chemotherapy with surgery reserved for those patients in whom disease has been stabilized or reduced such that an R_0 resection can be achieved.

Injury from Prehepatectomy Chemotherapy to the Nontumor Bearing Liver

Oxaliplatin- and irinotecan-based prehepatectomy chemotherapy has been shown to result in pathologic injury to the nontumor bearing liver. In an early study, Rubbia-Brandt et al *(40)* noted injury in the centrilobular zones of the liver characterized by severe sinusoidal dilation, erythrocyte congestion (with occasional extravasation in severe cases secondary to sinusoidal wall disruption), and associated perisinusoidal fibrosis and fibrotic venular occlusion associated with oxaliplatin. Nodular regenerative hyperplasia was occasionally associated with these lesions. Other investigators have since confirmed this association *(41–48)*. In an early study comprised of 37 patients, Fernanadez et al *(49)* noted that prehepatectomy irinotecan or oxaliplatin was associated with the development of nonalcoholic steatohepatitis (NASH) in the nontumor bearing liver compared to 5-FU-based chemotherapy and that obese individuals are more likely to develop NASH as compared to lean individuals. Pawlik et al *(45)* has also confirmed the association of prehepatectomy irinotecan treatment with steatosis and steatohepatitis which was independent of diabetes or BMI. There was no association between duration of treatment and development of steatosis in this study. Vauthey et al *(43)* have clarified this pathologic association by demonstrating that irinotecan was associated with steatohepatitis when compared to patients who did not receive prehepatectomy chemotherapy (20% vs. 4%, $p<0.001$, HR 8.3 [2.9–23.6]) and that this hepatic injury did not correlate with preoperative BMI.

The influence of this injury on morbidity and/or mortality after subsequent hepatic resection has not been consistently demonstrated. In a phase II trial including six cycles of FOLFOX4 or XELOX before hepatic resection, postoperative complications were only noted in 12% of patients with no mortality *(50)*. A second phase II trial, which incorporated bevacizumab with XELOX showed a postoperative complication rate of 21% *(51)*. However, larger studies have shown increased morbidity from prehepatectomy chemotherapy (Table 2). Aloia et al *(42)* noted that patients with regenerative nodular hyperplasia and hemorrhagic centrilobular necrosis had an increased transfusion requirement when compared to patients without these adverse pathologic findings ($p=0.04$). Nakano et al *(44)* noted that preoperative hepatic function (as measured by preoperative indocyanine green retention rate at 15 min) was reduced in patient receiving prehepatectomy oxaliplatin compared to other chemotherapeutic agents ($p=0.011$).

Table 2
Large studies evaluating the effects of prehepatectomy chemotherapy on morbidity/mortality after hepatic resection of colorectal liver metastases

Author	*Year*	*Treatment (n)*	*Morbidity*	*Mortality*	*Comments/conclusions*
Nordlinger et al *(139)*	2008	159 FOLFOX4 170 None	25% vs. 16% $p=0.04$	1% vs. 1%	–
Welsh et al *(140)*	2007	252 Chemotherapy 245 None	29% vs. 27% $p=0.34$	2% vs. 2% $p=1.0$	Chemotherapy patients had longer duration of surgery Patients receiving oxaliplatin had greater blood loss More respiratory morbidity and sepsis/abscess among chemo patients Interval from chemo to resection predicted postop morbidity Trend to increased complications with duration of chemo treatment Chemotherapy independently associated with morbidity (HR 5.5 [1.0–29.8], $p=0.046$)
Karoui et al *(41)*	2006	45 Chemotherapy 22 None	38% vs. 14% $p=0.03$	0% vs. 0%	All underwent major hepatectomy with prior portal vein embolization Similar operative duration and blood transfusion rate 11% vs. 0% incidence of transient hepatic failure ≥6 cycles of chemotherapy associated with morbidity (54% vs. 19%, $p=0.047$)
Aloia et al *(42)*	2006	65 FOLFOX/5FU-LV 17 None	20% vs. 6% $p=0.17$	0% vs. 0%	Rate of transfusion higher among chemotherapy patients Chemotherapy independently associated with >1 PRBCs transfused (HR 2.3 [2.0–4.3], $p=0.005$) ≥12 cycles of chemotherapy associated with higher reoperation rate (11% vs. 0%)
Vauthey et al *(43)*	2006	248 Chemotherapy 158 None			No difference in estimated blood loss or operative duration Steatohepatitis injury to nontumor bearing liver associated with post-operative mortality (15% vs. 2%, $p=0.001$, HR 10.5 [2.0–36.4]) Duration of chemotherapy not related to degree of hepatic injury

(continued)

Table 2
(continued)

Author	*Year*	*Treatment (n)*	*Morbidity*	*Mortality*	*Comments/conclusions*
Pawlik et al *(45)*	2007	153 Chemotherapy 59 None	35% vs. 31% $p=0.79$		No association between steatosis or degree of injury to nontumor bearing liver and morbidity No difference in postoperative mortality Overall rate of hepatic injury was low (<20%)
Sahajpal et al *(141)*	2007	53 Chemotherapy 43 None	37% vs. 51% $p=0.26$		No difference in operative duration and estimated blood loss Microscopic steatosis more common in chemotherapy patients (57% vs. 28%, $p=0.005$) No difference according to interval between chemotherapy and resection
Mehta et al *(47)*	2008	70 Oxaliplatin 60 Chemotherapy 43 None		3% vs. 2% vs. 9%	Oxaliplatin associated with higher blood transfusion and length of stay No difference in morbidity or mortality

However, oxaliplatin-based therapy itself did not increase morbidity after hepatic resection compared to other prehepatectomy treatments. They also found that sinusoidal injury was independently associated with the delivery of greater than six cycles of prehepatectomy oxaliplatin-based chemotherapy ($p=0.048$, HR 3.2 [1.0–10.1]). Among patients who underwent major hepatic resection, those with sinusoidal injury in the nontumor bearing liver had greater postoperative morbidity (40% vs. 6%, $p=0.026$). Patients who developed sinusoidal injury also had a shorter interval from the end of oxaliplatin based chemotherapy to resection compared to those who did not (mean 3.6 vs. 6.5 months, $p=0.048$). Vauthey et al *(43)* note that the presence of NASH was associated with an increased 90-day mortality (15% vs. 2%, $p=0.001$, HR 10.5 [2.0–36.4]) and death from postoperative liver failure (6% vs. 1%, $p=0.01$, HR 7.7 [1.3–47.7]) after partial hepatectomy. The reported influence of bevacizumab on the effects of irinotecan and/or oxaliplatin on morbidity after liver resection is inconsistent. Several studies show that (1) the addition of bevacizumab has no effect on steatohepatitis and may actually have a protective effect on the sinusoidal dilation caused by oxaliplatin while still yielding a greater tumor response compared to chemotherapy without bevacizumab, (2) the addition of bevacizumab to oxaliplatin/irinotecan does not affect morbidity after partial hepatectomy, and (3) the timing of discontinuation of bevacizumab may be important in affecting morbidity after hepatic resection *(52–55)*. In contrast, other studies suggest that bevacizumab may impair regeneration after portal vein embolization (PVO) in patients who require major hepatectomy to resect CLM .*(56)*.

While the safety of contemporary prehepatectomy chemotherapy for subsequent resection of CLM is still undetermined, it is clear from these above studies that prolonged durations of treatment (greater than 12 cycles) are associated with postoperative morbidity – particularly for major hepatectomy. By necessitating a larger liver remnant due to limited synthetic function in the nontumor bearing liver, hepatic injury from oxaliplatin or irinotecan-based chemotherapy may, functionally, render some disease (particularly multiple metastases or lesions near the major hepatic veins and/or portal pedicles, which require major hepatectomy for complete surgical extirpation) unresectable.

Use of Chemotherapy to Downsize Unresectable to Resectable Liver Disease

In addition to prolonging survival, *(57–59)* a key advantage to chemotherapy for unresectable CLM is that it has the potential to downsize hepatic lesions making resection a possibility. In the first BEATrial, the addition of bevacizumab to contemporary multiagent chemotherapy enabled 17% of patients initially presenting with unresectable hepatic disease to undergo partial hepatectomy *(60)*. Smaller prospective trials utilizing prolonged treatment with oxaliplatin or irinotecan-based chemotherapy have demonstrated resectability rates of 13–63% in initially unresectable patients, depending on the presence of EHD *(9,13,61–65)*. While the long-term outcomes of patients made eligible for resection by prehepatectomy chemotherapy are not as good as those for patients with initially resectable disease *(9)*, long-term survival exceeding that provided with chemotherapy alone is still achievable *(13,63,66)*. In the largest series reported to date of long-term survival after extirpation of previously unresectable hepatic disease, Adam et al *(67)* report a 5-year and 10-year overall survival of 33 and 27% among 148 patients with follow-up greater than 5 years and a "cure" rate of 16% (24/148 patients). Antibiologic agents may further increase those patients eligible for hepatic resection with CRLM refractory to conventional chemotherapeutics *(68)*.

Prehepatectomy Portal Venous Occlusion

PVO has been employed to broaden the criteria for resectability by increasing the volume and synthetic function of the future liver remnant *(13)*. Below a certain volume, the residual liver is not able to accomplish adequate synthetic, metabolic, and detoxifying functions – thus resulting in postoperative hepatic insufficiency. By redistributing portal venous blood flow to the future liver remnant, PVO induces apoptosis and atrophy in the occluded liver and cellular proliferation and hypertrophy in the nonoccluded liver *(69)*. The increase in volume of the nonoccluded liver can range from 20 to 56% *(70–74)*. This results in an increase in the ratio of future liver remnant volume to total liver volume (degree of hypertrophy) of 8–10% *(72)*. Most of the growth in the nonoccluded liver occurs within 3 weeks of PVO *(72)*. This hypertrophy improves liver function as measured by biliary excretion, increased albumin uptake, and improvement in postoperative liver function tests following extended hepatectomy compared to patients who did not undergo PVO *(13)*. The volume threshold of the future liver remnant at which to consider PVO is not established and is dependent on the degree of disease/injury in the nontumor bearing liver. While not agreed upon at all centers, reported contraindications to PVO include tumor invasion into the portal vein, uncorrectable coagulopathy, tumor extension into the future liver remnant, portal hypertension, and renal failure *(13)*. The degree of hypertrophy after PVO can be used to assess the risk of postoperative hepatic insufficiency after major liver resection *(69*75)*. Failure to achieve liver growth of at least 5% is associated with a high risk of complications after partial hepatectomy. Thus, PVO can be used as a barometer to gauge the ability of the future liver remnant (that may have been damaged by prehepatectomy chemotherapy) to regenerate after future liver resection *(72*76)*. In relatively rare situations (an initially small left lateral section with a tumor burden requiring an extended right hepatectomy for total surgical extirpation), PVO has been used in combination with prehepatectomy chemotherapy to achieve hypertrophy of a potential liver remnant and shrinkage in liver metastases to increase the likelihood of margin negative resection *(69)*. Despite the potential deleterious effects of chemotherapy to the nontumor bearing liver, several studies have shown no adverse outcomes on the hypertrophy of the nonoccluded liver due to chemotherapy *(73)*. Zorzi et al *(77)* demonstrate that the addition of bevacizumab to chemotherapy treatment before PVO does not alter subsequent liver hypertrophy. Specifically, there was no significant difference in future liver remnant volume or in the degree of hypertrophy of the future liver remnant (10.1%, 8.8%, 6.8%, $p=0.11$) between patients treated with oxaliplatin with ($n=26$) or without ($n=17$) bevacizumab and patients not receiving chemotherapy before PVO ($n=22$). Similarly, Covey et al *(71)* show no difference in the number of patients exhibiting less than 5% growth after PVO (6/57 vs. 4/43) or in the average growth of the nonoccluded liver (26±3% vs. 22±3%) between patients receiving/not receiving chemotherapy after PVO.

One key concern regarding PVO is that it may promote growth of CRLM in the occluded or nonoccluded portions of liver, thereby making an initially borderline resectable case unresectable *(75)*. Potential mechanisms of growth include alteration in the ratio of cytokines and growth factors in tissues surrounding liver tumors, increasing hepatic arterial blood flow in the occluded liver, which supplies liver metastases, and enhancing the cellular host response, thereby facilitating tumor growth and angiogenesis *(75)*. Some small case series have demonstrated growth of CRLM after PVO in both the occluded and nonoccluded liver that prevents subsequent resection *(75,78)*. However, these studies are all small, retrospective, and, importantly, do not include appropriate control groups consisting of patients who did not undergo PVO. Thus, tumor growth due to aggressive tumor biology without stimulation from PVO could not be excluded in these studies *(75)*. Moreover, small reports comparing long-term outcomes between patients who underwent major hepatic resection with and without preceding PVO demonstrate no difference in overall survival *(74,78,79)* with one study even showing a decreased intrahepatic recurrence rate associated with PVO *(79)*. Thus, the current evidence suggesting that PVO itself can lead to an increase in hepatic tumor growth that negatively impacts resectability or long-term survival is circumstantial at best and should not prevent the use of PVO when a small future liver remnant is anticipated.

Two-Stage Hepatectomy

At high volume centers with close interactions between medical and surgical oncologists, two-stage hepatectomy is a potentially effective resection strategy for selected patients with multiple, bilateral colorectal liver metastases that would otherwise be unresectable. A two-stage hepatectomy consists of an initial resection (with or without local ablative techniques) in one hemiliver (usually the left), with or without concomitant or staged contralateral PVO depending on the size of the anticipated liver remnant after complete surgical extirpation of disease. Systemic chemotherapy is often administered between hepatic resections to control tumor progression. A time interval between operations is crucial to ascertain the degree of hypertrophy of the nonoccluded liver and the response of disease to chemotherapy. If there is adequate hypertrophy and disease stability or response to chemotherapy, then final hepatic resection (usually of the right hemiliver) is performed to achieve complete extirpation *(69,75,80)*. This strategy relies on compensatory regeneration after the first partial hepatectomy, allowing the potential to perform the second hepatectomy safely with lower risk of postoperative hepatic insufficiency. Because the first stage entails a minor hepatectomy, simultaneous resection of primary disease may be performed.

The largest experience of two-stage hepatectomy is reported by Wicherts et al *(80)* in which 41/59 (69%) patients targeted for two-stage hepatectomy completed the second-staged resection. The remaining patients experienced disease progression, which precluded final resection. Mean number of metastases was 9.1±5.4 with a mean duration of 9 months between first and second hepatectomy, with 78% of patients requiring PVO before second hepatectomy. Nonhepatic- and hepatic-related morbidity after second hepatectomy was greater than after the first resection (29% vs. 7%, $p=0.01$ and 51% vs. 15%, $p=0.01$, respectively). This high morbidity rate after second-staged hepatectomy likely reflects (1) an increased rate of major hepatic resection and (2) hepatectomy after prolonged use of chemotherapy relative to first-staged hepatectomy and has been confirmed by other investigators *(81)*. Forty nine percent of patients had disease recurrence after a median follow-up of 24 months, with a 3-year disease-free survival of 26% and 3-year overall survival of 60%. Of note, the overall survival among patients who completed the two-staged hepatectomy was similar to other patients who had complete surgical extirpation of disease with a single-staged hepatectomy. Patients with disease progression after the first stage that precluded second-staged hepatectomy had a median survival of 11.4 months, similar to unresected patients. Chun et al, *(82)* Homayounfar et al, *(83)* and Jaeck et al *(84)* noted that 21/30 (70%), 19/24 (79%), and 25/33 (76%) patients successfully completed two-stage hepatectomy with similar survival outcomes among those who completed the second resection.

LONG-TERM OUTCOMES

Resection

Prospective trials and retrospective studies with long-term follow-up demonstrate survival benefits after resection CRLM. In the EORTC Intergroup 40983 randomized clinical trial of 364 total patients comparing outcomes between those treated with perioperative

FOLFOX4 and resection of CRLM compared to patients treated with partial hepatectomy and no chemotherapy, patients treated with chemotherapy and who ultimately underwent partial hepatectomy had a 3-year progression-free survival of 42% at a median follow-up of 3.9 years. In comparison, patients not treated with chemotherapy and who underwent partial hepatectomy had a 3-year progression free survival of 33% ($p=0.025$) *(85)*. A pooled analysis of the AURC 9002 and EORTC 40923 phase III randomized controlled trials evaluating the efficacy of bolus fluorouracil plus leucovorin after resection of CRLM demonstrated a median progression-free and overall survival of 27.9 and 62.2 months among 5-FU-treated patients compared to 18.8 and 47.3 months among patients treated with surgery alone. 5-FU treatment was independently associated with improved progression-free and overall survival on multivariate analysis *(86)*. After a 10-year follow-up of 612 patients treated without contemporary chemotherapeutics who underwent resection of CRLM at a single institution, Tomlinson et al *(87)* note a median overall disease-specific survival of 44 months after partial hepatectomy with a plateau in the survival curve after 10 years. One hundred two actual 10-year survivors were observed (corresponding to a minimum cure rate of 17%), and 98% of these patients were without evidence of disease at last follow-up. Of note, the authors stated that classically poor prognostic clinicopathologic factors, such as short disease-free interval (DFI), multiplicity of hepatic disease, large size of hepatic metastases, and bilobar disease were present among some of the long-term survivors. No patients with positive surgical resection margins were among the 10-year survivors. Similarly, Vigano et al *(88)* report the result of 10-year follow-up on 121 patients, none of which were treated with prehepatectomy chemotherapy or contemporary chemotherapeutics. Nineteen 10-year survivors were observed, resulting in an actual 10-year overall and recurrence-free survival of 15.7 and 10.4%, respectively. No recurrences were observed after 10 years, and no patients with positive surgical margins were among the 10-year survivors.

Survival after resection of CRLM has also been established by several contemporary retrospective resection series (Table 1). Results from these studies suggest several factors that may be associated with improved survival after partial hepatectomy including gender; patient age; primary tumor tumor/node stage, grade, and overall stage group; rectal primary; prehepatectomy CEA; DFI from primary tumor resection to diagnosis of liver metastases; hospital volume; EHD; size, number, volume, and/or satellitosis of liver metastases; bilobar hepatic disease; intraoperative blood transfusion; portal lymph node disease; margin status, anatomic resections; date of surgery; and posthepatectomy chemotherapy. In addition, Blazer et al *(89)* analyzed the pathologic response to prehepatectomy chemotherapy and long-term outcomes after surgical extirpation among 305 patients who underwent resection of CRLM. Five-year survival was improved among the 9% of patients who exhibited a complete pathologic response to prehepatectomy chemotherapy vs. 36% who exhibited a major response vs. 55% with a minor response (75% vs. 56% vs. 33%, $p<0.05$). This was also shown to be significant on multivariate analysis ($p<0.05$). Similarly, Gruenberger et al *(50)* demonstrated an improvement in recurrence-free and overall survival among patients with liver disease responsive to prehepatectomy XELOX or FOLFOX chemotherapy by radiologic imaging prior to subsequent hepatic resection. Recurrence-free survival was 24.7 vs. 8.2 vs. 3.0 months among patients with responding vs. stable vs. progressive disease ($p<0.004$). Similarly, overall survival was not reached vs. 21.2 vs. 12.2 months ($p=0.046$). Both of these associations remained significant on multivariate analysis.

The actuarial survival and factors associated with survival vary among studies (Table 1), precluding applicability of the results of any one of these series to other patient populations. Nonetheless, several groups have published prognostic models for long-term outcomes after resection of colorectal metastases that may also be used to guide the implementation and timing of multimodal treatment strategies *(90–94)*. In an effort to more accurately assess the specific value of each component, some groups have created prognostic nomograms to assess long-term outcomes after resection of CRLM *(95,96)*. As a critique to these proposed scoring systems, Zakaria et al *(94)* analyzed outcomes of 662 patients after partial hepatectomy for CRLM and found the correlation coefficients of three widely used scoring systems to be 0.53–0.56 (i.e., only slightly better than chance). Other problems of prognostic scoring systems include varied selection criteria (stringent to more liberal with improvements in safety of partial hepatectomy), differing quality of preoperative imaging over a long study period, and inadequate follow-up in the "test cohort." Moreover, most of these prognostic models have not been validated with independent data sets – thus, unrecognized selection biases, population differences, possible overfitting because of too few events, and differences in surgical and imaging techniques between institutions may limit the applicability of a model created at one institution to other populations *(94)*.

Ablation

Indications for radiofrequency ablation (RFA) include (1) unresectability of liver disease due to location, size, number, or patient comorbidity such that the hepatic reserve provided by the future liver remnant would not be sufficient for patient survival or (2) an adjunct to hepatic resection to clear the liver remnant of disease while preserving liver function *(13)*. While RFA does not provide comparable long-term survival to that provided by resection, outcomes after RFA are superior to that using systemic chemotherapy alone.

Large retrospective series demonstrate long-term survival after RFA. Siperstein et al *(1)* report the results of 292 RFAs in 235 patients over a 10 year period whose disease was considered unresectable secondary to poor response to chemotherapy or extensive comorbidities. Eighty percent of patients had progression of disease on chemotherapy prior to ablation and 24% had extrahepatic disease. Median overall survival after ablation was 24 months with actual 3-year and 5-year survival of 20.2% and 18.4%, respectively. Median disease-free survival was 6 months. Greater than three metastases, initial CEA levels, and treatment with postablation chemotherapy were associated with survival. Neither size nor presence of extrahepatic disease was prognostic. The authors note survival outcomes compared favorably to that of patients with unresectable disease unresponsive to chemotherapy not undergoing ablation. Reuter et al *(97)* compared 66 patients treated with RFA alone to 126 patients who underwent resection alone in which mode of treatment was left to the discretion of the operating surgeon. Patient demographics and clinicopathologic tumor characteristics were similar except that resected patients had larger lesions (mean 5.3 vs. 3.2 cm, $p<0.001$). RFA was associated with improved overall (71% vs. 46%, $p<0.001$), treatment site (17% vs. 2%, $p<0.0001$), lobar (42% vs. 3%, $p<0.0001$), and intrahepatic distant (33% vs. 14%, $p=0.002$) recurrence rates with no difference in extrahepatic recurrence or overall survival rates (median 27.0 vs. 36.4 months). In one of the largest comparative studies between resection and ablation, Abdalla et al *(98)* report the outcomes of 418 total patients treated over a 10-year interval in which 190 underwent hepatic resection alone, 101 underwent combined resection and ablation, 57 underwent ablation alone, and 70 were treated with systemic chemotherapy without direct hepatic treatment. RFA was performed in cases in which resection of all disease would leave too small a remnant to support hepatic function, and chemotherapy alone was performed when the hepatic disease was too extensive for curative therapy. Despite this treatment algorithm, the authors state that there was no difference in patient demographics or primary/liver tumor clinicopathologic characteristics between patient groups. On multivariable analysis, RFA with resection was associated with poorer recurrence-free (HR = 1.73 [1.19–2.51] $p = 0.004$) and overall (HR = 2.14 [1.28–3.59] $p = 0.004$) survival compared to resection alone. Similarly, RFA alone was associated with poorer recurrence-free (HR = 2.60 [1.84–3.68] $p < 0.0001$) and overall (HR = 2.79 [1.68–4.62] $p < 0.0001$) survival compared to resection. Comparing RFA alone to resection with RFA to resection alone, the use of RFA was associated with an increased risk of intrahepatic (44% vs. 28% vs. 11%, $p < 0.001$) and marginal (9% vs. 5% vs. 2%, $p = 0.02$) recurrence with no difference in extrahepatic recurrence (40% vs. 37% vs. 41%). Comparing any use of RFA vs. chemotherapy alone, RFA was associated with improved survival ($p = 0.002$), which maintained when comparing RFA alone to chemotherapy ($p = 0.005$). Thus, these investigators conclude that while long-term outcomes after RFA are inferior to that after resection, RFA can provide survival benefit over that provided by chemotherapy alone for metastatic disease confined to the liver. As a criticism to these comparative studies, Gleisner et al *(99)* using a propensity score methods model of analysis showed that differences in demographics, clinicopathologic tumor characteristics, and treatments prevent accurate comparisons between patients treated with hepatic resection versus those treated with resection and ablation, and that these differences were unable to support any causal comparisons about the differential treatment effect.

CONCLUSION

The criterion for resectability of CRLM has evolved from deemphasizing old standards that center on disease burden to a new paradigm, which focuses on what remains after potential extirpation. Recent studies have shown that the inability to achieve a 1-cm resection margin or the presence of resectable EHD are no longer contraindications to resection. Oxaliplatin and irinotecan based chemotherapy may serve to both augment the resectability of CRLM by shrinking previously unresectable lesions and hinder disease resectability via injury to the nontumor bearing liver. PVO and two-stage hepatectomy can be utilized in select patients to achieve complete surgical extirpation with sufficient liver remnant volume. Resection of CRLM provides the best long-term outcomes with ablation reserved for those patients in which resection is not possible or when complete surgical extirpation would result in an insufficient liver remnant. These developments underscore the need for the early involvement of hepatobiliary surgeons in the multidisciplinary care of patients with CRLM.

REFERENCES

1. Siperstein AE, Berber E, Ballem N, Parikh RT. Survival after radiofrequency ablation of colorectal liver metastases. *Ann Surg*. 2007;246:559–567.
2. Newland RC, Dent OF, Chapuis PH, et al. Clinicopathologically diagnosed residual tumour after resection for colorectal cancer: a 20-year prospective study. *Cancer*. 1993;72:1536–1542.
3. Vigano L, Ferrero A, Tesoriere RL, et al. Liver surgery for colorectal metastases: results after 10 years of follow-up, long-term survivors, late recurrences, and prognostic role of morbidity. *Ann Surg Oncol*. 2008;15(9):2458–2464.
4. Cady D, Monson DO, Swinton NW. Survival of patients after colonic resection for carcinoma with simultaneous liver metastases. *Surg Gynecol Obstet*. 1970;131:697–700.
5. Blumgart LH, Allison DJ. Resection and embolization in the management of secondary hepatic tumors. *World J Surg*. 1982;6:32–45.
6. Jatzko G, Wette V, Muller M, et al. Simultaneous resection of colorectal carcinoma and synchronous liver metastases in a district hospital. *Int J Colorectal Dis*. 1991;6:111–114.

7. Rougier P, Milan C, Lazorthes F, et al. Prospective study of prognostic factors in patients with unresected hepatic metastases from colorectal cancer. *Br J Surg*. 1995;82:1397–1400.
8. Stangl R, Altendorf-Hofmann A, Charnley RM, et al. Factors influencing the natural history of colorectal liver metastases. *Lancet*. 1994;343:1405–1410.
9. Adam R, Delvart V, Pascal G, et al. Rescue surgery for unresectable colorectal liver metastases downstaged by chemotherapy. *Ann Surg*. 2004;240:644–658.
10. Fortner JG, Silva JS, Cox EB, et al. Multivariate of a personal series of 247 patients with liver metastases from colorectal cancer. *Ann Surg*. 1984;199:317–324.
11. Yamamura T, Senda T, Akaishi O, et al. Comparative studies on treatment for liver metastases from colorectal cancer. *St Marianna Med J*. 1990;18:501–508.
12. Poston GJ, Figureas J, Giuliante F, et al. Urgent need for a new staging system in advanced colorectal cancer. *J Clin Oncol*. 2008;26:4828–4833.
13. Abdalla EK, Adam R, Bilchik AJ, et al. Improving resectablity of hepatic colorectal metastases: expert consensus statement. *Ann Surg Oncol*. 2006;13:1271–1280.
14. Cummings LC, Payes JD, Cooper GS. Survival after hepatic resection in metastatic colorectal cancer: a population-based study. *Cancer*. 2007;109:718–726.
15. Ekberg J, Tranberg KG, Andersson R, et al. Determinants of survival in liver resection for colorectal secondaries. *Br J Surg*. 1986;73:727–731.
16. Charnsangavej C, Clary B, Fong Y, et al. Selection of patients for resection of hepatic colorectal metastases: expert consensus statement. *Ann Surg Oncol*. 2006;13:1261–1268.
17. Pawlik TM, Schulick RD, Choti MA. Expanding criteria for resectability of colorectal liver metastases. *Oncologist*. 2008;13:51–64.
18. Figueras J, Burdio F, Ramos E, et al. Effect of subcentimeter nonpositive resection margin on hepatic recurrence in patients undergoing hepatectomy for colorectal liver metastases. Evidences from 663 liver resections. *Ann Oncol*. 2007;18:1190–1195.
19. Are C, Gonen M, Zazzali K, et al. The impact of margins on outcome after hepatic resection for colorectal metastases. *Ann Surg*. 2007;246:295–300.
20. Bodingbauer M, Tamandl D, Schmid K, et al. Size of surgical margin does not influence recurrence rates after curative liver resection for colorectal cancer liver metastases. *Br J Surg*. 2007; 94:1133–1138.
21. Pawlik TM, Scoggins CR, Zorzi D, et al. Effect of surgical margin status on survival and site of recurrence after hepatic resection of colorectal metastases. *Ann Surg*. 2005;241:715–724.
22. Konopke R, Kersting S, Makowiec F, et al. Resection of colorectal liver metastases: is a resection margin of 3 mm enough? *World J Surg*. 2008;32:2047–2056.
23. de Haas RJ, Wicherts DA, Flores E, et al. R1 resection by necessity for colorectal liver metastases: is it still a contraindication to surgery? *Ann Surg*. 2008;248:626–637.
24. Kokudo N, Miki Y, Sugai S, et al. Genetic and histological assessment of surgical margins in resected liver metastases from colorectal carcinoma: minimum surgical margins for successful resection. *Arch Surg*. 2002;137:833–840.
25. Ng JK, Urbanski SJ, Mangat N, et al. Colorectal liver metastases contract centripetally with a response to chemotherapy: a histomorphologic study. *Cancer*. 2008;112:362–371.
26. Sa Cunha A, Laurent C, Rault A, et al. A second liver resection due to recurrent colorectal liver metastases. *Arch Surg*. 2007;142:1144–1149.
27. Matsuda K, Hotta T, Uchiyama K, et al. Repeat reduction surgery after an initial hepatectomy for patients with colorectal cancer. *Oncol Rep*. 2007;18:189–194.
28. Nishio H, Hamady ZZ, Malik HZ, et al. Outcome following repeat liver resection for colorectal liver metastases. *Eur J Surg Oncol*. 2007;33:729–734.
29. Antoniou A, Lovegrove RE, Tinley HS, et al. Meta-analysis of clinical outcome after first and second liver resection for colorectal liver metastases. *Surgery*. 2007;141:9–18.
30. Thelen A, Jonas S, Benckert C, et al. Repeat liver resection for recurrent liver metastases from colorectal cancer. *Eur J Surg Oncol*. 2007;33:324–328.
31. Shaw IM, Rees M, Welsh FK, et al. Repeat hepatic resection for recurrent colorectal liver metastases is associated with favourable long-term survival. *Br J Surg*. 2006;93:457–464.

32. Adam R, Bismuth H, Castaing D, et al. Repeat hepatectomy for colorectal liver metastases. *Ann Surg*. 1997;225:51–60.
33. Pawlik TM, Vauthey JV. Surgical margin during hepatic surgery for colorectal liver metastases: complete resection not millimeters defines outcome. *Ann Surg Oncol*. 2008;15:677–679.
34. Elias D, Sideris L, Pocard M, et al. Results of R0 resection for colorectal liver metastases associated with extrahepatic disease. *Ann Surg Oncol*. 2004;11:274–280.
35. Elias D, Ouellet JF, Bellon N, et al. Extrahepatic disease does not contraindicate hepatectomy for colorectal liver metastases. *Br J Surg*. 2003;90:567–574.
36. Adam R, de Haas RJ, Wicherts DA, et al. Is hepatic resection justified after chemotherapy in patients with colorectal lymph node metastases and lymph node involvement? *J Clin Oncol*. 2008;26:3672–3680.
37. Miller G, Biernacki P, Kemeny NE, et al. Outcomes after resection of synchronous or metachronous hepatic and pulmonary colorectal metastases. *J Am Coll Surg*. 2007;205:231–238.
38. Shah SA, Haddad R, Al-Sukhni W, et al. Surgical resection for hepatic and pulmonary metastases from colorectal carcinoma. *J Am Coll Surg*. 2006;202:468–475.
39. Mineo TC, Ambrogi V, Tonini G, et al. Long term results after resection of simultaneous and sequential lung and liver metastases from colorectal carcinoma. *J Am Coll Surg*. 2003;197:386–391.
40. Rubbia-Brandt L, Audard V, Sartoretti P, et al. Severe hepatic sinusoidal obstruction associated with oxaliplatin-based chemotherapy in patients with metastatic colorectal cancer. *Ann Oncol*. 2004;15:460–466.
41. Karoui M, Penna C, Amin-Hashem M, et al. Influence of preoperative chemotherapy on the risk of major hepatectomy for colorectal liver metastases. *Ann Surg*. 2006;243:1–7.
42. Aloia T, Sebagh M, Plasse M, et al. Liver histology and surgical outcomes after preoperative chemotherapy with fluorouracil plus oxaliplatin in colorectal cancer liver metastases. *J Clin Oncol*. 2006;24:4983–4990.
43. Vauthey JN, Pawlik TM, Ribero D, et al. Chemothearpy regimen predicts steatohepatitis and an increase in 90-day mortality after surgery for hepatic colorectal metastases. *J Clin Oncol*. 2006;24:2065–2072.
44. Nakano H, Oussoultzoglou E, Rosso E, et al. Sinusoidal injury increases morbidity after major hepatectomy in patients with colorectal liver metastases receiving preoperative chemotherapy. *Ann Surg*. 2008;247:118–124.
45. Pawlik TM, Olino K, Gleisner AL, et al. Preoperative chemotherapy for colorectal liver metastases: impact on hepatic histology and postoperative outcome. *J Gastrointest Surg*. 2007;11:860–868.
46. Kandutsch S, Klinger M, Hacker S, et al. Patterns of hepatotoxicity after chemotherapy for colorectal cancer liver metastases. *Eur J Surg Oncol*. 2008;34(11):1231–1236.
47. Mehta NN, Ravikumar R, Coldham CA, et al. Effect of preoperative chemotherapy on liver resection for colorectal liver metastases. *Eur J Surg Oncol*. 2008;34:782–786.
48. Julie C, Lutz MP, Aust D, et al. Pathological analysis of hepatic injury after oxaliplatin-based neoadjuvant chemotherapy of colorectal cancer liver metastases: results of the EORTC Intergroup phase III study 40983. *2007 Gastrointestinal Cancers Symposium*, abstr 241; 2007.
49. Fernandez FG, Ritter J, Goodwin JW, et al. Effect of steatohepatitis associated with irinotecan or oxaliplatin pretreatment on resectability of hepatic colorectal metastases. *J Am Coll Surg*. 2005;200:845–853.
50. Gruenberger B, Scheithauer W, Punzengruber R, et al. Importance of response to neoadjuvant chemotherapy in potentially curable colorectal cancer liver metastases. *BMC Cancer*. 2008; 8:120–127.
51. Gruenberger G, Tamandl D, Schueller J, et al. Bevacizumab, capecitabine, and oxaliplatin as neoadjuvant therapy for patients with potentially curable metastatic colon cancer. *J Clin Oncol*. 2008;26:1830–1835.
52. Reddy SK, Morse MA, Hurwitz HI, et al. Addition of bevacizumab to irinotecan- and oxaliplatin-based preoperative chemotherapy regimens does not increase morbidity after resection of colorectal liver metastases. *J Am Coll Surg*. 2008;206:96–106.
53. Klinger M, Kandutsch S, Hacker S, et al. Patterns of hepatotoxicity after chemotherapy for colorectal cancer metastases. *J Clin Oncol*. 2008;226:abstr 4082.

54. Ribero D, Wang H, Donadon M, et al. Bevacizumab improves pathologic response and protects against hepatic injury in patients treated with oxaliplatin-based chemotherapy for colorectal liver metastases. *Cancer.* 2007;110:2761–2767.
55. Kesmodel SB, Ellis LM, Lin E, et al. Preoperative bevacizumab does not significantly increase postoperative complication rates in patients undergoing hepatic surgery for colorectal liver metastases. *J Clin Oncol.* 2008;26:5254–5260.
56. Aussilhou B, Faivre S, Lepille D, et al. Preoperative bevacizumab may impair liver hypertrophy of the future remnant liver after a portal vein occlusion in patients undergoing major resections of colorectal liver metastases. *J Clin Oncol.* 2008;26:abstr 4081.
57. Tournigand C, Andre T, Achille E, et al. FOLFIRI followed by FOLFOX or the reverse sequence in advanced colorectal cancer: a randomized GERCOR study. *J Clin Oncol.* 2004;22:229–237.
58. Hurwitz H, Fehrenbacher L, Novotny W, et al. Bevacizumab plus irinotecan, fluorouracil, and leucovorin for metastatic colorectal cancer. *New Engl J Med.* 2004;350:2335–2342.
59. Meyerhardt JA, Mayer RJ. Systemic therapy for colorectal cancer. *New Engl J Med.* 2005;352: 476–487.
60. Rivera F, Van Cutsem E, Kretzschmar A, et al. Preliminary efficacy of bevacizumab with first-line FOLFOX, XELOX, FOLFIRI, and monotherapy for mCRC: first BEATrial. *Ann Oncol.* 2007;18:abstr O-0025.
61. Tirelli U, Berretta M, Di Benedetto F, et al. Presurgical chemotherapy with FOLFOX4-regimen for patients with unresectable liver metastases from colorectal cancer. *J Clin Oncol.* 2008;26:abstr 15052.
62. Masi G, Loupakis F, Baldi G, et al. Outcome of initially unresectable metastatic colorectal cancer patients treated with first-line FOLFOXIRI followed by R0 surgical resection of metastases. *J Clin Oncol.* 2008;26:abstr 4074.
63. Wicherts DA, de Haas RJ, Adam R. Bringing unresectable liver disease to resection with curative intent. *Eur J Surg Oncol.* 2007;33:S42-S51.
64. Pozzo C, Basso M, Cassano A, et al. Neoadjuvant treatment of unresectable liver disease with irinotecan and 5-fluorouracil plus folinic acid in colorectal cancer patients. *Ann Oncol.* 2004;15:933–939.
65. Nuzzo G, Giuliante F, Ardito F, et al. Liver resection for primary unresectable colorectal metastases downsized by chemotherapy. *J Gastrointest Surg.* 2007;11:318–324.
66. Nordlinger B, Van Cutsem E, Rougier P, et al. Does chemotherapy prior to liver resection increase the potential for cure in patients with metastatic colorectal cancer? *Eur J Cancer.* 2007;43:2037–2045.
67. Adam R, Wicherts DA, de Haas RJ, et al. Patients with initially irresectable colorectal liver metastases: is there a possibility of cure by an oncosurgical approach? *J Clin Oncol.* 2008;26:abstr 4081.
68. Adam R, Aloia T, Levi F, et al. Hepatic resection after rescue cetuximab treatment for colorectal liver metastases previously refractory to conventional systemic therapy. *J Clin Oncol.* 2007;25: 4593–4602.
69. Clavien PA, Petrowsky H, DeOliveira ML, Graf R. Strategies for safer liver surgery and partial liver transplantation. *N Engl J Med.* 2007;356:1545–1559.
70. Capussotti L, Muratore A, Baracchi F, et al. Portal vein ligation as an efficient method of increasing the future liver remnant volume in the surgical treatment of colorectal liver metastases. *Arch Surg.* 2008;143:978–982.
71. Covey AM, Brown KT, Jarnagin WR, et al. Combined portal vein embolization and neoadjuvant chemotherapy as a treatment strategy for resectable hepatic colorectal metastases. *Ann Surg.* 2008;247:451–455.
72. Ribero D, Abdalla EK, Madoff DC, et al. Portal vein embolization before major hepatectomy and its effects on regeneration, resectablity, and outcome. *Br J Surg.* 2007;94:1386–1394.
73. Goere D, Farges O, Laporrier J, et al. Chemotherapy does not impair hypertrophy of the left liver after right portal vein obstruction. *J Gastrointest Surg.* 2006;10:365–370.
74. Linder P, Cahlin C, Friman S, et al. Extended right sided liver resection for colorectal liver metastases – impact of percutaneous portal venous embolisation. *Eur J Surg Oncol.* 2006;32:292–296.
75. de Graaf W, van den Esschert JW, van Lienden KP, van Gulik TM. Induction of tumor growth after pre-operative portal vein embolization: is it a real problem? *Ann Surg Oncol.* 2009;16(2): 423–430.

76. Abdalla EK. Commentary: Radiofrequency ablation for colorectal liver metastases: do not blame the biology when it is the technology. *Am J Surg*. 2009;197:737–739.
77. Zorzi D, Chin YS, Madoff DC, et al. Chemotherapy with bevacizumab does not affect liver regeneration after portal vein embolization in the treatment of colorectal liver metastases. *Ann Surg Oncol*. 2008;15:2765–2772.
78. Mueller L, Hillert C, Moller L, et al. Major hepatectomy for colorectal metastases: is preoperative portal occlusion an oncologic risk factor? *Ann Surg Oncol*. 2008;15:1908–1917.
79. Oussoultzoglou E, Bachelier P, Rosso E, et al. Right portal vein embolization before right hepatectomy for unilobar colorectal liver metastases reduces the intrahepatic recurrence rate. *Ann Surg*. 2006;244:71–79.
80. Wicherts DA, Miller R, de Haas RJ, et al. Long-term results of two-stage hepatectomy for irresectable colorectal cancer liver metastases. *Ann Surg*. 2008;248:994–1005.
81. Tanaka K, Shimada H, Matsuo K, et al. Regeneration after two-stage hepatectomy vs repeat resection for colorectal metastases recurrence. *J Gastrointest Surg*. 2007;11:1154–1161.
82. Chun YS, Vauthey JN, Ribero D, et al. Systemic chemotherapy and two-stage hepatectomy for extensive bilateral colorectal liver metastases: perioperative safety and survival. *J Gastrointest Surg*. 2007;11:1498–1505.
83. Homayounfar K, Liersch T, Schuetze G, et al. Two-stage hepatectomy (R0) with portal vein ligation – towards curing patients with extended bilobular colorectal liver metastases. *Int J Colorectal Dis*. 2009;24(4):409–418.
84. Jaeck D, Oussoultzoglou E, Rosso E, et al. A two-stage hepatectomy procedure combined with portal vein embolization to achieve curative resection for initially unresectable multiple and bilobar colorectal liver metastases. *Ann Surg*. 2004;240:1037–1051.
85. Nordlinger B, Sorbye H, Glimelius B, et al. Perioperative chemotherapy with FOLFOX4 and surgery versus surgery alone for resectable liver metastases from colorectal cancer (EORTC intergroup trial 40983): a randomised controlled trial. *Lancet*. 2008;371:1007–1016.
86. Mitry E, Fields ALA, Bleiberg H, et al. Adjuvant chemotherapy after potentially curative resection of metastases from colorectal cancer: a pooled analysis of two randomized trials. *J Clin Oncol*. 2008;26:4906–4911.
87. Tomlinson JS, Jarnagin WR, DeMatteo RP, et al. Actual 10-year survival after resection of colorectal liver metastases defines cure. *J Clin Oncol*. 2007;25:4575–4580.
88. Vigano L, Ferrero A, Tesoriere RL, Capussotti L. Liver surgery for colorectal metastases: results after 10 years of follow-up. Long-term survivors, late recurrences, and prognostic role of morbidity. *Ann Surg Oncol*. 2008;15:2458–2464.
89. Blazer DG III, Kishi Y, Muru DM, et al. Pathologic response to pre-operative chemotherapy: a new outcome end point after resection of hepatic colorectal metastases. *J Clin Oncol*. 2008;25:5344–5351.
90. Nordlinger B, Guiguet M, Vaillant JC, et al. Surgical resection of colorectal carcinoma metastases to the liver: a prognostic scoring system to improve case selection, based on 1568 patients. *Cancer*. 1996;77:1254–1262.
91. Fong Y, Fortner J, Sun RL, et al. Clinical score for predicting recurrence after hepatic resection for metastatic colorectal cancer: analysis of 1001 consecutive cases. *Ann Surg*. 1999;230: 309–321.
92. Iwatsuki S, Dvorchik I, Madariaga JR, et al. Hepatic resection for metastatic colorectal adenocarcinoma: a proposal of a prognostic scoring system. *J Am Coll Surg*. 1999;189:291–299.
93. Malik HZ, Prasad KR, Halazum KJ, et al. Preoperative prognostic score for predicting survival after hepatic resection of colorectal liver metastases. *Ann Surg*. 2007;246:806–814.
94. Zakaria S, Donohue JH, Que FG, et al. Hepatic resection for colorectal metastases: value for risk scoring systems? *Ann Surg*. 2007;246:183–191.
95. Kanemitsu Y, Kato T. Prognostic models for predicting death after hepatectomy in individuals with hepatic metastases. *World J Surg*. 2008;32:1097–1107.
96. Kattan MW, Gonen M, Jarnagin WR, et al. A nomogram for predicting disease-specific survival after hepatic resection for colorectal cancer. *Ann Surg*. 2008;247:282–287.
97. Reuter NP, Woodall CE, Scoggins CR, et al. Radiofrequency ablation vs. resection for hepatic colorectal metastases: therapeutically equivalent? *J Gastrointest Surg*. 2009;13(3):486–491.

98. Abdalla EK, Vauthey JN, Ellis LM, et al. Recurrence and outcomes following hepatic resection, radiofrequency ablation, and combined resection/ablation for colorectal liver metastases. *Ann Surg*. 2004;239:818–827.
99. Gleisner AL, Choti MA, Assumpcao L, et al. Colorectal liver metastases: recurrence and survival following hepatic resection, radiofrequency ablation, and combined resection-radiofrequency ablation. *Arch Surg*. 2008;143:1204–1212.
100. Hughes K, Scheele J, Sugarbaker PH. Surgery for colorectal cancer metastatic to the liver: optimizing the results of treatment. *Surg Clin North Am*. 1989;69:339–359.
101. Hughes KS, Rosenstein RB, Songhorabodi S, et al. Resection of the liver for colorectal carcinoma metastases: a multi-institutional study of long-term survivors. *Dis Colon Rectum*. 1988;31:1–4.
102. Doci R, Gennari L, Bignami P, et al. One hundred patients with hepatic metastases from colorectal cancer treated by resection: analysis of prognostic determinants. *Br J Surg*. 1991;78:797–801.
103. van Ooijen B, Wiggers T, Meijer S, et al. Hepatic resections for colorectal metastases in The Netherlands: a multi-institutional 10-year study. *Cancer*. 1992;70:28–34.
104. Hohenberger P, Schlag PM, Gerneth T, et al. Pre- and postoperative carcinoembryonic antigen determinations in hepatic resection for colorectal metastases: predictive value and implications for adjuvant treatment based on multivariate analysis. *Ann Surg*. 1994;219:135–143.
105. Jamison RL, Donohue JH, Nagorney DM, et al. Hepatic resection for metastatic colorectal cancer results in cure for some patients. *Arch Surg*. 1997;132:505–511.
106. Donato N, Dario S, Giovanni S, et al. Retrospective study on adjuvant chemotherapy after surgical resection of colorectal cancer metastatic to the liver. *Eur J Surg Oncol*. 1994;20:454–460.
107. Jenkins LT, Millikan KW, Bines SD, et al. Hepatic resection for metastatic colorectal cancer. *Am Surg*. 1997;63:605–610.
108. Ohlsson B, Stenram U, Tranberg KG. Resection of colorectal liver metastases: 25-year experience. *World J Surg*. 1998;22:268–277.
109. Cady B, Jenkins RL, Steele GD, et al. Surgical margin in hepatic resection for colorectal metastases: a critical and improvable determinant of outcome. *Ann Surg*. 1998;227:566–571.
110. Bakalakos EA, Kim JA, Young DC, et al. Determinants of survival following hepatic resection for metastatic colorectal cancer. *World J Surg*. 1998;22:399–405.
111. Kokudo N, Seki M, Ohta H, et al. Effects of systemic and regional chemotherapy after hepatic resection for colorectal metastases. *Ann Surg Oncol*. 1998;5:706–712.
112. Harms J, Obst T, Thorban S, et al. The role of surgery in the treatment of liver metastases for colorectal cancer patients. *Hepatogastroenterology*. 1999;46:2321–2328.
113. Ambiru S, Miyazaki M, Isono T, et al. Hepatic resection for colorectal metastases: analysis of prognostic factors. *Dis Colon Rectum*. 1999;42:632–639.
114. Harmon KE, Ryan JA, Biehl TR, et al. Benefits and safety of hepatic resection for colorectal metastases. *Am J Surg*. 1999;177:402–404.
115. Bradley AL, Chapman WC, Wright JK, et al. Surgical experience with hepatic colorectal metastasis. *Am Surg*. 1999;65:560–566.
116. Seifert JK, Bottger TC, Weigel TF, et al. Prognostic factors following liver resection for hepatic metastases from colorectal cancer. *Hepatogastroenterology*. 2000;47:239–246.
117. Choti MA, Sitzmann JV, Tiburi MF, et al. Trends in long-term survival following liver resection for hepatic colorectal metastases. *Ann Surg*. 2002;235:759–766.
118. Ercolani G, Grazi GL, Ravaioli M, et al. Liver resection for multiple colorectal metastases: influence of parenchymal involvement and total tumor volume, vs number or location, on long-term survival. *Arch Surg*. 2002;137:1187–1192.
119. Mala T, Bohler G, Mathisen O, et al. Hepatic resection for colorectal metastases: can preoperative scoring predict outcome? *World J Surg*. 2002;26:1348–1353.
120. Kato T, Yasui K, Hirai T, et al. Therapeutic results for hepatic metastases of colorectal cancer with special reference to effectiveness of hepatectomy: analysis of prognostic factors for 763 cases recorded at 18 institutions. *Dis Colon Rectum*. 2003;46:S22-S31.
121. Altendorf-Hofmann A, Scheele J. A critical review of the major indicators of prognosis after resection of hepatic metastases form colorectal carcinoma. *Surg Oncol Clin N Am*. 2003;12:165–192.
122. Scheele J, Stang R, Altendorf-Hofmann A, et al. Resection of colorectal liver metastases. *World J Surg*. 1995;19:59–71.

123. Laurent C, Cunha AS, Couderc P, et al. Influence of postoperative morbidity on long-term survival following liver resection for colorectal metastases. *Br J Surg*. 2003;90:1131–1136.
124. Nagashima I, Takada T, Matsuda K, et al. A new scoring system to classify patients with colorectal liver metastases: proposal of criteria to select candidates for hepatic resection. *J Hepatobiliary Pancreat Surg*. 2004;11:79–83.
125. Nicoli N, Casaril A, Mangiante G, et al. Surgical treatment for liver metastases from colorectal carcinoma: results of 228 patients. *Hepatogastroenterology*. 2004;51:1810–1814.
126. Schindl M, Wigmore SJ, Currie EJ, et al. Prognostic scoring in colorectal cancer liver metastasis: development and validation. *Arch Surg*. 2005;140:183–189.
127. Wei AC, Greig PD, Grant D, et al. Survival after hepatic resection for colorectal metastases: a 10-year experience. *Ann Surg Oncol*. 2006;13:668–676.
128. Tanaka K, Shimada H, Ueda M, et al. Long-term characteristics of 5-year survivors after liver resection for colorectal metastases. *Ann Surg Oncol*. 2007;14:1336–1346.
129. Tsai MS, Su YH, Ho MC, et al. Clinicopathological features and prognosis in resectable synchronous and metachronous colorectal liver metastasis. *Ann Surg Oncol*. 2007;14:786–794.
130. Figueras J, Torras J, Valls C, et al. Surgical resection of colorectal liver metastases in patients with expanded indications: a single-center experience with 501 patients. *Dis Colon Rectum*. 2007;50: 478–488.
131. Jonas S, Thelen A, Benckert C, et al. Extended resections of liver metastases from colorectal cancer. *World J Surg*. 2007;31:511–521.
132. Minagawa M, Yamamoto J, Kosuge T, et al. Simplified staging system for predicting the prognosis of patients with resectable liver metastasis: development and validation. *Arch Surg*. 2007;142:269–276.
133. Minagawa M, Makuuchi M, Torzilli G, et al. Extension of the frontiers of surgical indications in the treatment of liver metastases from colorectal cancer: long-term results. *Ann Surg*. 2000;231: 487–499.
134. Niu R, Yan TD, Zhu JC, et al. Recurrence and survival after hepatic resection with or without cryotherapy for liver metastases from colorectal carcinoma. *Ann Surg Oncol*. 2007;14:2078–2087.
135. Parks R, Gonen M, Kemeny N, et al. Adjuvant chemotherapy improves survival after resection of hepatic colorectal metastases: analysis of data from two continents. *J Am Coll Surg*. 2007;204:753–763.
136. Shah SA, Bromberg R, Coates A, et al. Survival after liver resection for metastatic colorectal carcinoma in a large population. *J Am Coll Surg*. 2007;205:676–683.
137. Rees M, Tekkis PP, Welsh FKS, et al. Evaluation of long-term survival after hepatic resection for metastatic colorectal cancer. *Ann Surg*. 2008;247:125–135.
138. Reddy SK, Broadwater G, Niedzwiecki D, et al. Multiagent chemotherapy for isolated colorectal liver metastases: a single-institution analysis. *J Gastrointest Surg*. 2009;13:74–84.
139. Nordlinger B, Sorbye H, Glemelius B, et al. Perioperative chemotherapy with FOLFOX4 and surgery versus surgery alone for respectable liver metastases from colorectal cancer (EORTC Intergroup trial 40983): a randomized controlled trial. *Lancet*. 2008;371:1007–1016.
140. Welsh FKS, Tilney HS, Tekkis PP, et al. Safe liver resection following chemotherapy for colorectal liver metastases is a matter of timing. *Br J Cancer*. 2007;96:1037–1042.
141. Sahajpal A, Vollmer CM, Dixon E, et al. Chemotherapy for colorectal cancer prior to liver resection for colorectal cancer hepatic metastases does not adversely affect peri-operative outcomes. *J Surg Oncol*. 2007;95:22–27.

9 Surgical Pathology

Nicholas P. West and Philip Quirke

INTRODUCTION

Pathologists play a critical role in the multidisciplinary management of rectal cancer by providing valuable information to the surgeon, radiologist, medical and radiation oncologists. They have contributed considerably to the improvement in rectal cancer outcomes by the identification of the importance and frequency of circumferential resection margin (CRM) involvement, the importance of planes of surgery and the identification of the major issues involved in abdominoperineal excision (APE) for low rectal cancer. This has led to fundamental changes in surgical, oncological and radiological practice over the last 20 years. Pathologists continue to lead the way in the identification of novel predictive markers, which could allow targeted therapy directed at the biology of an individual tumour. Pathologists also continue to make advances in the use of digital and three-dimensional pathology, which will reform the way rectal cancer specimens are handled in the modern digital age.

THE ROLE OF THE PATHOLOGIST IN THE MODERN MULTIDISCIPLINARY TEAM

Traditionally, the role of the pathologist in the management of rectal cancer was to confirm the diagnosis of invasive malignancy to the surgeon and indicate the stage of disease to determine an accurate prognosis. Over recent years, the modern treatment of rectal cancer has changed, focusing on a multidisciplinary team approach where the pathologist has a much wider role and closely interacts with all members of the team.

From: *Current Clinical Oncology: Rectal Cancer*,
Edited by: B.G. Czito and C.G. Willett, DOI: 10.1007/978-1-60761-567-5_9,

Interaction with Surgeons

There is now a wide body of evidence from both randomised clinical trials and large observational studies showing that CRM involvement is associated with an increased risk of local disease recurrence and poorer survival *(1–7)*. It is now customary for the pathologist to indicate to the surgeon whether the CRM of the resection specimen is involved by tumour, as this may influence the selection of adjuvant therapy. The frequency of CRM involvement is obviously dependent on the stage of disease but is also significantly influenced by the quality of surgery; hence, it is also important to report the plane of mesorectal dissection followed by the surgeon. Classifying the plane of dissection in this manner has been shown to predict local disease recurrence and survival *(8,9)* and can therefore be relayed to the surgical team as a marker of surgical quality.

Interaction with Medical and Radiation Oncologists

An increasing number of rectal cancer patients now receive pre-operative (neoadjuvant) radiotherapy, which may be given in combination with various chemotherapeutic agents. It is important that the oncologist is made aware of the degree of response to such therapy, which can be indicated by a qualitative tumour regression grade. Studies have shown that cases with either a complete or marked response to neoadjuvant therapy have an improved prognosis *(10)*.

Following primary surgery, further adjuvant therapy may be indicated if the pathologist identifies CRM involvement *(11,12)* or lymph node metastases *(13–16)* to reduce the likelihood of local disease recurrence. There is also increasing evidence that stage II (lymph node negative), CRM negative patients with other high risk factors, e.g. extra-mural vascular invasion (EMVI), perforation, peritoneal involvement and extensive extra-mural spread, have a poorer outcome *(17)* and may benefit from additional therapy *(16)*.

While the role of the pathologist in the identification of poor prognostic factors is reasonably well established, recent research has revealed a potential role in the identification of novel predictive markers of response to therapy. So far, the only accepted marker is in patients with activating k-ras mutations who do not benefit from anti-epidermal growth factor receptor agents such as panitumumab and cetuximab *(18)*. Other possible predictive markers, which require further evaluation, include b-raf mutations, *(19)* PI3K mutations, PTEN loss of expression, EGF-r polysomy and amplification of EGF-r detected by FISH.

Interaction with Radiologists

In many centres, rectal cancer patients routinely undergo magnetic resonance imaging (MRI) of the pelvis prior to surgery to accurately stage the tumour and ensure complete resection is possible. Other important prognostic factors that can be determined from the MRI include likelihood of CRM positivity, *(20,21)* depth of extra-mural spread, *(22,23)* lymph node involvement, *(24,25)* EMVI *(24,26)* and peritoneal involvement *(24)*. From the resection specimen, the pathologist can then provide feedback on the accuracy of such image interpretation and on the prediction of the completeness of excision. The ability of the radiologist to predict outcome has been confirmed by Martling et al who demonstrated that radiologically determined CRM positive tumours have a similar poor outcome to that seen on histology *(27)*.

Other Roles of the Pathologist

In addition to the management of individual patients, the pathologist has the duty of ensuring that pathological reports are adequately archived and that full and accurate data are submitted to the relevant cancer registry and screening programme, if one exists. This facilitates accurate audit of all colorectal services including pathology, radiology, oncology and surgery and enables high quality research to be undertaken on a large number of cases.

HISTOPATHOLOGICAL REPORTING OF RECTAL CANCER

It is essential that the final report issued by the pathologist for rectal cancer resection specimens should be carefully written and accurate. A failure to report key pathological features can result in understaging the disease. This could result in inappropriate selection of adjuvant therapy for a given patient and therefore poorer outcomes. The use of proforma reporting is highly recommended and has been shown to significantly improve both the standard and completeness of pathological reporting *(28–31)*. A template for proforma reporting is provided in the recent United Kingdom Royal College of Pathologists (RCPath) dataset for colorectal cancer for both resection specimens (http://www.rcpath.org/resources/worddocs/G049ColorectalDatasetAppendixC-Sep07.doc) and local excisions (http://www.rcpath.org/resources/worddocs/G049ColorectalDatasetAppendixD-Sep07.doc) along with the evidence for the inclusion of specific data *(32)*. This dataset has been approved by all relevant professional bodies within the UK, i.e. the Association of Coloproctology of Great Britain and Ireland, the National Cancer Research Institute Colorectal Cancer Subcommittee and the Pathology Section of the British Society of Gastroenterology and has been validated in routine clinical practice *(33)*. Equivalent guidelines for cancers detected in a bowel cancer screening programme are also available (http://www.cancerscreening.nhs.uk/bowel/publications/nhsbcsp01.pdf) and European guidelines are currently under development.

Macroscopic Dissection of the Rectal Cancer Resection Specimen

Rectal cancer resection specimens should be carefully dissected to a uniform standard to ensure all relevant prognostic information is identified both at the time of dissection and subsequent histological reporting. A protocol was developed at the University of Leeds in the 1980s, *(34)* which has now been widely adopted around the world including into the RCPath dataset *(32,35)*.

Ideally, the specimen should be promptly received from the operating theatre in a fresh and un-opened state. If there is likely to be a delay in specimen handling, it should be placed either in the refrigerator overnight or straight into formalin fixative for longer periods. Surgeons should be strongly discouraged from opening specimens prior to pathological evaluation unless absolutely essential, as this may impair the proper assessment of CRM involvement. It is particularly important to protect the anterior aspect of the specimen as the anterior CRM is the most frequently involved margin by tumour due to the thinness of the anterior mesorectum and, additionally, peritoneal involvement frequently occurs in the anterior paracolic gutters.

Once received by the pathologist, the specimen should be carefully inspected and palpated to identify the location of the tumour. The anterior peritonealised surface can then be opened longitudinally proximal to the tumour segment, leaving 1–2 cm of normal bowel intact above the tumour (Fig. 1). If fresh tissue is required for research purposes/tissue bank

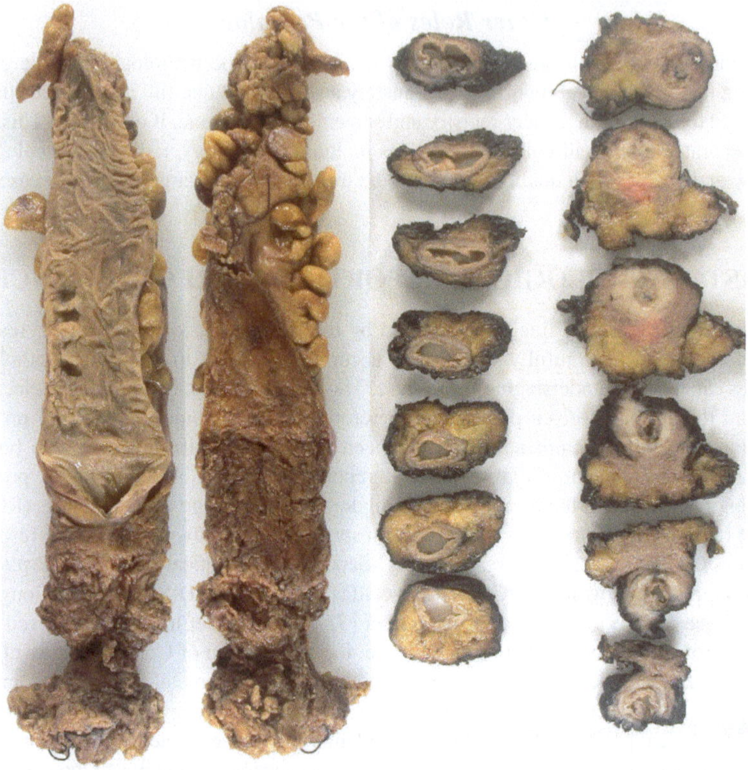

Fig. 1. Digital photographs of the front, back and cross-sectional slices of a post-fixation abdominoperineal excision specimen. Note the specimen has been opened anteriorly to the level of the peritoneal reflection to aid fixation.

archiving, it can easily be taken at this time under direct observation using a scalpel, provided that the tumour is of sufficient size to allow subsequent staging. Opening the specimen in this way facilitates formalin penetration and therefore adequate tumour fixation. Alternatively, the lumen of the specimen can be inflated with formalin to prevent specimen disruption. It is essential that the tumour segment is not opened at any stage to preserve the CRM/serosa and to facilitate serial cross-sectional slicing. We also advocate not opening the non-peritonealised surface of the specimen distal to the tumour to ensure that the CRM remains intact. If fixation of the distal portion is a concern, tissue paper can be passed through the tumour segment (if traversable) to aid formalin diffusion. The specimen can then be loosely pinned to a cork board and immersed in a large volume of formalin fixative for a minimum of 48 h.

Following adequate fixation, the specimen should be carefully inspected prior to any further dissection. It is useful to take digital photographs at this stage to document the front and rear aspects of the specimen (Fig. 1). All photographs of the macroscopic specimen should be stored in a digital archive and used in multidisciplinary team meetings to provide evidence of the quality of surgery, feedback to individual clinicians and trainees and can be utilised in research projects. Important features to identify on the intact specimen are the presence of extra-rectal tissues, e.g. posterior vaginal wall and prostate gland, perforation of the specimen and the quality of the surgery.

The quality of surgery is assessed by determining the plane of mesorectal dissection and has now been incorporated into the most recent edition of the RCPath dataset *(32)*. Good quality surgery is judged to be in the *mesorectal plane* when the surgeon dissects immediately outside the layer of mesorectal fascia surrounding the mesorectum. This results in a bulky, smooth fascial-lined specimen with only very minor surface irregularities. Intermediate quality surgery is termed the *intra-mesorectal plane* when the surgeon enters the mesorectum in areas resulting in large defects that do not extend to the underlying muscularis propria. Poor quality surgery is known as the *muscularis propria plane* when the mesorectal defects are so extensive that they expose areas of muscularis propria. This results in the CRM being formed by the smooth muscle layer of the bowel with no mesorectal fat to protect the margin from extramural tumour extension. Occasionally such defects can actually enter the muscle layer, submucosa or even the lumen of the specimen resulting in an intra-operative perforation. There is now a growing body of evidence from randomised clinical trials to show that such a grading system cannot only predict CRM involvement but also local disease recurrence and patient survival *(8,9)*. The Medical Research Council CR07 trial has shown that the quality of surgery can be improved through feedback to surgeons leading to a significant reduction in CRM involvement *(9)*. Early evidence suggests that a similar quality grading system may also be important in predicting survival for higher tumours within the colon *(36)*.

Communications between the rectal lumen and the outside of the specimen should be documented and can be caused by either tumour perforation or surgical intra-operative disruption. Tumour perforation into the peritoneal cavity is associated with increased local disease recurrence and poorer survival *(37,38)*. Tumour perforation is defined as a visible defect into the lumen of the specimen at the level of the tumour and above the peritoneal reflection. Such cases should always be classified in the TNM staging system as pT4. Intra-operative defects into the lumen of the specimen made by the surgeon at the time of specimen removal and which are located below the peritoneal reflection should be classified as muscularis propria plane surgery. Although TNM staging does not accept that perforations can occur below the peritoneal reflection, we believe that if such defects lie at the level of the tumour they should also staged as pT4, as a similar poor prognosis can be expected in these patients.

Once the plane of surgery has been determined and any perforations described, the mesorectum should be inked over the entire CRM to allow accurate histological measurement of the distance from the tumour to this margin. Alternatively, painting the surgical margin can be performed at the time of specimen receipt and can facilitate later dissection as it ensures that the ink firmly adheres to the specimen. It is important that the inking process does not cover the peritoneal surface as this complicates the histological assessment and may lead to inaccurate staging. Tumour that has broken through the peritoneal surface is given a higher disease stage than tumour at the CRM. It is important to remember that involvement of the peritoneal surface is not CRM positivity as this is not a surgically created margin.

The specimen should then be serially sliced from the distal margin at 3–4 mm intervals to a level just above the tumour. A long, sharp and clean knife is essential to ensure that complete slices of the recommended thickness are produced. Regular replacement of the knife is a small price to pay in the overall treatment of this disease and difficult laboratory staff and managers should be reminded of this fact. The cross-sectional slices should be laid out in order and further digital photographs taken to ensure that the macroscopic appearance of the tumour and its relationship to the CRM is recorded (Fig. 1). Important features to document at this stage of the dissection are the position of the tumour (anterior, lateral,

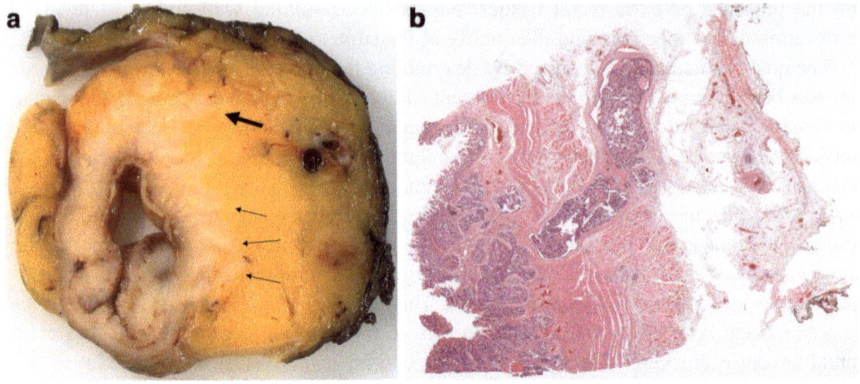

Fig. 2. (**a**) Areas suspicious for extra-mural vascular invasion on a macroscopic slice (*arrows*), which appear as serpiginous extensions of tumour arising from the muscularis propria. (**b**) Histological confirmation of extra-mural vascular tumour extension within a large vein.

circumferential, etc.), maximum tumour dimension, the relationship to the anterior peritoneal reflection (above, straddling or below) and in the case of APEs, the distance from the dentate line and distal margin.

As a minimum, it is recommended that five blocks of the tumour are taken, in particular focussing on areas, which will assess the nearest CRM and peritoneal surface. Areas suspicious for EMVI should also be adequately sampled (Fig. 2). These can be recognised as serpiginous extensions of tumour arising from the muscularis propria. It is not necessary to submit the longitudinal resection margin (or doughnuts) if the tumour is more than 30 mm away although this can be sampled as a representative block of background bowel if desired. It may be necessary to subsequently submit these margins if the tumour is shown histologically to be very infiltrative, a pure signet ring form, undifferentiated or to have extensive vascular invasion.

It is important that all lymph nodes identified within the specimen are submitted for histological examination, not just the minimum recommended number of 12. A failure to identify lymph node metastases by incomplete sampling may prevent patients from receiving appropriate adjuvant therapy and may negatively impact long-term survival *(39)*. The mean number of lymph nodes retrieved by pathologists has substantially improved in the UK from around six per specimen in the 1990s to around 15–18 in the best centres today *(39)*. The node nearest to the vascular tie (high-tie or apical node) should be blocked separately as involvement of this node confers a higher Dukes stage and is associated with poorer survival *(40)*. If any node appears close to the CRM, the inked margin should be included with the sample in the correct orientation to enable accurate measurement and determine whether this margin is involved.

The remaining specimen should be retained in the pathology department until after the final pathology report has been released and the case discussed at the multidisciplinary team meeting in case the pathologist needs to revisit the specimen. Common reasons for revisiting after initial histological assessment include failure to find tumour following neoadjuvant therapy (see later section) and to supplement the lymph node yield.

Histological Reporting of the Rectal Cancer Resection Specimen

All items on the RCPath minimum dataset *(32)* should be searched for and accurately reported. In addition to traditional grading and staging the tumour, factors such as CRM involvement, EMVI and peritoneal involvement are all very important and may dictate further adjuvant treatment.

Within the UK, pathologists are advised to use the fifth version of TNM for staging purposes rather than the more recent sixth edition. It is possible that the fourth version of TNM is the optimum system but due to ongoing clinical trials it was decided to use TNM5 until the TNM committee revised key changes such as the definitions of lymph nodes and vascular invasion. TNM5 *(41)* created the "3 mm rule" where all tumour deposits equal to or greater than 3 mm in dimension were counted as involved lymph nodes and all deposits smaller than this were considered to represent discontinuous tumour extensions. While this was not an evidence-based decision, TNM6 *(42)* created a further change whereby all "smooth" nodules in the perirectal fat were counted as involved lymph nodes, and all irregular nodules were counted as vascular invasion. On review, it was felt that TNM6 was too subjective, and it was the decision of the RCPath minimum dataset to stay with TNM5 *(39,43)*.

It is now well recognised that involvement of the non-peritonealised resection margin or CRM is associated with a worse patient outcome. It is generally accepted from clinical trial evidence that CRM involvement is defined as tumour cells within 1 mm of the inked surface although the Dutch TME study has suggested a cut off of 2 mm *(4)*. This suggestion was based on a small number of cases, and adequate data do not currently exist to support this position. CRM involvement can either be through direct spread, discontinuous spread, intravenous extension, perineural infiltration or lymphatic involvement with all showing a similar poor prognosis *(44)*. Tumour within a lymph node situated less than 1 mm from the CRM is currently also recommended as a positive margin, but further evidence is needed to support this position.

The prognostic significance of EMVI is well established *(45)*. It is expected that a meticulous pathologist would find EMVI in over 30% of the cases they report *(17)* although in routine practice this figure is highly variable. Its significance is especially important at institutions that may consider further adjuvant therapy for such patients, so a lack of identification could impact on patient survival. EMVI is defined in the RCPath dataset as "tumour within extra-mural endothelium-lined spaces that are either surrounded by a rim of muscle or contain red blood cells" *(32)*. The pathologist may strongly suspect EMVI if non-continuous tumour is seen adjacent to an artery with no accompanying vein and can be confirmed with further levels and/or elastin tissue stains if necessary. We do not accept the TNM6 definition, which states that "irregular tumour nodules situated in the mesorectum are counted as vascular invasion."

Peritoneal involvement is defined as tumour cells breaching the serosal layer of the bowel to lie either on its surface or within the peritoneal cavity and can lead to subsequent intra-peritoneal cavity disease *(46)*. It is important that CRM positivity is distinguished from peritoneal involvement as this would not denote a pT4 stage (unless adjacent structures are involved) and would be a risk factor for local rather than intra-peritoneal recurrence.

REPORTING RECTAL CANCER RESECTIONS FOLLOWING NEOADJUVANT THERAPY

Increasing numbers of rectal cancer patients now receive pre-operative (neoadjuvant) radiotherapy either alone or in combination with chemotherapy. This is associated with a variable degree of tumour regression, which ranges from no response through to a complete pathological response where no viable tumour cells remain. Patients with CRM negative

Table 1
The different tumour regression grading (TRG) systems commonly used in clinical practice. Note the similarity of the Mandard *(47)* and Bouzourene *(49)* methods and how the numbering system contrasts with that used in the Dworak *(48)* and Rodel *(10)* systems

TRG	*Mandard/Bouzourene*	*TRG*	*Dworak/(Rodel)*
1	No residual tumour	0	No regression
2	Rare residual tumour cells	1	Dominant tumour mass with obvious fibrosis (<25% of tumour mass)
3	Fibrosis outgrowing residual tumour	2	Dominantly fibrotic changes with few tumour cells (25–50% of tumour mass)
4	Residual cancer outgrowing fibrosis	3	Very few tumour cells in fibrotic tissue (>50% of tumour mass)
5	Absence of regressive changes	4	No tumour cells, only fibrotic mass

tumours, which have undergone either complete or marked regression, have been shown to do better than those that have not markedly regressed *(10)*. This requires confirmation from further studies but unfortunately to date there has been a lack of standardisation in the reporting of the degree of tumour regression, especially in large clinical trials.

A 5-point grading system for tumour regression was initially developed by Mandard for oesophageal cancer, *(47)* and modified systems have been used for rectal cancer patients including studies by Dworak, *(48)* Bouzourene *(49)* and Rodel *(10)*. Unfortunately, these systems do not run in parallel and can cause confusion for both pathologists and clinicians if a numeric grade is given (Table 1). The grade determined is subjective and therefore open to considerable inter-observer variation *(50,51)*. In addition to the above problems, there is little evidence to show that lesser degrees of tumour regression benefit the patient; therefore, in routine practice, we advocate the use of a simple three point descriptive scale to avoid confusion. This should grade tumours into those showing a *complete pathological response* (see below for definition), *minimal residual tumour* or *no marked response*. However, in clinical trials, the full 5-point system should be used.

The rate of complete pathological response often varies considerably between different studies due to the lack of a robust standard definition. In tumours that exhibit a complete or near-complete response, it may be difficult to macroscopically detect any residual tumour. Obviously, the number of blocks taken and the number of levels cut on each block will influence the complete pathological response rate. We prefer to use the method of the capecitabine, oxaliplatin, radiotherapy and excision (CORE) study, *(52,53)* which recommends that at least five blocks should be taken from the area of prior tumour involvement. If after histological examination no tumour is detected then the entire area of suspicion should be submitted for histological examination. If again no tumour can be detected, three deeper levels should be cut on each block. If this still fails to identify residual tumour, only then can it be recorded as a complete pathological response.

REPORTING LOW RECTAL CANCER RESECTION SPECIMENS

Low rectal cancer (within 6 cm of the anal verge) may be treated by an APE if it is not possible to achieve coloanal anastomosis, if the tumour is advanced or if poor defaecatory function is expected. It is generally accepted that around 20% of rectal cancers will require an APE. Overall rates of APE have significantly fallen in the UK from 29% in 1996 to 21% in 2004 *(54)* but remain highly variable between United Kingdom National Health Service Trusts, ranging from 8.5 to 52.6% *(55)*. This wide variation in the frequency of APE is considered to be unacceptable, and it is thought that the APE rate can be used as an indirect measure of surgical quality.

In APE surgery, the anal canal and a variable amount of perianal skin are removed in continuity with the rectum resulting in a permanent colostomy for the patient. This operation is well recognised to carry a worse clinical outcome with higher local recurrence and poorer survival when compared to cancers of the middle and upper rectum treated by anterior resection *(38,56,57)*. This is believed to be due to the high rates of CRM involvement and intra-operative perforation with standard APE surgery. These in turn are caused by the combination of a reduction in tissue volume in the lower mesorectum and the technical difficulties associated with operating deep in the pelvis via an abdominal approach *(58)*. Recently, surgeons in Sweden and Poland have presented improved results with more radical APE operations termed "extended abdominoperineal resection" *(59)* and "abdominosacral resection" *(60)*. Both of these procedures closely resemble the original Miles operation described in 1908, *(61)* which involves removal of the levator ani muscles in continuity with the mesorectum via a perineal approach. This has the advantage of producing a more cylindrical APE specimen, providing more tissue to protect the CRM compared to a standard specimen, which often displays a classic surgical "waist" (Fig. 3)*(62)*. Also, if the prone jack-knife position is

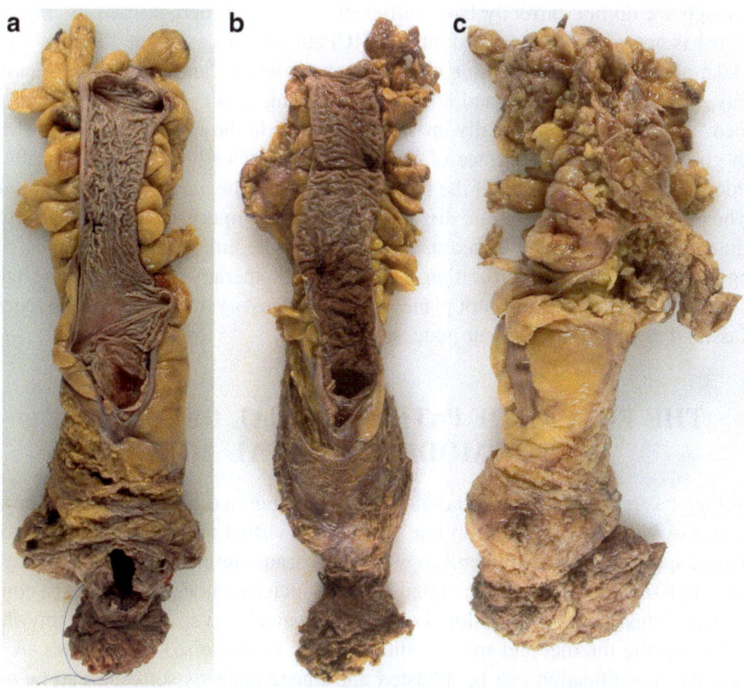

Fig. 3. The three proposed grades for assessing the quality of abdominoperineal excision surgery. (**a**) *Intra-muscular/sub-mucosal plane*: standard excision with a large anterior intra-operative perforation. (**b**) *Sphincteric plane*: standard excision showing the classic "waist" in the distal rectum as the plane of resection follows the mesorectum right down onto the sphincter muscles. (**c**) *Extra-levator plane*: cylindrical excision showing attached levator muscles and tip of the coccyx resulting in loss of the distal "waist".

Table 2
The high rate of CRM positivity and intra-operative perforations seen in standard abdominoperineal excision (APE) compared to the extra-levator cylindrical method, which is similar to that obtained with anterior resection. The figures quoted are from recent studies by West et al *(58)* and Nagtegaal et al *(38)*

	Standard APE		*Cylindrical APE*		*Anterior resection*	
	CRM positive (%)	*Perforated (%)*	*CRM positive (%)*	*Perforated (%)*	*CRM positive (%)*	*Perforated (%)*
West et al *(58)*	40.6	22.8	14.8	3.7	–	–
Nagtegaal et al *(38)*	30.4	13.7	–	–	10.7	2.5

used for the perineal phase, the surgeon can actually visualise the dissection, thus further reducing the incidence of intra-operative perforations (Table 2).

APE specimens can be graded in a similar manner to the mesorectal dissection (Fig. 3), *(38)* although we do not currently have sufficient evidence to demonstrate its importance; hence, this has not yet been integrated into the RCPath minimum dataset. "Radical" surgery should take place in the *extra-levator plane* where the levator ani muscles are removed in continuity with the mesorectum and anal canal resulting in a cylindrical specimen. Well-performed "standard" surgery usually involves dissection in the *sphincteric plane* where the excision goes down onto the surface of the sphincter muscles but does not actually enter them. Poor quality surgery occurs if the surgeon operates in the *intra-muscular/sub-mucosal plane* when the sphincter muscles are disrupted. With such surgery, the CRM may be formed by the internal sphincter or sub-mucosa, or even worse the lumen may actually be entered resulting in an intra-operative perforation. The Dutch radiotherapy and total mesorectal excision trial had no cases of extra-levator plane surgery, and just over one-third of the specimens were classified as intra-muscular/sub-mucosal *(38)*.

THE FUTURE OF PATHOLOGICAL REPORTING IN THE MODERN DIGITAL AGE

Pathology has recently followed radiology into the modern digital age, and we now have the facilities to view tissue slides "on line" and create virtual three-dimensional models of macroscopic specimens. Virtual microscopy involves scanning glass slides containing tissue sections at high resolution to create a digital image, which can then be viewed on a computer monitor. The virtual slides can be stored on a departmental server and viewed anywhere in the world using the Internet and specific slide viewing software *(63)*. The slides are easily navigated, the magnification can be adjusted and image analysis software can be used to quantify specific measures. At present these techniques are rarely seen outside of a research environment but can be used to automate the scoring of tissue microarrays, *(64)* facilitate clinical trials and enable widespread slide distribution of slides in external quality assessment schemes. While early studies showed virtual microscopy to be slower than conventional light microscopy for routine diagnosis, *(65)* later studies have shown that when using a powerwall interface, virtual slides can be just as efficient *(66)*. In Leeds, we currently have

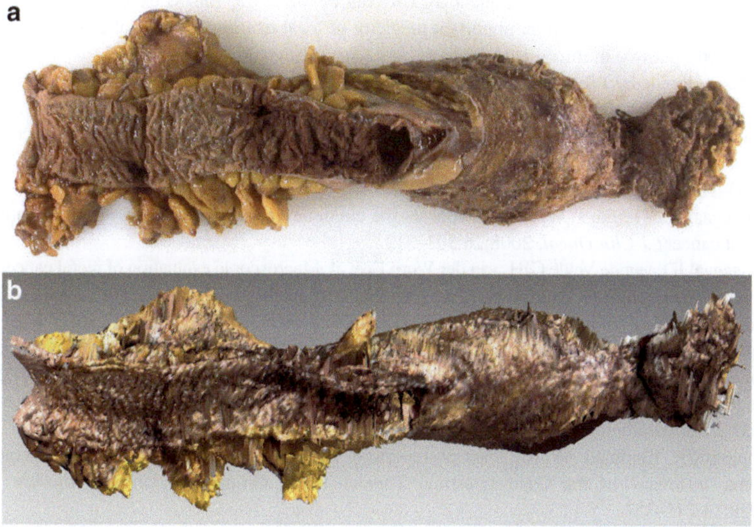

Fig. 4. A potential use for three-dimensional scanning photography in rectal cancer histopathology. (**a**) Two-dimensional digital photograph of an abdominoperineal excision specimen taken at the time of specimen dissection. (**b**) Three-dimensional virtual recreation of the same specimen, which can be manipulated to create virtual cross sectional slices and serves as a permanent specimen record.

over 3,000 cases scanned covering all areas of histopathology, which are all freely available to view via our website (http://www.virtualpathology.leeds.ac.uk).

Three-dimensional scanning photography can be used to create a virtual model of the macroscopic specimen prior to dissection, which can then be re-visited long after the original specimen has been destroyed (Fig. 4). In Leeds, we have photographed a series of rectal cancer resection specimens by scanning prior to serial slicing using the Minolta VI-910 non-contact digitiser. From these scans, three-dimensional colour digital images can be produced and analysed using specific computer software. Such virtual specimens can be serially sliced and the amount of mesorectum removed at various levels quantitated *(67)*. This may well have an important role in the future audit of rectal cancer surgery where we can look at the volume of mesorectum present on the pre-operative MRI scan and compare it to what was actually excised by the surgeon from the scanned virtual specimen.

REFERENCES

1. Quirke P, Durdey P, Dixon MF, Williams NS. Local recurrence of rectal adenocarcinoma due to inadequate surgical resection: histopathological study of lateral tumour spread and surgical excision. *Lancet*. 1986;2:996–999.
2. Adam IJ, Mohamdee MO, Martin IG, et al. Role of circumferential margin involvement in the local recurrence of rectal cancer. *Lancet*. 1994;344:707–711.
3. Ng IOL, Luk ISC, Yuen ST. Surgical lateral clearance in resected rectal carcinomas. A multivariate analysis of clinicopathological features. *Cancer*. 1993;71:1972–1976.

4. Nagtegaal ID, Marijnen CA, Kranenbarg EK, van de Velde CJ, van Krieken JH. Circumferential margin involvement is still an important predictor of local recurrence in rectal carcinoma: not one millimeter but two millimeters is the limit. *Am J Surg Pathol*. 2002;26:350–357.
5. Wibe A, Rendedal PR, Svensson E, et al. Prognostic significance of the circumferential resection margin following total mesorectal excision for rectal cancer. *Br J Surg*. 2002;89:327–334.
6. Martling A, Singnomklao T, Holm T, Rutqvist LE, Cedermark B. Prognostic significance of both surgical and pathological assessment of curative resection for rectal cancer. *Br J Surg*. 2004;91: 1040–1045.
7. Nagtegaal ID, Quirke P. What is the role for the circumferential margin in the modern treatment of rectal cancer? *J Clin Oncol*. 2008;26:303–312.
8. Nagtegaal ID, van de Velde CJH, van der Worp E, et al. Macroscopic evaluation of rectal cancer resection specimen: clinical significance of the pathologist in quality. *J Clin Oncol*. 2002;20:1729–1734.
9. Quirke P, Sebag-Montefiore D, Steele R, et al. Local recurrence after rectal cancer resection is strongly related to the plane of surgical dissection and is further reduced by preoperative short course radiotherapy. Preliminary results of the MRC CR07 trial. *J Clin Oncol*. 2006;24s:A3512.
10. Rodel C, Martus P, Papadoupolos T, et al. Prognostic significance of tumour regression after preoperative chemoradiotherapy for rectal cancer. *J Clin Oncol*. 2005;23:8688–8696.
11. Thomas PR, Lindblad AS. Adjuvant postoperative radiotherapy and chemotherapy in rectal carcinoma: a review of the Gastrointestinal Tumour Study Group experience. *Radiother Oncol*. 1988;13:245–252.
12. Medical Research Council Rectal Cancer Working Party. Randomised trial of surgery alone versus surgery followed by radiotherapy for mobile cancer of the rectum. *Lancet*. 1996;348:1610–1614.
13. Moertel CG, Fleming TR, MacDonald JS, et al. Fluorouracil plus levamisole as effective adjuvant therapy after resection of stage III colon carcinoma: a final report. *Ann Intern Med*. 1995;122:321–326.
14. Andre T, Boni C, Mounedji-Boudiaf L, et al. Oxaliplatin, fluorouracil, and leucovorin as adjuvant treatment for colon cancer. *N Engl J Med*. 2004;350:2343–2351.
15. Twelves C, Wong A, Nowacki MP, et al. Capecitabine as adjuvant treatment for stage III colon cancer. *N Engl J Med*. 2005;352:2696–2704.
16. QUASAR Collaborative Group. Adjuvant chemotherapy versus observation in patients with colorectal cancer: a randomised study. *Lancet*. 2007;370:2020–2029.
17. Quirke P, Morris E. Reporting colorectal cancer. *Histopathology*. 2007;50:103–112.
18. Amado RG, Wolf M, Peeters M, et al. Wild-type KRAS is required for panitumumab efficacy in patients with metastatic colorectal cancer. *J Clin Oncol*. 2008;26:1626–1634.
19. Di Nicolantonio F, Martini M, Molinari F, et al. Wild-type *BRAF* is required for response to panitumumab or cetuximab in metastatic colorectal cancer. *J Clin Oncol*. 2008;26(35):5705–5712; published online Nov 10th.
20. Group MS. Diagnostic accuracy of preoperative magnetic resonance imaging in predicting curative resection of rectal cancer: prospective observational study. *Br Med J*. 2006;333:779–784.
21. Purkayastha S, Tekkis PP, Athanasiou T, Tilney HS, Darzi AW, Heriot AG. Diagnostic precision of magnetic resonance imaging for preoperative prediction of the circumferential margin involvement in patients with rectal cancer. *Colorectal Dis*. 2006;9:402–411.
22. Brown G, Richards CJ, Newcombe RG, et al. Rectal carcinoma: thin-section MR imaging for staging in 28 patients. *Radiology*. 1999;211:215–222.
23. Mercury Study Group. Extramural depth of tumor invasion at thin-section MR in patients with rectal cancer: results of the MERCURY study. *Radiology*. 2007;243:132–139.
24. Brown G, Richards CJ, Bourne MW, et al. Morphologic predictors of lymph node status in rectal cancer with use of high-spatial-resolution MR imaging with histopathologic comparison. *Radiology*. 2003;227:371–377.
25. Brown G, Radcliffe AG, Newcombe RG, Dallimore NS, Bourne MW, Williams GT. Preoperative assessment of prognostic factors in rectal cancer using high-resolution magnetic resonance imaging. *Br J Surg*. 2003;90:355–364.
26. Smith NJ, Barbachano Y, Norman AR, Swift RI, Abulafi AM, Brown G. Prognostic significance of magnetic resonance imaging-detected extramural vascular invasion in rectal cancer. *Br J Surg*. 2008;95:229–236.

27. Martling A, Holm T, Bremmer S, Lindholm J, Cedermark B, Blomqvist L. Prognostic value of preoperative magnetic resonance imaging of the pelvis in rectal cancer. *Br J Surg*. 2003;90:1422–1428.
28. Cross SS, Feeley KM, Angel CA. The effect of four interventions on the informational content of histopathology reports of resected colorectal carcinomas. *J Clin Pathol*. 1998;51:481–482.
29. Rigby K, Brown SR, Lakin G, Balsitis M, Hosie KB. The use of a proforma improves colorectal cancer pathology reporting. *Ann R Coll Surg Engl*. 1999;81:401–402.
30. Branston LK, Greening S, Newcombe RG, et al. The implementation of guidelines and computerised forms improves the completeness of cancer pathology reporting. The CROPS project: a randomised controlled trial in pathology. *Eur J Cancer*. 2002;38:764–772.
31. Beattie GC, McAdam TK, Elliott S, Sloan JM, Irwin ST. Improvement in quality of colorectal cancer pathology reporting with a standardized proforma – a comparative study. *Colorectal Dis*. 2003;5:558–562.
32. Williams GT, Quirke P, Shepherd N. *Standards and datasets for reporting cancers: Dataset for colorectal cancer*. 2nd ed. London: The Royal College of Pathologists; 2007.
33. Maughan NJ, Morris E, Forman D, Quirke P. The validity of the Royal College of Pathologists' colorectal cancer minimum dataset within a population. *Br J Cancer*. 2007;97:1393–1398.
34. Quirke P, Dixon MF. The prediction of local recurrence in rectal adenocarcinoma by histopathological examination. *Int J Colorectal Dis*. 1988;3:127–131.
35. Quirke P, Williams GT. *Minimum dataset for colorectal cancer histopathology reports*. London: The Royal College of Pathologists; 1998.
36. West NP, Morris EJA, Rotimi O, Cairns A, Finan PJ, Quirke P. Pathology grading of colon cancer surgical resection and its association with survival: a retrospective observational study. *Lancet Oncol*. 2008;9:857–865.
37. Eriksen MT, Wibe A, Syse A, Haffner J, Wiig JN, on behalf of the Norwegian Rectal Cancer Group and the Norwegian Gastrointestinal Cancer Group. Inadvertent perforation during rectal cancer resection in Norway. *Br J Surg*. 2004;91:210–216.
38. Nagtegaal ID, Van de Velde CJH, Marijnen CAM, van Krieken JHJM, Quirke P. Low rectal cancer: a call for a change of approach in abdominoperineal resection. *J Clin Oncol*. 2005;23:9257–9264.
39. Quirke P, Williams GT, Ectors N, Ensari A, Piard F, Nagtegaal I. The future of the TNM staging system in colorectal cancer: time for a debate? *Lancet Oncol*. 2007;8:651–657.
40. Gabriel WB, Dukes C, Bussey HJR. Lymphatic spread in cancer of the rectum. *Br J Surg*. 1935;23:395–413.
41. Sobin LH, Wittekind C. *UICC TNM classification on malignant tumours*. 5th ed. New York: Wiley Liss; 1997.
42. Sobin LH, Wittekind C. *UICC TNM classification on malignant tumours*. 6th ed. New York: Wiley Liss; 2002.
43. Howarth SM, Morgan JM, Williams GT. The new (6th edition) TNM classification of colorectal cancer – a stage too far. *Gut*. 2004;53:a21-a22.
44. Birbeck K, Macklin CP, Tiffin NJ, et al. Rates of circumferential resection margin involvement vary between surgeons and predict outcomes in rectal cancer surgery. *Ann Surg*. 2002;235:449–457.
45. Talbot IC, Ritchie S, Leighton MH, Hughes AO, Bussey HJ, Morson BC. The clinical significance of invasion of veins by rectal cancer. *Br J Surg*. 1980;67:439–442.
46. Shepherd NA, Baxter KJ, Love SB. The prognostic importance of peritoneal involvement in colonic cancer: a prospective evaluation. *Gastroenterology*. 1997;112:1096–1102.
47. Mandard AM, Dalibard F, Mandard JC, et al. Pathologic assessment of tumor regression after preoperative chemoradiotherapy of esophageal carcinoma. Clinicopathologic correlations. *Cancer*. 1994;73:2680–2686.
48. Dworak O, Keilholz L, Hoffmann A. Pathological features of rectal cancer after preoperative radiochemotherapy. *Int J Colorectal Dis*. 1997;12:19–23.
49. Bouzourene H, Bosman FT, Seelentag W, Matter M, Coucke P. Importance of tumor regression assessment in predicting the outcome in patients with locally advanced rectal carcinoma who are treated with preoperative radiotherapy. *Cancer*. 2002;94:1121–1130.
50. Wheeler JMD, Warren BF, Mortensen Mc NJ, et al. Quantification of histologic regression of rectal cancer after irradiation: a proposal for a modified staging system. *Dis Colon Rectum*. 2002;45:1051–1056.

51. Ryan R, Gibbons D, Hyland JMP, et al. Pathological response following long-course neoadjuvant chemoradiotherapy for locally advanced rectal cancer. *Histopathology*. 2005;47:141–146.
52. Sebag-Montefiore D, Brown G, Rutten H, et al. An international phase II study of capcitabine, oxaliplatin, radiotherapy and excision (CORE) in patients with MRI-defined locally advanced rectal adenocarcinoma. Interim results. *Eur J Cancer*. 2005;3s:170.
53. Rutten H, Sebag-Montefiore D, Glynne-Jones R, et al. Capecitabine, oxaliplatin, radiotherapy, and excision (CORE) in patients with MRI-defined locally advanced rectal adenocarcinoma: results of an international multicenter phase II study. *J Clin Oncol*. 2006;24s:A3528.
54. Tilney HS, Heriot AG, Purkayastha S, et al. A national perspective on the decline of abdominoperineal resection for rectal cancer. *Ann Surg*. 2008;247:77–84.
55. Morris E, Quirke P, Thomas JD, Fairley L, Cottier B, Forman D. Unacceptable variation in abdominoperineal excision rates for rectal cancer – time to intervene? *Gut*. 2008;57:1690–1697; published online June 5th.
56. Wibe A, Syse A, Anderson E, et al. Oncological outcomes after total mesorectal excision for cure for cancer of the lower rectum: anterior vs. abdominoperineal resection. *Dis Colon Rectum*. 2004;47:48–58.
57. Marr R, Birbeck K, Garvican J, et al. The modern abdominoperineal excision: the next challenge after total mesorectal excision. *Ann Surg*. 2005;242:74–82.
58. West NP, Finan PJ, Anderin C, Lindholm J, Holm T, Quirke P. Evidence of the oncologic superiority of cylindrical abdominoperineal excision for low rectal cancer. *J Clin Oncol*. 2008;26:3517–3522.
59. Holm T, Ljung A, Haggmark T, Jurell G, Lagergren J. Extended abdominoperineal resection with gluteus maximus flap reconstruction of the pelvic floor for rectal cancer. *Br J Surg*. 2007;94:232–238.
60. Bebenek M, Pudelko M, Cisarz K, et al. Therapeutic results in low-rectal cancer patients treated with abdominosacral resection are similar to those obtained by means of anterior resection in mid- and upper-rectal cancer cases. *Eur J Surg Oncol*. 2007;33:320–323.
61. Miles WE. A method of performing abdomino-perineal excision for carcinoma of the rectum and of the terminal portion of the pelvic colon. *Lancet*. 1908;2:1812–1813.
62. Salerno G, Chandler I, Wotherspoon A, Thomas K, Moran B, Brown G. Sites of surgical wasting in the abdominoperineal specimen. *Br J Surg*. 2008;95:1147–1154.
63. Treanor D, Waterhouse M, Lewis F, Quirke P. A virtual slide library for histopathology. *J Pathol*. 2007;213(S1):27A.
64. Wright A, Magee D, Quirke P, Treanor D. Automated scoring of tissue microarrays using virtual slides. *J Pathol*. 2008;216(S1):S33.
65. Treanor D, Quirke P. The virtual slide and conventional microscope – a direct comparison of their diagnostic efficiency *J Pathol*. 2007;213(S1):7A.
66. Treanor D, Jordan-Owers N, Hodrien J, Wood J, Ruddle R, Quirke P. A virtual reality powerwall compared to the conventional light microscope: results of a pilot study. *J Pathol*. 2008;216(S1):S43.
67. West N, Quirke P. An evaluation of mesorectal tissue volume using three dimensional digital imaging. *J Pathol*. 2007;213(S1):31A.

10 Chemotherapy: Concurrent Delivery with Radiation Therapy

Jean-François Bosset, Christophe Borg, Philippe Maingon, Gilles Crehange, Stéphanie Servagi-Vernat, and Mathieu Bosset

In 1958, Heidelberger et al *(1)* demonstrated that the addition of 5-fluorouracil (5-FU) enhanced the effect of radiation on transplanted animal tumors. Ten years later, Moertel et al *(2)* reported that this effect translated into an increased overall survival in patients with unresectable gastrointestinal cancer. This pioneering clinical study began the development of chemoradiotherapy (CRT) in the adjuvant setting of rectal cancer.

The main objective of radiosensitization in the clinic is to enhance local control *(3)*. A gain in survival might be expected if the local effect is dramatically improved *(4,5)*. However, CRT may also increase the effects of radiation on rapidly dividing cells of normal tissues within the irradiated volume, especially small bowel. The severity of acute treatment-related toxicity is related to the irradiated volume, the radiotherapy technique and scheme, the type of concurrently delivered drug, its delivery modality, and dosage. If acute toxicity surpasses tolerability levels, it may compromise radiation dose intensity and hamper treatment efficacy. Late toxicity is expressed by slowly dividing cells of normal tissues such as capillary endothelium and connective tissues. It is related to the total dose of radiotherapy, the fractional dose, and select concurrently delivered drugs as bleomycin, methotrexate, and anthracyclines. Late toxicity may occur from a few months to many years following treatments *(6)*.

Clinical research on postoperative CRT was initiated in the USA in the mid-1970s. At that time, 5-year overall survival following curative rectal cancer resection (commonly performed by blunt dissection) was about 45%, and patients with stage II–III (pT3N0, pTxN+) disease had 5-year rates local and distant recurrence rates of about 30–40%, respectively *(7,8)*. The primary advantage of postoperative treatments was an optimal selection of patients based on

From: *Current Clinical Oncology: Rectal Cancer*,
Edited by: B.G. Czito and C.G. Willett, DOI: 10.1007/978-1-60761-567-5_10,

pathologic criteria, excluding patients with early-stage disease and those discovered to have distant metastases at surgery.

Adjuvant treatment schemes were designed using one of two sequences: a pure CRT regimen in which 5-FU-based chemotherapy was delivered concurrently with pelvic radiotherapy (50 Gy over 5 weeks) or delivery of adjuvant chemotherapy following CRT or both before and after CRT.

In 1990, on the basis of the results of two randomized trials that demonstrated improved survival with postoperative CRT in comparison with surgery or with postoperative radiotherapy alone, postoperative CRT was recommended in the USA for patients with stage II–III rectal cancer *(9–12)*.

Subsequent trials aimed to optimize the two sequences. It was shown that delivering 5-FU by protracted venous infusion during radiotherapy further reduced distant metastasis and improved overall survival *(13)* and that 5-FU delivered by bolus injection was as efficient as modulating 5-FU with leucovorin and levamisole *(14,15)*.

In the early investigation of this approach, grade 3 and higher acute toxicities were observed in up to 60% of patients, leading to treatment interruption and early death in 35 and 5% of patients, respectively *(16)*. Refinement in radiotherapy techniques, reduction in the number of chemotherapy courses, and introduction of quality assurance procedures *(17)* increased both treatment compliance and reduced rates of treatment related deaths, which remained at about 1% *(13)*.

Late adverse effects included radiation enteritis (4%), small bowel obstruction (5%), and anastomotic stricture (5%) *(18)*. Chronic diarrhea was observed in up to 40% of patients and anorectal sphincter dysfunction in up to 60% *(19)*.

In the late 1980s, the publication of the first randomized trial results of adjuvant combined modality therapy from the USA and the demonstration that moderate dose preoperative radiotherapy improved treatment-related outcomes prompted the development of preoperative CRT *(16)*.

After properly defining the dose of 5-FU dose that could be safely delivered with leucovorin concurrent with pelvic radiotherapy, *(20)* the European Organization for Research and Treatment of Cancer (EORTC) Radiotherapy Group initiated a four-arm randomized trial (study 22921) assessing the value of adding chemotherapy to preoperative radiotherapy as well as the value of postoperative chemotherapy versus none in patients with cT3-cT4, resectable tumors. The concurrent and postoperative chemotherapy regimen consisted of 5-FU-leucovorin, and the radiotherapy dose was 45 Gy given over 5 weeks. Adding chemotherapy to preoperative radiotherapy increased grade 3+ acute toxicity (7.4% vs 13.9%) but did not compromise surgical resection or increase postoperative morbidity/mortality *(21)*. Tumors in the CRT groups were smaller (downsizing effect) ($p<10^{-4}$), more frequently achieved pathologic complete response (13.7% vs 5.3%) ($p<10^{-4}$), had less advanced pT and pN stages (downstaging effect) ($p<10^{-3}$), and had less lymphatic, venous, and perineural invasion ($p<10^{-3}$) *(22)*. However, there was no survival difference between the groups that received chemotherapy preoperatively ($p=0.84$) and those that received chemotherapy postoperatively ($p=0.12$). The 5-year cumulative rate of local recurrence was 17.1% in the radiotherapy group and decreased to 8.5% in the groups that received chemotherapy ($p=0.002$). The 5-year distant metastasis rate was approximately 35% in both treatment groups. Late side effects were moderate: grade 2+ diarrhaea was encountered in 10% and fecal incontinence in 9% of patients. Colostomy was required in 2% of patients and 1.4% required surgery for small bowel obstruction *(23)*.

A companion trial conducted in France by the Fondation Francophone de Cancérologie Digestive (FFCD 9203 trial) was an exact reproduction of EORTC 22921 with the exception

Table 1
Five-year results of preoperative CRT in cT3-4 rectal cancer: randomized studies

Trials	*No. of patients*	*Local recurrence (%)*	*Distant metastases (%)*	*Overall survival (%)*
German[25]	823	6	36	75
EORTC[23]	1,011	8.7	35	65
FFCD[24]	762	8.1	–	67

that all patients received postoperative chemotherapy. Similar results concerning acute toxicity, tumor effect, and local control were observed *(24)*.

While these two trials were being conducted, a German study randomized patients to preoperative CRT or postoperative CRT using 5-FU alone *(25)*. This study demonstrated that patients in the preoperative arm experienced less acute and late toxic effects, with lower rates of local recurrence (6% vs 13%). In a subgroup of patients initially deemed to require abdominoperineal resection, preoperative CRT appeared to increase the chance of sphincter sparing surgery. The primary outcomes of these three trials are reported in Table 1.

Results of these pivotal trials have led to 5-FU-based preoperative CRT being considered as standard treatment in cT3-cT4, resectable rectal cancers. Using this treatment approach with TME, the 5-year local recurrence rate is now approaching 5%, a rate unexpected 15 years ago in locally advanced rectal cancer. However, this approach has not significantly impacted the rate of distant metastasis development and therefore appears insufficient to further increase survival. In the EORTC trial, postoperative chemotherapy had no detectable impact on treatment-related outcomes on the group of patients as a whole, although only 42.5% of patients planned to receive postoperative chemotherapy actually received such with respect to dose and timing. The main reasons for this were that postoperative complications delayed treatment and/or patient refusal because they judged adjuvant chemotherapy too burdensome. Despite this poor adherence, an unplanned exploratory analysis of patients undergoing R0 resection showed a significant increase in disease-free survival in patients whose tumors were downstaged to ypT0-2 as compared to those with ypT3-4 following preoperative radiotherapy or preoperative CRT *(26,27)*. However, these results should not necessarily be interpreted that because downstaging was achieved that chemotherapy was of benefit, but instead may simply suggest that the same inherent, unknown tumor factors that favored downstaging also led to a benefit from postoperative chemotherapy. FU-based adjuvant chemotherapy is certainly inadequate for all patients, and other chemotherapy regimens should be evaluated.

The ability to predict tumor response to preoperative CRT could result in considerable clinical benefit. It may allow patients with poorly or nonresponding tumors to be spared from useless and toxic treatment and allow consideration of alternative or more intense treatment strategies. Several promising predictive biomarkers of response have been identified, including p21, spontaneous apoptosis, and sequencing of the p53 gene *(28–30)*. Microarray gene expression profiling has been shown to predict response with both sensitivity and specificity of approximately 80% *(31,32)*. The combination of tumor epidermal growth factor receptor (EGFR) negativity and vascular endothelial growth factor (VEGF) positivity appears to be a strong indicator of high resistance to radiotherapy *(33)*.

Perfusion indexes (PI) and apparent diffusion coefficient (ADC) are parameters obtained from dynamic magnetic resonance imaging (dMRI) that are associated with tumor microcirculation and tumor necrosis, respectively. Using tumor size reduction and/or pathological downstaging as endpoints, a significant effect of preoperative CRT was observed in patients whose tumors exhibited low PI and ADC as measured by dMRI preceding treatment *(34,35)*. All of these potential predictive markers need validation through prospective studies to establish their respective clinical benefit before they can be recommended for routine use in clinical practice.

The ability to accurately assess tumor and nodal response following preoperative CRT is another endpoint that may increasingly challenge the traditional approach of 'radical' resection (i.e., sphincter sparing resection in lieu of abdominoperineal resection; simple local excision or to no surgery at all in lieu of standard rectal resection). However, clinical response following CRT does not accurately predict pathological response. Among 6–20% of patients judged to have a clinical complete response, 75–95% still had tumor present at pathologic examination of the surgical specimen *(36,37)*. Additionally, transrectal ultrasound has limited accuracy in this regard *(38,39)*. MRI accurately assesses T and N complete response in about 70% of patients following CRT, although this is still may not be sufficient enough with regard to adopting more conservative surgical approaches *(40,41)*. Results with PET are conflicting and require further evaluation *(42–44)*. Thus, presently, there is no reliable method to facilitate reappraisal of the originally planned surgical approach preceding preoperative CRT *(45)*.

Due to the effects of preoperative treatment on tumor and draining nodes, standard prognostic factors, such as pTN, may not be appropriate for predicting outcomes. An analysis of patients undergoing rectal resection in the EORTC trial showed that the following factors were independently significant predictors of local recurrence, disease-free, and overall survival: sphincter sparing surgery (as opposed to APR), uninvolved circumferential radial margins (CRM); downstaging to ypT0-2 and to ypN0 *(46)*. CRM involvement has been also recognized as an important prognostic determinant in other studies *(47)*. These tumor and treatment-related factors should be introduced to stratify patients in clinical trials assessing adjuvant therapies.

Studies investigating the significance and prognostic value of molecular biomarkers have provided valuable information. Caspase-3 activity has been shown to predict local recurrence in stage III patients treated with surgery alone *(48)*. High intratumoral thymidilate synthase gene expression in the residual tumor is predictive of lower survival following preoperative CRT *(49)*. Adding chemotherapy to preoperative radiotherapy decreases COX-2 upregulation, proliferation, and increases peritumoral fibroinflammatory reaction, which have been linked with downstaging and suggests a role of immunity in good-responding patients *(50)*.

Researchers have initiated clinical trials aiming to further improve upon the effects of preoperative CRT, using tumor sterilization (ypT0) as an endpoint *(51)*. Substituting oral fluoropyrimidine (capecitabine, UFT) for 5-FU has shown good tolerability profiles, with treatment-related effects to those seen with 5-FU *(52–54)*. Combination of drugs (capecitabine+oxaliplatin; 5-FU-LV+irinotecan) showed ypT0 rates possibly higher than those obtained with single drug therapy *(55–57)*. Cetuximab alone or combined with other drug has been tested *(58,59)*. A randomized phase III French study has compared a regimen using capecitabine with 45 Gy RT to a regimen of capecitabine/oxaliplatin with 50 Gy RT, with a primary endpoint of rates of ypT0 specimens. Results are pending *(60)*.

A Pan-European randomized study is currently comparing preoperative CRT with capecitabine to preoperative CRT with capecitabine and oxaliplatin in resectable T3-4 or N+ tumors, with corresponding postoperative adjuvant chemotherapy with capecitabine or with capecitabine and oxaliplatin *(61)*.

Studies are also in progress evaluating bevacizumab, a monoclonal antibody that targets angiogenesis, in combination with preoperative CRT. In a preliminary study, beyond promising tumor downsizing, bevacizumab was shown to directly induce tumor cell apoptosis, decrease tumor vascularization, and to decrease viable circulating endothelial cells *(62)*. A phase I study in the USA evaluating bevacizumab, oxaliplatin, and capecitabine with radiation therapy showed good tolerability and encouraging response rates *(63)*. An ongoing randomized phase II study from France is comparing preoperative CRT regimens including PVI 5-FU and bevacizumab versus the same regimen following up-front chemotherapy including bevacizumab with FOLFOX in high risk T3N0/N+ patients as selected by pretherapy MRI (INOVA study) *(64)*.

With regard to the advances in surgery, questions have arisen regarding the need for preoperative CRT in all patients with T3N0 or N+ disease. Retrospective analysis of data from patients enrolled onto five adjuvant US trials showed 5-year survival rates of 74–85% and local recurrence rates of 5–11% in a group of patients with pT3N0 and pT1-2 N1 disease, whether postoperative chemotherapy or postoperative CRT was used *(65)*. Historically, the extent of extramural tumor spread (EMS) has been identified as a strong predictor for outcome *(66)*. In patients undergoing curative resection, those with pT3N0 disease and EMS$\leq$5 mm had 5-year survival and local recurrence rates of 85 and 5.5%, respectively, whereas those with EMS>5 mm and/or nodal involvement had significantly lower survival and higher local recurrence rates *(67)*. Thus, trimodality therapy may be excessive in some subsets of patients, and determination of the amount of EMS and nodal involvement would be helpful in treatment decision-making. MRI may correctly identify EMS extent in approximately 85% of patients *(68)* but for nodal disease, accuracy is less than 80%. In patients with a cT3N0 cancer in the mid-rectum assessed by endorectal ultrasonography or MRI followed by preoperative CRT, 22% still had undetected, involved mesorectal lymph nodes in the resected specimen, suggesting an even larger percentage would be understaged and require postoperative CRT, which is less effective and more toxic *(69)*. Despite possible overtreatment in some patients, preoperative CRT should be offered to all patients with cT3N0 disease *(70)*. This is also the position of the American College of Radiology *(71)*.

Future research efforts should be made to properly evaluate and reduce toxicities of preoperative CRT. In the EORTC trial, 10% and 9% of patients suffered from late grade 2 diarrhea and fecal incontinence, respectively. These toxicities were scored by attending physicians and may not have reflected the true reality. Pietrzak et al *(72)* evaluated quality of life, anorectal and sexual function in a randomized trial that compared preoperative short-course radiotherapy (5×5 Gy) to preoperative CRT (same scheme as in EORTC 22921). Evaluating 118 patients who underwent sphincter sparing surgery by dedicated questionnaires approximately 1 year following surgery, they showed that two-thirds of patients had anorectal function impairment in both arms, leading to quality of life alterations in 20% of patients. A similar study was conducted in 150 patients who underwent sphincter conservation in the EORTC study. Four years following surgery, 21% suffered from chronic diarrhea and 67% declared some forms of anal incontinence (at least one episode per week). Both toxicities had a significant negative impact on quality of life *(73)*.

Reducing the amount of small bowel irradiated by using three-dimensional conformal radiotherapy or intensity-modulated delivery of radiotherapy *(74)* and excluding the anal sphincter from the treated volume for tumors located in the mid-rectum *(75)* are both measures to reduce toxicity. With the implementation of TME, the sites of local recurrences have changed, preferentially located in the low pelvis, the presacral region and at or close to the anastomosis. Partial resection of the mesorectum for tumors located in the upper part of the rectum may be responsible for some local recurrences *(76,77)*. These new findings should prompt radiation oncologists to revise the pelvic volumes to be treated (Figs. 1 and 2).

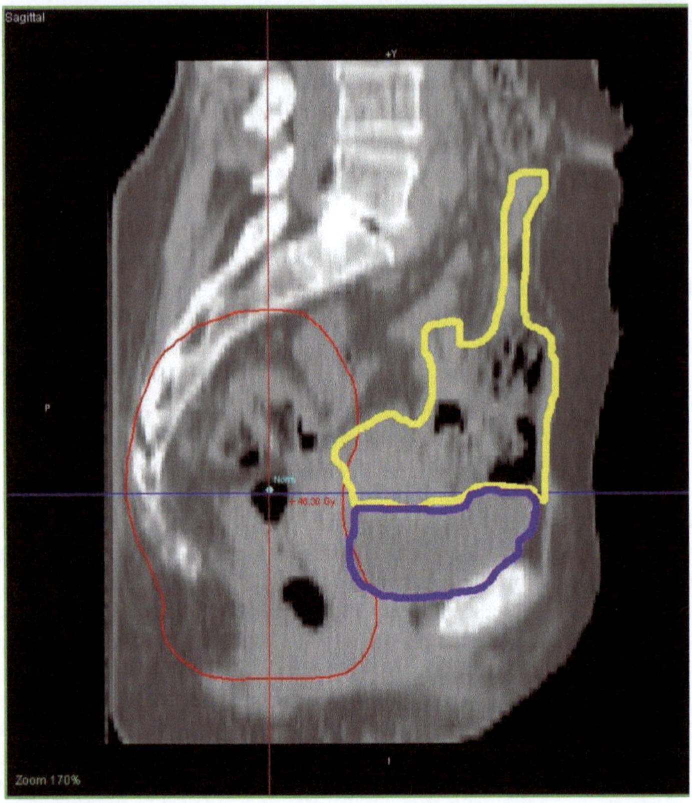

Fig. 1. Lateral view of the treated volume for a T3N+ mid-rectal cancer. The *red line* encompasses the volume receiving 45 Gy, the *yellow line* encompasses small bowel, and the *purple line* encompasses the bladder.

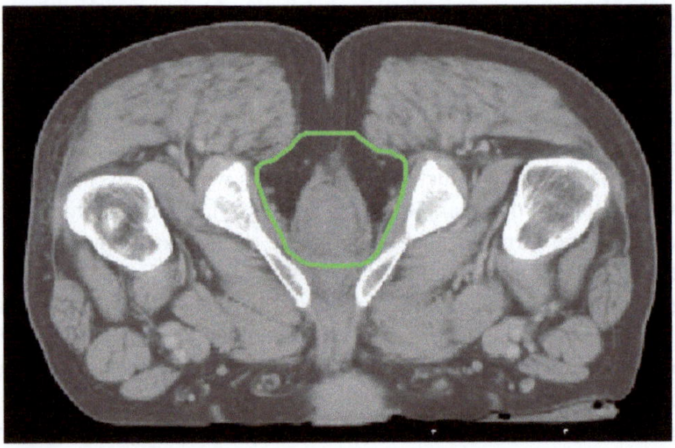

Fig. 2. Axial slice of a planning CT for a patient with T3N+ adencarcinoma of the distal rectum. An abdominoperineal resection is planned. The *green line* encompasses the ischiorectal fossa that should be included in the treatment volume.

Studies from tumor registries have already shown that the survival of patients with rectal cancer has significantly improved during the last 15 years, in parallel to the implementation of TME and preoperative treatments *(78,79)*. In parallel to clinical research, translational research should be conducted to further improve upon the outcome of rectal cancer patients and to more precisely define which groups of patients need more or less intensive preoperative treatments.

REFERENCES

1. Heidelberger C, Griesbach L, Montag BJ, et al. Studies on fluorinated pyrimidines. II. Effects on transplanted tumors. *Cancer Res.* 1958;18:305–317.
2. Moertel CG, Childs DS, Reitemeier RJ, Colby MY, Holbrook MA. Combined 5-fluorouracil and supervoltage radiation therapy of locally unresectable gastrointestinal cancer. *Lancet.* 1969;2:865–867.
3. Vokes EE. Combined modality therapy of solid tumors. *Lancet.* 1997;349:4–6.
4. Suit HD. Local control and patient survival. *Int J Radiat Oncol Biol Phys.* 1992;23:653–660.
5. Tubiana M. The role of local treatment in the cure of cancer. *Eur J Cancer.* 1992;28A:2061–2069.
6. Bosset JF, Marty M, Pavy JJ. Combinaisons radiothérapie et chimiothérapie. Applications aux radiochimiothérapies concomitantes. *Bull Cancer.* 1993;80:317–326.
7. Galandiuk S, Wieand HS, Moertel CG, et al. Patterns of recurrence after curative resection of carcinoma of the colon and rectum. *Surg Gynecol Obstet.* 1992;174:27–32.
8. Minsky BD, Mies C, Recht A, Rich TA, Chaffey JT. Resectable adenocarcinoma of the rectosigmoid and rectum. I. Patterns of failure and survival. *Cancer.* 1988;61:1408–1416.
9. Gastrointestinal Tumor Study Group. Prolongation of the disease-free interval in surgically treated rectal carcinoma. *N Engl J Med.* 1985;312:1465–1472.
10. Douglas HO, Moertel CG, on behalf of the Gastrointestinal Tumor Study Group. Survival after postoperative combination treatment of rectal cancer. *N Engl J Med.* 1986;315:1294–1296.
11. Krook JE, Moertel CG, Gunderson LL, et al. Effective surgical adjuvant therapy for high-risk rectal carcinoma. *N Engl J Med.* 1991;324:709–715.
12. National Institute of Health Consensus Conference. Adjuvant therapy for patients with colon and rectal cancer. *JAMA.* 1990;264:1444–1449.
13. O'Connell MJ, Martenson JA, Wieand HS, et al. Improving adjuvant therapy of rectal cancer by combining protracted-infusion fluorouracil with radiation therapy after curative surgery. *N Engl J Med.* 1994;331:502–507.
14. Tepper JE, O'Connell MJ, Niedzwiecki D, et al. Adjuvant therapy in rectal cancer: analysis of stage, sex, and local control – final report of Intergroup 0114. *J Clin Oncol.* 2002;20:1744–1750.
15. Smalley SR, Benedetti JK, Williamson SK, et al. Phase III trial of fluorouracil-based chemotherapy regimens plus radiotherapy in postoperative adjuvant rectal cancer: GI INT 0144. *J Clin Oncol.* 2006;24:3542–3547.
16. Bosset JF, Horiot JC. Adjuvant treatment in the curative management of rectal cancer: a critical review of the results of clinical randomised trials. *Eur J Cancer.* 1993;29A:770–774.
17. Martenson JA, Urias R, Smalley M, et al. Radiation therapy quality control in a clinical trial of adjuvant treatment for rectal cancer. *Int J Radiat Oncol Biol Phys.* 1995;32:51–55.
18. Ooi BS, Tjandra JJ, Green MD. Morbidities of adjuvant chemotherapy and radiotherapy for resectable rectal cancer. *Dis Colon Rectum.* 1999;42:403–418.
19. Kollmorgen CF, Meagher AP, Wolff BG, Pemberton JH, Martenson JA, Ilstrup DM. The long-term effect of adjuvant postoperative chemoradiotherapy for rectal carcinoma on bowel function. *Ann Surg.* 1994;220:676–682.
20. Bosset JF, Pavy JJ, Hamers HP, et al. Determination of the optimal dose of 5-fluorouracil when combined with low dose D, L-Leucovorin and irradiation in rectal cancer: results of three consecutive phase II studies. *Eur J Cancer.* 1993;29A:1406–1410.
21. Bosset JF, Calais G, Daban A, et al. Preoperative chemoradiotherapy versus preoperative radiotherapy in rectal cancer patients: assessment of acute toxicity and treatment compliance. Report of

the 22921 randomised trial conducted by the EORTC Radiotherapy Group. *Eur J Cancer.* 2004;40:219–224.
22. Bosset JF, Calais G, Mineur L, et al. Enhanced tumorocidal effect of chemotherapy with preoperative radiotherapy for rectal cancer: preliminary results EORTC 22921. *J Clin Oncol.* 2005;23: 5620–5627.
23. Bosset JF, Collette L, Calais G, et al. Chemotherapy with preoperative radiotherapy in rectal cancer. *N Engl J Med.* 2006;355:1114–1123.
24. Gerard JP, Conroy T, Bonnetain F, et al. Preoperative radiotherapy with or without concurrent fluorouracil and leucovorin in T3–4 rectal cancers: results of FFCD 9203. *J Clin Oncol.* 2006;24: 4620–4625.
25. Sauer R, Becker H, Hohenberger W, et al. Preoperative versus postoperative chemoradiotherapy for rectal cancer. *N Engl J Med.* 2004;351:1731–1740.
26. Collette L, Bosset JF, Den Dulk M, et al. Patients with curative resection of cT3-4 rectal cancer after preoperative radiotherapy or radiochemotherapy: does anybody benefit from adjuvant fluorouracil-based chemotherapy? A trial of the European Organisation for Research and Treatment of Cancer Radiation Oncology Group. *J Clin Oncol.* 2007;25:4379–4386.
27. Collette L, Bosset JF. Adjuvant chemotherapy following neoadjuvant therapy of rectal cancer: the type of neoadjuvant therapy (chemoradiotherapy or radiotherapy) may be important for selection of patients by Fietkau R, Klauthke G. *J Clin Oncol.* 2008;26:508–509.
28. Smith FM, Reynolds JV, Miller N, Stephens RB, Kennedy MJ. Pathological and molecular predictors of the response of rectal cancer to neoadjuvant radiochemotherapy. *Eur J Cancer Surg.* 2005;32:55–64.
29. Rebischung C, Gerard JP, Gayet J, Thomas G, Hamelin R, Laurent-Puig P. Prognostic value of p53 mutations in rectal carcinoma. *Int J Cancer.* 2002;100:131–135.
30. Rödel C, Grabenbauer GG, Papadopoulos T, et al. Apoptosis as a cellular predictor for histopathologic response to neoadjuvant radiochemotherapy in patients with rectal cancer. *Int J Radiat Oncol Biol Phys.* 2002;52:294–303.
31. Ghadimi BM, Grade M, Difilippantonio MJ, et al. Effectiveness of gene expression profiling for response prediction of rectal adenocarcinomas to preoperative chemoradiotherapy. *J Clin Oncol.* 2005;23:1826–1838.
32. Kim IJ, Lim SB, Kang HC, et al. Microarray gene expression profiling for predicting complete response to preoperative chemoradiotherapy in patients with advanced rectal cancer. *Dis Colon Rectum.* 2007;50:1342–1353.
33. Zlobec I, Vuong T, Compton CC, et al. Combined analysis of VEGF and EGFR predicts complete tumour response in rectal cancer treated with preoperative radiotherapy. *Br J Cancer.* 2008;98: 450–456.
34. Dzik-Jurasz A, Domenig C, George M, et al. Diffusion MRI for prediction of response of rectal cancer to chemoradiation. *Lancet.* 2002;360:307–308.
35. DeVries AF, Kremsen C, Hein PA, et al. Tumor microcirculation and diffusion predict therapy outcome for primary rectal carcinoma. *Int J Radiat Oncol Biol Phys.* 2003;56:958–965.
36. Hiotis SP, Weber SM, Cohen AM, et al. Assessing the predictive value of clinical complete response to neoadjuvant therapy for rectal cancer: an analysis of 488 patients. *J Am Coll Surg.* 2002;194:131–136.
37. Guillem JG, Chessin DB, Shia J, et al. Clinical examination following preoperative chemoradiation for rectal cancer is not a reliable surrogate end point. *J Clin Oncol.* 2005;23:3475–3479.
38. Fleshman JW, Myerson RJ, Fry RD, et al. Accuracy of transrectal ultrasound in predicting pathologic stage of rectal cancer before and after preoperative radiation therapy. *Dis Colon Rectum.* 1992;35:823–829.
39. Vanagunas A, Lin DE, Stryker SJ. Accuracy of endoscopic ultrasound for restaging rectal cancer following neoadjuvant chemoradiation therapy. *Am J Gastroenterol.* 2004;99:109–112.
40. Hoffmann KT, Rau B, Wust P, et al. Restaging of locally advanced carcinoma of the rectum with MR imaging after preoperative radio-chemotherapy plus regional hyperthermia. *Strahlenther Onkol.* 2002;178:386–392.

41. Koh DW, Chau I, Tait D, Wotherspoon A, Cunningham D, Brown G. Evaluating mesorectal lymph nodes in rectal cancer before and after neoadjuvant chemoradiation using thin-section T2-weighted magnetic resonance imaging. *Int J Radiat Oncol Biol Phys*. 2008;71:456–461.
42. Guillem JG, Puig-La Caille Jr J, et al. Prospective assessment of primary rectal cancer response to preoperative radiation and chemotherapy using 18-fluorodeoxyglucose positron emission tomography. *Dis Colon Rectum*. 2000;43:18–24.
43. Kristiansen C, Loft A, Berthelsen AK, et al. PET/CT and histopathologic response to preoperative chemoradiation therapy in locally advanced rectal cancer. *Dis Colon Rectum*. 2007;51:21–25.
44. Calvo FA, Domper M, Matute R, et al. 18F-FDG positron emission tomography staging and restaging in rectal cancer treated with preoperative chemoradiation. *Int J Radiat Oncol Biol Phys*. 2004;58:528–535.
45. Bosset JF. Distal rectal cancer: sphincter-sparing is also a challenge for the radiation oncologist. *Radiother Oncol*. 2006;80:1–3.
46. den Dulk M, Collette L, van de Velde CJH, et al. Quality of surgery in T3-4 rectal cancer: involvement of circumferential resection margin not influenced by preoperative treatment. Results from EORTC trial 22921. *Eur J Cancer*. 2007;43:1821–1828.
47. Gosens MJEM, Klaassen RA, Tan-Go I, et al. Circumferential margin involvement is the crucial prognostic factor after multimodality treatment in patients with locally advanced rectal carcinoma. *Clin Cancer Res*. 2007;13:6617–6623.
48. de Heer P, de Bruin EC, Klein-Kranenbarg E, et al. Caspase-3 activity predicts local recurrence in rectal cancer. *Clin Cancer Res*. 2007;13:5810–5815.
49. Liersch T, Langer C, Ghadimi BM, et al. Lymph node status and *TS* gene expression are prognostic markers in stage II/III rectal cancer after neoadjuvant fluorouracil-based chemoradiotherapy. *J Clin Oncol*. 2006;24:4062–4068.
50. Debucquoy A, Libbrecht L, Roobrouck V, Goethals L, McBride W, Haustermans K. Morphological features and molecular markers in rectal cancer from 95 patients included in the European Organisation for Research and Treatment of Cancer 22921 trial: prognostic value and effects of preoperative radio (chemo)therapy. *Eur J Cancer*. 2008;44:791–797.
51. Capirci C, Valentini V, Cionini L, et al. Prognostic value of pathologic complete response after neoadjuvant therapy in locally advanced rectal cancer: long-term analysis of 566 ypCR patients. *Int J Radiat Oncol Biol Phys*. 2008;72:99–107.
52. Dunst J, Reese T, Sutter T, et al. Phase I trial evaluating the concurrent combination of radiotherapy and capecitabine in rectal cancer. *J Clin Oncol*. 2002;20:3983–3991.
53. Fernandez-Martos C, Aparicio J, Bosch C, et al. Phase II multicenter study of preoperative oral uracil and tegafur (UFT) and concomitant radiotherapy in operable rectal cancer: final results with 3 years of follow-up. *J Clin Oncol*. 2004;22:3016–3022.
54. Das P, Lin EH, Bhatia S, et al. Preoperative chemoradiotherapy with capecitabine versus protracted infusion 5-fluorouracil for rectal cancer: a matched-pair analysis. *Int J Radiat Oncol Biol Phys*. 2006;66:1378–1383.
55. Hartley A, Ho KF, McConkey C, et al. Pathological complete response following preoperative chemoradiotherapy in rectal cancer: analysis of phase II/III trials. *Br J Radiol*. 2005;78:934–938.
56. Sebag-Montefiore D, Glynne-Jones R, Falk S, et al. A phase I/II study of oxaliplatin when added to 5-fluorouracil and leucovorin and pelvic radiation in locally advanced rectal cancer: a Colorectal Clinical Oncology Group (CCOG) study. *Br J Cancer*. 2005;93:993–998.
57. Glynne-Jones R, Falk S, Maughan TS, et al. A phase I/II study of irinotecan when added to 5-fluorouracil and leucovorin and pelvic radiation in locally advanced rectal cancer: a Colorectal Clinical Oncology Group study. *Br J Cancer*. 2007;96:551–558.
58. Rödel C, Arnold D, Hipp M, et al. Phase I-II trial of cetuximab, capecitabine, oxaliplatin, and radiotherapy as preoperative treatment in rectal cancer. *Int J Radiat Oncol Biol Phys*. 2008;70:1081–1086.
59. Hofheinz RD, Horisberger K, Woernle C, et al. Phase I trial of cetuximab in combination with capecitabine weekly irinotecan, and radiotherapy as neoadjuvant therapy for rectal cancer. *Int J Radiat Oncol Biol Phys*. 2006;66:1384–1390.

60. Phase III randomized study of neoadjuvant chemoradiotherapy comprising radiotherapy and capecitabine with versus without oxaliplatin followed by total mesorectal excision in patients with resectable stage II or III rectal cancer. Registered in ClinicalTrials.gov NCT00227747. http://www.cancer.gov/clinicaltrials/FRE-FNCLCC-ACCORD-12/0405/.
61. Phase III randomized study of neoadjuvant chemoradiotherapy and adjuvant chemotherapy comprising capecitabine with versus without oxaliplatin in patients with locally advanced rectal cancer. Registered in ClinicalTrials.gov NCT00766155. http://www.cancer.gov/clinicaltrials/EORTC-40054/.
62. Willett CG, Boucher Y, Duda DG, et al. Direct evidence that the VEGF-specific antibody bevacizumab has antivascular effects in human rectal cancer. *Nat Med.* 2004;10:145–147.
63. Czito BG, Bendell JC, Willett CG, et al. Bevacizumab, oxaliplatin and capecitabine with radiation therapy in rectal cancer: phase I trial results. *Int J Radiat Oncol Biol Phys.* 2007;68:472–478.
64. Essai randomisé de phase II évaluant l'efficacité et la tolérance de deux stratégies néoadjuvantes avec bevacizumab, visant à optimiser le traitement de patients atteints d'un cancer rectal localement avancé nouvellement diagnostiqué. Protocole ML 19202 INOVA (http://www.roche-trials.com/patient/trials/trial110697.html/); 2007. Coordinator JF Bosset, jean-francois.bosset@univ-fcomte.fr
65. Gunderson LL, Sargent DJ, Tepper JE, et al. Impact of T and N stage and treatment on survival and relapse in adjuvant rectal cancer: a pooled analysis. *J Clin Oncol.* 2004;10:1785–1796.
66. Dukes CE, Bussey JH. The spread of cancer and its effect on prognosis. *Cancer.* 1958;12:309–320.
67. Merkel S, Mansmann U, Siassi M, Papadopoulos T, Hohenberger W, Hermanek P. The prognostic inhomogeneity in pT3 rectal carcinomas. *Int J Colorectal Dis.* 2001;16:298–304.
68. Brown G, Daniels IR. Preoperative staging of rectal cancer: the MERCURY research project. *Recents Results Cancer Res.* 2005;165:58–74.
69. Guillem JG, Diaz-Gonzalez JA, Minsky BD, et al. cT3N0 rectal cancer: potential overtreatment with preoperative chemoradiotherapy is warranted. *J Clin Oncol.* 2008;26:368–373.
70. Kachnic LA, Hong TS, Ryan DP. Rectal cancer at the crossroads: the dilemma of clinically staged T3, N0, M0 disease. *J Clin Oncol.* 2008;26:350–351.
71. Suh WW, Blackstock AB, Herman J, et al. ACR appropriateness criteria on resectable rectal cancer. *Int J Radiat Oncol Biol Phys.* 2008;70:1427–1430.
72. Pietrzak L, Bujko K, Nowacki MP, et al. Quality of life, anorectal and sexual functions after preoperative radiotherapy for rectal cancer: report of a randomised trial. *Radiother Oncol.* 2007;84:217–225.
73. Mercier M, Pasquet P, Puyraveau M, et al. Evaluation of the sphincter function and quality of life in French patients with rectal cancer who entered the EORTC 22921 study. *Eur J Cancer Suppl.* 2005;3:171.
74. Urbano MTG, Henrys AJ, Adams EJ, et al. Intensity-modulated radiotherapy in patients with locally advanced rectal cancer reduces volume of bowel treated to high dose levels. *Int J Radiat Oncol Biol Phys.* 2006;65:907–916.
75. Bujko K, Bujko M, Pietrzak L. Clinical target volume for rectal cancer: in regard to Roels et al. (Int J Radiat Oncol Biol Phys 2006;65:1129–1142). *Int J Radiat Oncol Biol Phys.* 2007;68:313–316.
76. Syk E, Torkzad MR, Blomqvist L, Ljungqvist O, Glimelius B. Radiological findings do not support lateral residual tumour as a major cause of local recurrence of rectal cancer. *Br J Surg.* 2006;93:113–119.
77. Yu TK, Bhosale PR, Crane CH, et al. Patterns of locoregional recurrence after surgery and radiotherapy or chemoradiation for rectal cancer. *Int J Radiat Oncol Biol Phys.* 2008;71:1175–1180.
78. den Dulk M, Krijnen P, Marijnen CAM, et al. Improved overall survival for patients with rectal cancer since 1990: the effects of TME surgery and preoperative radiotherapy. *Eur J Cancer.* 2008;44:1710–1716.
79. Paganelli E, Danzon A, Bosset JF, et al. Improvement in survival of patients with rectal cancer in France and French guidelines. A population-based study of period 1984–2003. *Eur J Cancer.* 2010.

11 Chemotherapy: Adjuvant and Neoadjuvant Approaches

Rachel Wong, David Cunningham, and Ian Chua

Despite constituting approximately 25% of all diagnosed colorectal cancers, as opposed to colon cancer, there are relatively few large randomized controlled trials definitively supporting the use of adjuvant chemotherapy in the treatment of nonmetastatic rectal cancer. The optimal management of localized rectal cancer mandates a multidisciplinary approach to treatment. The main goals of treating nonmetastatic rectal cancer are achieving local control, particularly since local recurrence is associated with significant morbidity and mortality, as well as preventing distant recurrence.

Although routine use of total mesorectal excision (TME) and/or neoadjuvant short-course radiotherapy or long-course chemoradiotherapy have resulted in improved local recurrence rates, they have had little impact on overall survival (OS) *(1–6)*. Only the Swedish Rectal Cancer trial has reported an improvement in OS (38% for radiotherapy vs. 30% for non-irradiated patients; $p=0.008$) *(7)*. The failure of improvements in local recurrence rates to correspond to significant improvements in OS outcomes for rectal cancer patients may, at least in part, be due to the presence of micrometastatic disease resulting in incurable distant relapse. Therefore, in theory, adjuvant chemotherapy to eradicate micrometastatic disease should result in improved survival outcomes. Another approach to treatment currently under evaluation in patients with high-risk rectal cancer is the addition of neoadjuvant chemotherapy as a prelude to long-course chemoradiation, TME, and adjuvant chemotherapy.

WHO SHOULD RECEIVE ADJUVANT CHEMOTHERAPY?

In colon cancer, adjuvant treatment recommendations are predominantly based on the histopathologic characteristics of the postoperative specimen – this is, principally based upon the presence or absence of lymph node involvement. Additional features to be considered in the decision to deliver adjuvant chemotherapy (as in the case of stage II colon tumors) include the

From: *Current Clinical Oncology: Rectal Cancer,*
Edited by: B.G. Czito and C.G. Willett, DOI: 10.1007/978-1-60761-567-5_11,

total number of lymph nodes examined, T stage, degree of differentiation, and the presence or absence of extramural venous or lymphatic invasion. In rectal cancer, however, many patients will receive neoadjuvant therapy, frequently in the form of long-course chemoradiation therapy. The pathological downstaging often associated with long-course chemoradiation means that relying on histopathologic characteristics of the surgical specimen alone runs the risk of undertreating the disease. Therefore, the decision to recommend adjuvant chemotherapy to rectal cancer patients is usually based on the preoperative staging, which may include digital rectal examination alongside radiological staging techniques such as endorectal ultrasound (ERUS) or magnetic resonance imaging (MRI). These staging techniques do, however, have their limitations, particularly in their ability to accurately identify nodal disease. Generally, ERUS and MRI can be regarded as complementary investigations *(8)*. ERUS is particularly useful in assessing early T1–T2 tumors, but less so for bulky, fixed tumors. The German CAO/ARO/AIO-94 study evaluating preoperative versus postoperative chemoradiation therapy used ERUS for staging. In the group assigned to postoperative chemoradiation, 18% of patients had histologically confirmed TNM stage I disease despite preoperative ERUS staging indicating either a T3 or T4, or node-positive tumor *(6)*. On the other hand, there is increasing evidence defining the circumferential resection margin (CRM) as an important prognostic marker. The MERCURY study demonstrated that MRI evidence of tumor within ≤1 mm of the mesorectal fascia strongly predicts for CRM involvement and that MRI can accurately stage degree of extramural spread *(9)*. As a result of this study, pelvic MRI is being increasingly used as a method of assessing both the initial resectability of the tumor, and determining whether neoadjuvant therapy is indicated.

WHAT IS THE EVIDENCE FOR ADJUVANT CHEMOTHERAPY IN RECTAL CANCER PATIENTS?

The 1990 United States (US) National Institute for Health (NIH) Consensus Guidelines recommended postoperative sequential 5-fluorouracil (5FU)-based chemotherapy and chemoradiotherapy for stage II and III rectal cancer *(10)*. Studies such as the Gastrointestinal Tumor Study Group (GITSG) GI-7175 trial had demonstrated survival benefits for postoperative combined-modality therapy, and the National Surgical Adjuvant Breast and Bowel Project (NSABP) R-01 study for postoperative chemotherapy *(11,12)*.

In the NSABP R-01 study, 555 patients with resected rectal cancer (Dukes B and C) were randomized to no further treatment (184 patients), postoperative adjuvant chemotherapy with 5FU, semustine, and vincristine (MOF) (187 patients), or postoperative radiation therapy (184 patients) *(11)*. Compared to surgery alone, adjuvant chemotherapy resulted in a statistically significant improvement in both disease-free survival (DFS, $p=0.006$) and OS ($p=0.05$). Interestingly, when analyzed according to sex, the benefit in terms of both 5-year DFS (29% vs. 47%; $p<0.001$) and OS (37% vs. 60%; $p=0.001$) was restricted to males, with younger males (<65 years) deriving the most benefit. Females had worse OS if treated with MOF chemotherapy. Postoperative radiotherapy did not improve DFS or OS, although local recurrence rates were reduced when compared to surgery alone.

Subsequently, the NSABP R-02 trial, which was designed to evaluate the role of adjuvant radiotherapy in addition to chemotherapy, randomized male patients to four treatment arms (5FU/leucovorin, 5FU/leucovorin and radiotherapy, MOF or MOF and radiotherapy), whereas female patients were only randomized to receive 5FU/leucovorin with or without radiotherapy. Males treated with 5FU/leucovorin had better DFS ($p=0.009$), but not OS ($p=0.17$) compared to those treated with MOF *(13)*. The MOF regimen is now obsolete.

In another study of high-risk rectal cancer patients, the North Central Cancer Treatment Group (NCCTG) 79-47-51 study, combined modality adjuvant therapy consisting of semustine-5FU chemotherapy plus 5FU-based chemoradiation resulted in a statistically significant 34% (95% CI, 12–50%; $p=0.0016$) reduction in the risk of recurrence and a 29% (95% CI, 7–45%; $p=0.025$) reduction in the risk of death when compared to adjuvant radiation therapy alone *(14)*. With no chemotherapy-alone or chemoradiation-alone arms in this trial for comparison, it is impossible to determine what degree of benefit associated with combined-modality therapy is attributable to chemotherapy alone or to chemoradiation therapy.

A pooled analysis of five phase III North American adjuvant rectal cancer studies evaluated the impact of T and N stage and postoperative treatment on both DFS and OS *(15)*. Eligible patients had intermediate to high-risk rectal cancer (T3-4/N0, T1-2/N1-2 or T3-4/N1-2) and, apart from the 179 patients randomized to the surgery-alone arm of NSABP-01, were treated with surgery followed by adjuvant treatment with either radiation therapy, chemoradiation therapy, chemoradiation therapy and maintenance chemotherapy, or chemotherapy alone. Compared to surgery alone and adjuvant radiotherapy alone, chemoradiation therapy, chemotherapy and the combination of chemoradiation therapy and maintenance chemotherapy resulted in significantly improved OS ($p<0.001$). These data support the rationale for the use of systemic chemotherapy in the treatment of rectal cancer.

Increasing evidence supports the administration of either short-course radiotherapy or long-course chemoradiotherapy in the preoperative rather than postoperative setting where appropriate *(6,16,17)*. Despite a paucity of clinical trials specifically addressing the role of adjuvant chemotherapy for rectal cancer patients following preoperative radiotherapy or chemoradiotherapy and TME, most clinicians continue to recommend adjuvant chemotherapy to stage II and III disease.

The Netherlands adjuvant colorectal cancer project prospectively randomized resected stage II and III colorectal cancer patients to 12 months of bolus 5FU and levamisole or observation *(18)*. Of the 1,029 patients randomized, 299 had rectal cancer. Just over half of the patients (167/299) with rectal cancer also received adjuvant radiation therapy. The trial was closed early due to the emergence of data from other trials in support of adjuvant chemotherapy for colorectal cancer. Although there was a significant improvement in OS (65% vs. 55%; $p=0.007$) and a 21% relative reduction in the risk of relapse for the whole cohort at 5 years, analysis of the rectal cancer subgroup showed a nonsignificant trend toward overall and/or recurrence-free survival with adjuvant chemotherapy. Radiation therapy did not appear to impact on the effectiveness of adjuvant therapy. Of note, only 68 rectal cancer patients (46%) randomized to adjuvant chemotherapy completed the 12 month course, mainly due to toxicity.

The four arm European Organization for Research and Treatment of Cancer (EORTC) 22921 trial randomized 1,011 patients with T3 or T4 rectal cancer to: preoperative radiotherapy, preoperative chemoradiotherapy, preoperative radiotherapy and postoperative chemotherapy, and preoperative chemoradiotherapy and postoperative chemotherapy, with a primary endpoint of OS *(19)*. Systemic chemotherapy consisted of bolus 5FU and leucovorin. The initial analysis reported a nonsignificant trend toward improved 5-year overall and DFS between the groups of patients receiving adjuvant chemotherapy and those that did not. Five-year OS improved from 63.2 to 67.2% ($p=0.12$) and DFS from 52.2 to 58.2% ($p=0.13$) with the administration of adjuvant chemotherapy. Again, a significant proportion of patients did not complete the assigned therapy. Twenty-seven percent of patients assigned to postoperative chemotherapy did not commence treatment, and of those who did commence adjuvant chemotherapy, only 43% completed more than 95% of the planned dose of 5FU without delay. Additionally, a lower dose of 5FU was used compared to other adjuvant chemotherapy regimens and only four cycles of treatment were planned. Of note, compared to preoperative radiotherapy alone, any form of systemic chemotherapy (administered as part of long-course preoperative chemoradiotherapy, as adjuvant chemotherapy or as both) significantly reduced local recurrence rates ($p=0.002$ for any chemotherapy arm vs. radiotherapy alone).

The authors subsequently published an unplanned subgroup analysis on the 785 patients treated within EORTC 22921 who achieved an R0 resection, evaluating the effect of adjuvant chemotherapy on DFS and OS. In this exploratory analysis, patients achieving significant downstaging (ypT0-2 tumors) appeared to benefit from adjuvant chemotherapy in terms of DFS (HR 0.64: 95% CI, 0.45–0.91; $p=0.013$) and OS (HR 0.64: 95% CI, 0.42–0.96; $p=0.030$) *(20)*. On the other hand, patients without significant downstaging (ypT3-4 tumors) did not appear to benefit from adjuvant chemotherapy, with HR for DFS and OS of 1.18 (95% CI, 0.89–1.57; $p=0.244$) and 1.19 (95% CI, 0.84–1.68; $p=0.337$), respectively. From this exploratory analysis, the authors concluded that for patients who do not achieve tumor downstaging with neoadjuvant radiotherapy or chemoradiation therapy, adjuvant 5FU and leucovorin may be an ineffective treatment. These patients may benefit from more intensive chemotherapy regimens such as FOLFOX (folinic acid/5FU/oxaliplatin); however, there are currently no phase III data to support this hypothesis.

The preliminary results of another study, which randomized patients with T3/T4 tumors to 6 months of adjuvant chemotherapy (bolus 5FU/leucovorin) or observation following neoadjuvant chemoradiotherapy and surgery, did not show a significant survival benefit with chemotherapy. At the time of reporting, survival was 67.5% in the adjuvant chemotherapy group and 63.5% in the control group *(21)*. Again, a significant number of patients did not complete the assigned adjuvant chemotherapy.

Other retrospective studies evaluating the role of adjuvant chemotherapy in patients who have received neoadjuvant chemoradiotherapy also suggest a benefit, although reports on which patient subgroups were most likely to gain from adjuvant chemotherapy vary between studies *(22–24)*.

The QUASAR (*Qu*ick *A*nd *S*imple *A*nd *R*eliable) trial was designed to evaluate the role of adjuvant 5FU with high or low-dose folinic acid, levamisole or both in the treatment of colorectal patients. Patients were categorized as "certain" – patients whom clinicians felt were certain to benefit from adjuvant chemotherapy or "uncertain" – patients for whom the indication for adjuvant chemotherapy was unclear *(25,26)*. The 3,239 patients for whom the role of adjuvant chemotherapy was unclear were randomized to adjuvant chemotherapy or observation. Results of this component of the trial were recently published. Although the overwhelming majority of patients had stage II colorectal cancer, 29% of recruited patients had primary rectal tumors. Patients were allowed pre- or postoperative radiotherapy, but not chemoradiation therapy. In the intent-to-treat analysis, compared to observation, adjuvant chemotherapy significantly reduced the risk of recurrence and the risk of death to 0.78 (95% CI, 0.67–0.91; $p=0.001$) and 0.82 (95% CI, 0.70–0.95; $p=0.008$), respectively. For the rectal cancer subgroup, the relative risk of recurrence with chemotherapy compared to observation was 0.68 (95% CI, 0.52–0.88; $p=0.004$) and the relative risk of death was 0.77 (95% CI, 0.54–1.00; $p=0.05$) *(26)*.

Together, these data (summarized in Tables 1 and 2) provide some evidence to support the use of adjuvant 5FU-based chemotherapy in both stage II and stage III rectal cancer with improved survival and recurrence rates compared to surgery alone and surgery with radiotherapy. However, the true benefit of adjuvant chemotherapy following preoperative chemoradiotherapy and TME remains uncertain, with few randomized controlled trials specifically designed to address this question. Additionally, the conflicting results from available studies (which are often retrospective and heterogeneous in terms of preoperative treatment) and

Table 1
Selected randomized trials evaluating the role of adjuvant chemotherapy in nonmetastatic rectal cancer

Study	*Treatment*	*N*	*Results*
No neoadjuvant therapy given:			
GITSG GI-7175 (*12*)	Surgery alone	58	Study closed early. 24% survival benefit for CRT compared to surgery alone ($p=0.005$)
	Chemotherapy (MF)	48	
	RT alone	50	
	CRT (5FU)	46	
NSABP R-01 (*11*)	Surgery alone	184	Improvement in DFS and OS with MOF chemotherapy, but benefit restricted to males
	Chemotherapy (MOF)	187	
	RT alone	184	Radiation alone improved LR rates (not significant) but not DFS or OS
NCCTG 79-47-51 (*14*)	Chemotherapy (MF) and CRT (5FU)	104	Combined modality treatment significantly reduce rates of recurrence (both local and distant) and death ($p=0.025$) compared to radiation alone
	RT alone	100	
NCCTG 86-47-51 (*27*)	Chemotherapy (MF) and CRT (bolus 5FU)	112	PVI 5FU improved time to relapse ($p=0.01$) and survival ($p=0.005$)
	Chemotherapy (MF) and CRT (PVI 5FU)	114	No additional benefit from semustine (arms closed after interim analysis)
	Chemotherapy (5FU) and CRT (bolus 5FU)	220	
	Chemotherapy (5FU) and CRT (PVI 5FU)	214	
INT 0114 (*28*)	5FU and CRT (5FU)	421	No significant difference in DFS or OS between the four treatment groups. All bolus regimens
	5FU/LV and CRT (5FU/LV)	425	
	5FU/Lev and CRT (5FU)	426	
	5FU/LV/Lev and CRT (5FU/LV)	424	
NSABP R-02 (*13*)	5FU/LV	245	Addition of RT improved LR rates from 13% to 8% (HR 0.57; $p=0.02$) but did not improve DFS ($p=0.90$) or OS ($p=0.89$)
	5FU/LV and RT	242	
	MOF (males only)	103	Better DFS (but not OS) with 5FU/LV compared to MOF in males
	MOF and RT (males only)	104	
NACCP (*18*)	5FU + lev	514	OS and DFS improvement with adjuvant chemotherapy for entire cohort 299 rectal cancer patients recruited. 167/299 also received adjuvant RT
	Observation	515	Rectal cancer subgroup: nonsignificant trend toward benefit seen

N number of patients, *RT* radiotherapy, *CRT* chemoradiation, *DFS* disease free survival, *OS* overall survival, *LR* local recurrence, *HR* hazard ratio, *PVI* protracted venous infusion, *MF* semustine/5-fluorouracil, *MOF* semustine/vincristine/5-fluorouracil, *5FU* 5-fluorouracil, *LV* leucovorin, *lev* levamisole

Table 2
Selected randomized trials evaluating the role of adjuvant chemotherapy in early-stage rectal cancer

Study	*Treatment*	*N*	*Results*
Neoadjuvant therapy mandated or allowed:			
EORTC 22921 *(19)*	Preoperative RT	252	Trend toward improved 5-year DFS 0.87 (0.72–1.04), $p=0.13$ and OS HR 0.85 (0.68–1.04), $p=0.12$ with adjuvant chemotherapy
	Preoperative CRT (5FU/LV)	253	
	Preoperative RT and postoperative chemotherapy (5FU/LV)	253	Significant reduction in LR rates with addition of systemic chemotherapy compared to RT alone, regardless of timing ($p=0.002$)
	Preoperative CRT (5FU/LV) and postoperative chemotherapy (5FU/LV)	253	
Cionini *(21)*	Preoperative CRT and postoperative chemotherapy (5FU/LV)	326	Preliminary results available in abstract form only. No significant benefit in terms of relapse rates or OS for adjuvant chemotherapy. Less than half of patients completed the assigned chemotherapy
	Preoperative CRT	309	
QUASAR -certain *(25)*	5FU/low-dose LV	2,463	Total 4,927 patients enrolled and randomized in a 2 by 2 factorial fashion
	5FU/high-dose LV	2,464	
	5FU/LV + levamisole	2,429	
	5FU/LV + placebo	2,434	No extra benefit for high-dose LV over low-dose LV No benefit for levamisole over placebo in terms of disease recurrence or survival
QUASAR -uncertain *(26)*	Chemotherapy (fluoropyrimidine-based)	1,622	OS and DFS improvement with adjuvant chemotherapy for entire cohort. 948 rectal cancer patients recruited. Neoadjuvant RT and postoperative RT allowed. Significantly improved OS and DFS in subgroup analysis
	Observation	1,617	

N number of patients, *RT* radiotherapy, *CRT* chemoradiation, *DFS* disease free survival, *OS* overall survival, *LR* local recurrence, *HR* hazard ration, *5FU* 5-fluorouracil, *LV* leucovorin

poor compliance with the proposed adjuvant chemotherapy schedule (often due to toxicity) makes interpretation of the data challenging. In the UK, the CHRONICLE study (chemotherapy or no chemotherapy in clear margins after neoadjuvant chemoradiation in locally advanced rectal cancer) was a randomized phase III trial designed to compare observation to adjuvant capecitabine plus oxaliplatin in patients with locally advanced rectal cancer with clear margins following neoadjuvant chemoradiation therapy. The study was closed to recruitment in April 2008 after recruiting only 113 of the targeted 800 patients and therefore is unlikely to have the statistical power to answer this question.

WHAT ARE THE OPTIMAL DRUGS TO USE?

A further question that arises when considering adjuvant chemotherapy is which regimen to use. The NCCTG 86-47-51 established not only that infusional 5FU was superior to bolus 5FU when used as part of chemoradiation therapy but also that there was no significant difference in terms of local relapse, DFS, or OS for the combination of semustine and bolus 5FU when compared to single agent 5FU administered at a higher dose *(27)*. Consequently, the majority of future trials evaluating adjuvant chemotherapy were conducted using nonsemustine-containing fluoropyrimidine-based therapies, predominantly bolus 5FU/leucovorin (Mayo, Roswell Park) or bolus 5FU/levimasole regimens.

The Intergroup 0114 study did not demonstrate a difference in survival outcomes between patients treated with leucovorin- or levamisole-containing chemotherapy regimens over bolus 5FU alone *(28)*. Within the QUASAR study, of the 4,927 patients considered by clinicians to be "certain" to benefit from adjuvant chemotherapy, approximately one-third had rectal cancer *(25)*. Radiotherapy for rectal cancer was permitted, with preoperative therapy preferred over postoperative treatment. Overall, the results of QUASAR indicate that for colorectal cancer patients receiving adjuvant 5FU-based chemotherapy, compared to low-dose leucovorin, high dose leucovorin did not improve recurrence rates (odds ratio 1.00; 95% CI 0.91–1.09; $p=0.94$), or survival (odds ratio 1.04; 95% CI 0.94–1.15; $p=0.43$). Similarly, the addition of levamisole to 5FU/leucovorin did not impact on disease recurrence (odds ratio 1.07; 95% CI 0.97–1.17; $p=0.16$) or OS (odds ratio 1.10; 95% CI 1.00–1.22; $p=0.06$) compared to placebo. In the subgroup analyses, there was no difference in outcomes for rectal patients for both comparisons, thereby establishing bolus 5FU/leucovorin (high or low dose) as the standard adjuvant regimen.

In the adjuvant treatment of colon cancer and in the treatment of metastatic colorectal cancer, infusional 5FU and oral capecitabine have since been demonstrated to be at least equivalent to bolus 5FU/leucovorin, with differing and arguably more tolerable toxicity profiles *(29–31)*. Additional data favoring non-bolus 5FU regimens in the adjuvant treatment of rectal cancer was obtained from a multicentre study conducted in the UK comparing 6 months of bolus 5FU/leucovorin with 12 weeks of protracted venous infusion (PVI) 5FU (300 mg/m^2/day) as adjuvant treatment for colorectal cancer *(32)*. Patients with rectal cancer were allowed to have either preoperative or postoperative radiotherapy. Initial results at a median follow-up of 19.8 months reported a significant improvement in relapse-free survival (RFS: log-rank $p=0.023$) with PVI 5FU but not OS. Rectal cancer patients had significantly less relapses if treated with PVI 5FU ($p=0.007$). In the multivariate analysis, rectal cancer patients had significantly better RFS if treated with PVI 5FU ($p=0.043$) and there was a trend toward worse survival when these patients were treated with bolus 5FU/leucovorin ($p=0.08$) *(33)* (HR 0.66; 95% CI 0.43–1.03; $p=0.0697$). These initial findings prompted the investigators to extend the study to recruit additional rectal cancer patients to further explore this observation. Including the expanded cohort, at a median follow-up of 5 years, there was no significant difference in 5-year relapse-free survival (HR 0.8; 95% CI 0.62–1.04; $p=0.10$) or OS (HR 0.79; 95% CI 0.61–1.03; $p=0.083$) amongst all eligible patients. Those who commenced adjuvant therapy within 8 weeks of surgery had a significant survival advantage ($p=0.0044$). Among the 323 rectal cancer patients recruited, at a median follow-up of 55 months, RFS remained significantly better (HR 0.63; 95% CI 0.43–0.94; $p=0.0246$). In particular, rectal cancer patients randomized to PVI 5FU had a significantly lower rate of distant failures compared to those receiving bolus 5FU/leucovorin (14% vs. 23%; $p=0.03$). The trend toward improved OS observed in the initial cohort persisted (HR 0.66; 95% CI 0.43–1.03; $p=0.0697$). In terms of toxicity, infusional 5FU was associated with significantly less diarrhea, stomatitis, nausea and vomiting, alopecia, lethargy, and neutropenia (all with $p<0.0001$).

Infusional 5FU and oral capecitabine regimens have therefore been widely accepted as alternative adjuvant treatment options to bolus 5FU regimens for rectal cancer patients.

Oral UFT (combined tegafur and leucovorin) was also shown to have equivalent efficacy to bolus 5FU in the NSABP C06 trial *(34)*. Despite this, UFT is not licensed for this indication in the USA. In Japan, several trials have evaluated the role UFT in the adjuvant treatment of rectal cancer with results in favor of adjuvant therapy in terms of DFS, OS and rates of local recurrence *(35)*. These promising results must be interpreted with caution before routine use outside an Asian population, as they have not yet been reproduced in a Western population.

In the meantime, extrapolating from the results of colon cancer trials, such as MOSAIC (Multicenter International Study of Oxaliplatin/5-Fluorouracil/Leucovorin in the Adjuvant Treatment of Colon Cancer) and NSABP C07, oxaliplatin is being increasingly used in the adjuvant treatment of rectal cancer, both in routine practice and clinical trials *(36,37)*. Nevertheless, adding oxaliplatin to pre-operative fluoropyrimidine-based chemoradiation did not improve complete pathological response (an important prognostic factor in rectal cancer) in two recently reported randomised controlled trials *(38, 39)*. Presently, there are no available data from clinical trials to support the use of biological agents in combination with chemotherapy in the adjuvant treatment of colorectal cancer. The results of several ongoing trials are awaited, but in the meantime, the use of biological agents in this setting should be confined to clinical trials.

WHAT IS THE ROLE OF NEOADJUVANT CHEMOTHERAPY?

It is increasingly accepted that high risk, locally advanced rectal cancer should be treated with long-course chemoradiation therapy, TME surgery, and adjuvant chemotherapy. An alternative management approach that continues to be explored is the use of neoadjuvant chemotherapy as a prelude to, or even instead of, chemoradiation therapy.

The rationale behind this approach is multifactorial. Firstly, early treatment of micrometastatic disease may result in improved systemic control and survival. By using this approach, systemic treatment can usually be commenced within 1–2 weeks of the treatment decision and not delayed by local treatments, which may require complex planning and may themselves cause delays to (or omission altogether of) adjuvant systemic treatment due to their own inherent toxicities. Secondly, administration of chemotherapy with the primary tumor in situ provides an in vivo demonstration of chemosensitivity or resistance. This may allow early identification of patients unlikely to benefit from standard treatment regimens and who therefore require more intensive treatment. Additionally, neoadjuvant chemotherapy may induce early relief of tumor-related symptoms, result in tumor downstaging, and potentially increase the rate of sphincter-preserving surgery. In selected cases, administration of neoadjuvant chemotherapy could possibly avoid the need for chemoradiation therapy altogether. Potential advantages of omitting chemoradiation therapy if significant downstaging occurs are the avoidance of short and long-term toxicity, in particular the preservation of fertility and sexual function/potency, and possibly reduced surgical complications since radiotherapy-associated fibrosis and tissue friability may be technically challenging to the surgeon.

On the other hand, possible disadvantages of the neoadjuvant chemotherapy approach are the risk of disease progression prior to surgery, the risk of tumor-related complications such as bleeding, perforation or obstruction, and treatment-related morbidity and mortality.

CURRENT EVIDENCE FOR THE ROLE OF NEOADJUVANT CHEMOTHERAPY

The feasibility of delivering neoadjuvant chemotherapy was first demonstrated in a study published by Chua et al in 2003 *(40)*. The study was designed to evaluate a 12-week course of neoadjuvant chemotherapy administered as 5FU (300 mg/m^2/day as a protracted venous infusion) and mitomycin C (7 mg/m^2 bolus weeks 1 and 6). This was followed by long-course chemoradiotherapy (45 Gy+5.4–9 Gy boost+infused 5FU 200 mg/m^2/day), surgery and postoperative chemotherapy (using the same schedule as neoadjuvant chemotherapy). Patients were determined to have locally advanced rectal cancer by a multidisciplinary team after assessment by digital rectal examination and radiological imaging (CT or MRI). Of the 36 patients recruited, 65% had improvement or resolution of symptoms during neoadjuvant chemotherapy. Radiological response rates using the World Health Organization Criteria were 28% (95% CI, 14–45%) following neoadjuvant chemotherapy and increased to 81% post chemoradiation. Thirty-four patients proceeded to surgical resection and R0 resection was achieved in 82% of these patients. Compared to baseline T and N stage, 25 (73.5%) of the patients proceeding to surgery had tumor downstaging. Median PFS and OS were 27.2 months and 66.4 months, respectively.

Therefore, this study demonstrated that it was possible to administer neoadjuvant chemotherapy to patients with locally advanced rectal cancer. Reassuringly, the majority of patients had rapid symptom resolution, no progression of primary lesions occurred during chemotherapy, and the toxicity associated with this approach was both predictable and manageable.

Subsequent studies have evaluated the role of neoadjuvant oxaliplatin-based chemotherapy regimens. Results from the first 77 eligible patients recruited to the EXPERT (oxaliplatin (*E*loxatin), capecitabine (*X*eloda) and *pre*operative *r*adio*t*herapy followed by TME for the treatment of patients with MRI-defined poor-risk rectal cancer) study have been published *(29)*. Poor-risk rectal cancer was defined as: tumor within ≤1 mm of mesorectal fascia (i.e., CRM threatened or involved); T3 tumors at/below levators (i.e., low-lying tumors); tumors extending ≥5 mm into peri-rectal fat; T4 tumors; or T1-4 N2 tumors. Patients were treated with four cycles of oxaliplatin (130 mg/m^2 day 1) and capecitabine (2,000 mg/m^2/day in two divided doses days 1–14). Cycles were repeated every 3 weeks. Chemoradiotherapy consisted of 45 Gy in 25 fractions followed by 9 Gy in five fractions, administered concurrently with capecitabine (1,650 mg/m^2/day). Postoperative chemotherapy (capecitabine 2,500 mg/m^2/day) was also administered.

As seen in the previous study, the majority of patients reported an improvement in symptoms. Complete resolution of symptoms was reported at a median of 32 days from the commencement of chemotherapy. The radiological response rate, assessed by pelvic MRI, was 88% (95% CI, 78–95%) following neoadjuvant chemotherapy and increased to 97% (95% CI, 90–100%) after neoadjuvant chemoradiation. A complete radiological response was noted in 4% of patients after initial chemotherapy and 20% of patients after chemoradiation. Again there were no episodes of progressive disease during neoadjuvant chemotherapy. Of the 67 patients who proceeded to TME, R0 resections were achieved in all bar one patient (99%). Pathological complete remission was seen in 16 patients (24%; 95% CI, 14–36%; or 21%; 95% CI, 12–32% by intent to treat analysis, and only residual microscopic foci were observed in a further 32 patients. Compared to baseline T and N stage on MRI, 76% of resected patients had downstaging of the primary tumor in terms of T stage, N stage or both. At a median follow-up time of 23 months, the 1-year failure- free survival rate was 87% (95% CI, 77–93%) and 1-year OS was 95% (95% CI 87–98%). Median survival for the entire cohort of patients has not yet been reached. Of note, the initial protocol was revised after a clinically significant number of cardiac/thromboembolic events, including three mortalities, were noted. No further grade 5 cardiac/thromboembolic events occurred after this modification. Recently, long term results from EXPERT study have been published for the entire 105-patients-population *(41)*. Radiological response rates after neoadjuvant chemotherapy and chemoradiation were 74% and 89% respectively. Twenty-one (20%) patients had pathological complete response. Five-year progression free and overall survival rates were 64% and 75% respectively.

A third nonrandomized study conducted in Spain compared the pathological outcomes of two consecutively treated groups of patients receiving either neoadjuvant UFT-based chemoradiotherapy (62 patients) or two cycles of FOLFOX chemotherapy prior to UFT-based chemoradiotherapy (52 patients) *(42)*. A significantly higher proportion of patients treated with neoadjuvant FOLFOX achieved either T downstaging of two or more levels (44%: $p=0.029$) or were pT_0 or $pT_{0\text{-}1}$ (tumor limited to the mucosa) at surgery. Table 3 summarizes the radiological and pathological response rates observed in these this and the preceding two studies.

The neoadjuvant chemotherapy treatment strategy is now under further evaluation in a number of clinical trials. The EXPERT-C trial, a multinational randomized phase II study conducted in the United Kingdom, Spain and Sweden, has completed recruitment. This study is comparing neoadjuvant oxaliplatin and capecitabine followed by capecitabine-based chemoradiation therapy, TME surgery and adjuvant oxaliplatin and capecitabine with the same chemotherapy and chemoradiotherapy regimens plus the epidermal growth factor receptor antibody, cetuximab. Additionally, in Spain, another randomized phase II trial designed to assess the impact of neoadjuvant chemotherapy with oxaliplatin and capecitabine prior to oxaliplatin–capecitabine chemoradiation therapy and surgery in patients with high-risk rectal cancer reported neoadjuvant chemotherapy to have a better safety and higher dose-intensity of systemic treatment compared to post-operative chemotherapy after pre-operative chemoradiation *(43)*.

In the USA, an additional ongoing study is evaluating the combination of FOLFOX chemotherapy and bevacizumab administered as neoadjuvant treatment as a potential substitute for radiation therapy in the treatment of patients with locally advanced rectal cancer.

Table 3
Radiological and pathological responses: results from trials evaluating neoadjuvant chemotherapy in rectal cancer

Author	*N*	*Neoadjuvant chemotherapy*	*Radiation with concurrent*	*Radiological response*	*R0 resection*	*pCR*	*pT0-1*
Chua *(38)*	36	5FU PVI+ Mitomycin-C ×12 weeks	5FU PVI	Post neoadjuvant chemo: 27.8% Post chemoradiation: 80.6%	77%	3%	11%
Chua *(41)*	105	Oxaliplatin	Capecitabine	Post neoadjuvant chemo: 74% Post Chemoradiation: 89%	89%	20%	27%
Calvo *(39)*	52	FOLFOX 4 ×2 cycles	Tegafur	NR	NR	29%	44%

N number of patients, *5FU* 5-Fluorouracil, *PVI* protracted venous infusion, *FOLFOX* Folinic acid/5FU/oxaliplatin, *NR* not reported, *pCR* pathological complete remission

CONCLUSION

The definitive role of chemotherapy in the treatment of nonmetastatic rectal cancer is yet to be determined. Changes to management approaches and refinement of staging, surgical techniques, and radiation schedules over the past few decades have resulted in a lack of consistency in what was considered standard treatment across many clinical trials. Furthermore, the advances seen in the treatment of colon cancer are often extrapolated to rectal cancer despite a lack of supporting data. Given the disappointing impact of radiotherapy, chemoradiotherapy and TME on rates of systemic failure and OS, despite improvements in rates of local control, it seems logical that systemic treatment in the form of either adjuvant or neoadjuvant chemotherapy with a view to eradicating micrometastases may be the mechanism by which better long-term outcomes can be achieved. Although compliance with adjuvant treatment regimens in this setting is often poor, most frequently, due to toxicity from definitive treatment, there is growing literature to support the use of adjuvant fluoropyrimidine-based chemotherapy for patients with locally advanced, nonmetastatic rectal cancer. The role of newer chemotherapeutic agents and other drugs, such as monoclonal antibodies, is under evaluation in clinical trials.

For now, neoadjuvant chemotherapy cannot be adopted into routine practice, and its use should remain within the context of clinical trials. However, it has been demonstrated that this treatment strategy is feasible and appears to be a successful method to downstage tumors. This is an increasingly important finding, particularly for those tumors with threatened circumferential margins at the outset that are known to have particularly poor outcomes. Also of interest is the potential to substitute neoadjuvant chemotherapy for neoadjuvant chemoradiotherapy, thus avoiding the short- and long-term toxicities associated chemoradiation therapy. Whether or not this will be achievable by the incorporation of newer systemic agents into neoadjuvant chemotherapy regimens remains to be seen.

REFERENCES

1. Gerard A, Buyse M, Nordlinger B, et al. Preoperative radiotherapy as adjuvant treatment in rectal cancer. Final results of a randomized study of the European Organization for Research and Treatment of Cancer (EORTC). *Ann Surg*. 1988;208(5):606–614.
2. Gerard JP, Conroy T, Bonnetain F, et al. Preoperative radiotherapy with or without concurrent fluorouracil and leucovorin in T3-4 rectal cancers: results of FFCD 9203. *J Clin Oncol*. 2006;24(28):4620–4625.
3. Heald RJ, Moran BJ, Ryall RD, Sexton R, MacFarlane JK. Rectal cancer: the Basingstoke experience of total mesorectal excision, 1978–1997. *Arch Surg*. 1998;133(8):894–899.
4. Kapiteijn E, Marijnen CA, Nagtegaal ID, et al. Preoperative radiotherapy combined with total mesorectal excision for resectable rectal cancer. *N Engl J Med*. 2001;345(9):638–646.
5. Martling A, Holm T, Rutqvist LE, et al. Impact of a surgical training programme on rectal cancer outcomes in Stockholm. *Br J Surg*. 2005;92(2):225–229.
6. Sauer R, Becker H, Hohenberger W, et al. Preoperative versus postoperative chemoradiotherapy for rectal cancer. *N Engl J Med*. 2004;351(17):1731–1740.
7. Folkesson J, Birgisson H, Pahlman L, Cedermark B, Glimelius B, Gunnarsson U. Swedish rectal cancer trial: long lasting benefits from radiotherapy on survival and local recurrence rate. *J Clin Oncol*. 2005;23(24):5644–5650.
8. Skandarajah AR, Tjandra JJ. Preoperative loco-regional imaging in rectal cancer. *ANZ J Surg*. 2006;76(6):497–504.
9. MERCURY Study Group. Diagnostic accuracy of preoperative magnetic resonance imaging in predicting curative resection of rectal cancer: prospective observational study. *BMJ*. 2006;333(7572):779.

10. NIH consensus conference. Adjuvant therapy for patients with colon and rectal cancer. *JAMA.* 1990;264(11):1444–1450.
11. Fisher B, Wolmark N, Rockette H, et al. Postoperative adjuvant chemotherapy or radiation therapy for rectal cancer: results from NSABP protocol R-01. *J Natl Cancer Inst.* 1988;80(1):21–29.
12. Thomas PR, Lindblad AS. Adjuvant postoperative radiotherapy and chemotherapy in rectal carcinoma: a review of the Gastrointestinal Tumor Study Group experience. *Radiother Oncol.* 1988;13 (4):245–252.
13. Wolmark N, Wieand HS, Hyams DM, et al. Randomized trial of postoperative adjuvant chemotherapy with or without radiotherapy for carcinoma of the rectum: national surgical adjuvant breast and bowel project protocol R-02. *J Natl Cancer Inst.* 2000;92(5):388–396.
14. Krook JE, Moertel CG, Gunderson LL, et al. Effective surgical adjuvant therapy for high-risk rectal carcinoma. *N Engl J Med.* 1991;324(11):709–715.
15. Gunderson LL, Sargent DJ, Tepper JE, et al. Impact of T and N stage and treatment on survival and relapse in adjuvant rectal cancer: a pooled analysis. *J Clin Oncol.* 2004;22(10):1785–1796.
16. Adjuvant radiotherapy for rectal cancer. A systematic overview of 8,507 patients from 22 randomised trials. *Lancet.* 2001;358(9290):1291–1304.
17. Frykholm GJ, Glimelius B, Pahlman L. Preoperative or postoperative irradiation in adenocarcinoma of the rectum: final treatment results of a randomized trial and an evaluation of late secondary effects. *Dis Colon Rectum.* 1993;36(6):564–572.
18. Taal BG, Van Tinteren H, Zoetmulder FA. Adjuvant 5FU plus levamisole in colonic or rectal cancer: improved survival in stage II and III. *Br J Cancer.* 2001;85(10):1437–1443.
19. Bosset JF, Collette L, Calais G, et al. Chemotherapy with preoperative radiotherapy in rectal cancer. *N Engl J Med.* 2006;355(11):1114–1123.
20. Collette L, Bosset JF, den Dulk M, et al. Patients with curative resection of cT3–4 rectal cancer after preoperative radiotherapy or radiochemotherapy: does anybody benefit from adjuvant fluorouracil-based chemotherapy? A trial of the European Organisation for Research and Treatment of Cancer Radiation Oncology Group. *J Clin Oncol.* 2007;25(28):4379–4386.
21. Cionini L, Manfredi B, Sainato A, et al. Randomized study of postoperative chemotherapy (CT) after preoperative chemoradiation (CTRT) in locally advanced rectal cancer (LARC). Preliminary results. *Eur J Cancer.* 2001;37(suppl 6):S300.
22. Chan AK, Wong A, Jenken D, Heine J, Buie D, Johnson D. Is postoperative adjuvant chemotherapy necessary in locally advanced rectal cancers after preoperative chemoradiation. *Int J Radiat Oncol Biol Phys.* 2004;60((suppl 1):S297.
23. Crane C, Thames H, Skibber J, et al. 5-FU based adjuvant chemotherapy given after neoadjuvant chemoradiation improves survival only among responders (abstract). *Eur J Cancer.* 2001;37(suppl 6): S271.
24. Fietkau R, Barten M, Klautke G, et al. Postoperative chemotherapy may not be necessary for patients with ypN0-category after neoadjuvant chemoradiotherapy of rectal cancer. *Dis Colon Rectum.* 2006;49(9):1284–1292.
25. QUASAR Collaborative Group. Comparison of flourouracil with additional levamisole, higher-dose folinic acid, or both, as adjuvant chemotherapy for colorectal cancer: a randomised trial. *Lancet.* 2000;355(9215):1588–1596.
26. Quasar Collaborative Group, Gray R, Barnwell J, et al. Adjuvant chemotherapy versus observation in patients with colorectal cancer: a randomised study. *Lancet.* 2007;370(9604):2020–2029.
27. O'Connell MJ, Martenson JA, Wieand HS, et al. Improving adjuvant therapy for rectal cancer by combining protracted-infusion fluorouracil with radiation therapy after curative surgery. *N Engl J Med.* 1994;331(8):502–507.
28. Tepper JE, O'Connell M, Niedzwiecki D, et al. Adjuvant therapy in rectal cancer: analysis of stage, sex, and local control – final report of intergroup 0114. *J Clin Oncol.* 2002;20(7):1744–1750.
29. Chau I, Brown G, Cunningham D, et al. Neoadjuvant capecitabine and oxaliplatin followed by synchronous chemoradiation and total mesorectal excision in magnetic resonance imaging-defined poor-risk rectal cancer. *J Clin Oncol.* 2006;24(4):668–674.
30. Mayer RJ. Oral versus intravenous fluoropyrimidines for advanced colorectal cancer: by either route, it's all the same. *J Clin Oncol.* 2001;19(21):4093–4096.

31. Twelves C, Wong A, Nowacki MP, et al. Capecitabine as adjuvant treatment for stage III colon cancer. *N Engl J Med.* 2005;352(26):2696–2704.
32. Chau I, Norman AR, Cunningham D, et al. A randomised comparison between 6 months of bolus fluorouracil/leucovorin and 12 weeks of protracted venous infusion fluorouracil as adjuvant treatment in colorectal cancer. *Ann Oncol.* 2005;16(4):549–557.
33. Saini A, Norman AR, Cunningham D, et al. Twelve weeks of protracted venous infusion of fluorouracil (5-FU) is as effective as 6 months of bolus 5-FU and folinic acid as adjuvant treatment in colorectal cancer. *Br J Cancer.* 2003;88(12):1859–1865.
34. Lembersky BC, Wieand HS, Petrelli NJ, et al. Oral uracil and tegafur plus leucovorin compared with intravenous fluorouracil and leucovorin in stage II and III carcinoma of the colon: results from National Surgical Adjuvant Breast and Bowel Project Protocol C-06. *J Clin Oncol.* 2006;24(13):2059–2064.
35. Casado E, Pfeiffer P, Feliu J, Gonzalez-Baron M, Vestermark L, Jensen HA. UFT (tegafur-uracil) in rectal cancer. *Ann Oncol.* 2008;19(8):1371–1378.
36. Andre T, Boni C, Mounedji-Boudiaf L, et al. Oxaliplatin, fluorouracil, and leucovorin as adjuvant treatment for colon cancer. *N Engl J Med.* 2004;350(23):2343–2351.
37. Wolmark N, Wieand S, Kuebler PJ, Colangelo L, O'Connell MJ, Yothers G. A phase III trial comparing FULV to FULV+oxaliplatin in stage II or III carcinoma of the colon: Survival results of NSABP Protocol C-07. *J Clin Oncol.* 2008;26 (May 20 suppl; abstr LBA 4005).
38. Gerard JP, Azria D, Gourgou-Bourgade S, et al. Comparison of two neoadjuvant chemoradiotherapy regimens for locally advanced rectal cancer: results of the phase III trial ACCORD 12/0405-Prodige 2. *J Clin Oncol.* 2010;28:1638–1644.
39. Aschele C, Pinto C, Cordio S, et al. Preoperative fluorouracil (FU)-based chemoradiation with and without weekly oxaliplatin in locally advanced rectal cancer: Pathologic response analysis of the Studio Terapia Adiuvante Retto (STAR)-01 randomized phase III trial. *J Clin Oncol* (Meeting Abstracts) 27:CRA40082009.
40. Chau I, Allen M, Cunningham D, et al. Neoadjuvant systemic fluorouracil and mitomycin C prior to synchronous chemoradiation is an effective strategy in locally advanced rectal cancer. *Br J Cancer.* 2003;88:1017–1024.
41. Chua YJ, Barbachano Y, Cunningham D, et al. Neoadjuvant capecitabine and oxaliplatin before chemoradiotherapy and total mesorectal excision in MRI-defined poor-risk rectal cancer: a phase 2 trial. *Lancet Oncol.* 2010;11:241–248.
42. Calvo FA, Serrano FJ, Diaz-Gonzalez JA, et al. Improved incidence of pT0 downstaged surgical specimens in locally advanced rectal cancer treated with induction oxaliplatin plus 5-fluorouracil and preoperative chemoradiaiton. *Ann Oncol.* 2006;17(7):1103–1110.
43. Fernandez-Martos C, Pericay C, Aparicio J, et al. Phase II, randomized study of concomitant chemoradiotherapy followed by surgery and adjuvant capecitabine plus oxaliplatin (CAPOX) compared with induction CAPOX followed by concomitant chemoradiotherapy and surgery in magnetic resonance imaging-defined, locally advanced rectal cancer: Grupo cancer de recto 3 study. *J Clin Oncol.* 2010;28:859–865.

41. Twelves C, Wong A, Nowacki MP, et al. Capecitabine as adjuvant treatment for stage III colon cancer. N Engl J Med. 2005;352(26):2696–[illegible]

42. Chau I, Norman AR, Cunningham D, et al. A [illegible]

12 Chemotherapy: Metastatic Disease

Kathryn M. Field and John R. Zalcberg

BACKGROUND AND EPIDEMIOLOGY

Colorectal cancer (CRC) is the second most common malignancy in the Western world and the fourth most common malignancy globally. The lifetime risk in developed nations for both men and women is approximately 6% *(1)*. This may be higher depending on an individual's family history of bowel cancer. Rectal cancer is less common than colon cancer, with around one-third of all CRCs arising in the rectum. The incidence has been slowly decreasing over the last 1–2 decades *(2)*. Males are more likely to develop the disease than females, with males carrying a lifetime risk of rectal cancer of approximately 1 in 27 and females 1 in 50 *(3)*. The median age at diagnosis is approximately 71 years *(4)*.

At presentation, approximately 20% of patients have stage IV (M1, metastatic) disease. A significant proportion of stage II or III tumors will ultimately progress to stage IV disease *(4,5)*. With the introduction of new therapies and improved surgical techniques, the death rate from CRC continues to decline at approximately 1.8% per year. However, the 5-year survival rate for stage IV disease remains approximately 7% *(6)*. Although less common than colon cancer, rectal cancer carries a worse overall prognosis at every stage of the disease *(6)* (Table 1). Whether this is a result of biological differences in colon versus rectal tumors remains relatively unknown and is a point of great interest in current translational research. Notably, there are no phase III trials of chemotherapy in metastatic disease which include only patients with rectal cancer, with all large-scale chemotherapy trials including patients with both colon and rectal cancer. This may change in the near future given the relatively new recognition that rectal cancer does not simply differ from colon cancer by its physical location, blood supply and method of presentation, but also by fundamental tumor biology.

Rectal cancer most commonly metastasizes to the liver and lung. Unlike colon cancer, rectal cancer is equally as likely to metastasize to the lungs as the liver, *(7)* accounting for

From: *Current Clinical Oncology: Rectal Cancer*,
Edited by: B.G. Czito and C.G. Willett, DOI: 10.1007/978-1-60761-567-5_12,

Table 1
Rectal cancer vs. colon cancer: relative 5-year survival rate

	Relative 5-year survival rate (6)	
Stage at diagnosis	*Colon (%)*	*Rectum (%)*
I	93	88
II	90	76
III	59	56
IV	5–7	5–7

the recommendation of routine chest imaging at the time of diagnosis *(8)*. The reason for this pattern of spread is thought to be due to the differing blood supply of the rectum, which drains via the mesenteric-portal system and internal iliac veins into both the portal venous and systemic venous systems, respectively *(9)*. Cerebral metastases are rare but are beginning to be seen more commonly with improved long-term survival and the ability to control metastatic disease at other sites. Bone metastases are also relatively uncommon except in long-term survivors. Peritoneal carcinomatosis may occur from trans-coelomic spread and generally carries a poor prognosis *(10)*.

Many trials enroll younger and fitter patients than may be seen in routine clinical practice. CRC is primarily a disease of the elderly, with 40% of cases occurring in patients over 75 years of age *(11)*. It can thus be difficult to extrapolate results from clinical trials to the elderly population as it is well-known that older patients are poorly represented in many clinical trials *(12)*. As only approximately 22% of patients in clinical trials are older than 65 years, and a mere 8–13% older than 70 years, it is difficult to simply apply data concerning regimens and doses from clinical trials to a more elderly population *(13)*. Due to this relative lack of evidence, clinical judgment is paramount, balancing efficacy against toxicity that may relate to age-related changes in drug metabolism. Nevertheless, available evidence demonstrates similar survival benefits for chemotherapy in patients over 70 years with metastatic CRC, and manageable toxicities that may be marginally higher than in the younger population. Choosing the most appropriate chemotherapy strategy should preferably be directed more by performance status and comorbidities than chronologic age itself.

CHEMOTHERAPY FOR CRC: A HISTORICAL PERSPECTIVE

Chemotherapy for the treatment of cancer really only commenced in the second half of the twentieth century *(14)*. Despite its somewhat inauspicious beginnings (the discovery of chemotherapy occurred as the result of investigation into chemical warfare agents during World War II), chemotherapy drugs, both alone and in combination, have resulted in significant improvements in outcomes, and even cures, for many patients with various malignancies.

With respect to colon and rectal cancer, 5-fluorouracil (5FU) was synthesized as a pyrimidine analog in the late 1950s after the observation that uracil (a pyrimidine base) was present in higher concentrations in tumor tissue compared with normal tissue *(15)*. In many respects, therefore, the development of 5FU was one of the very first examples of targeted therapy (the use of a drug which is specific for a molecule or pathway critical to the survival and proliferation of cancer cells). Fluoropyrimidines, including both systemic 5FU and oral prodrugs, remain the cornerstone of chemotherapy for CRC. In 1983, Charles Moertel, a pioneer in the use of fluoropyrimidines for this disease *(16,17)* wrote somewhat despondently "...none of our approaches for any stage of this disease can be regarded as optimal for clinical practice or even as having any established benefit" *(18)*. Nevertheless, as increasing efficacy was observed once 5FU was combined with adjuncts, dosing strategies changed, and combination therapies introduced, the work of Moertel and others has clearly improved survival outcomes for patients with both early and advanced stages of CRC.

It was not until the early 1990s that results from a number of small randomized trials in metastatic CRC demonstrated clear evidence of a survival benefit with chemotherapy compared with best supportive care. A meta-analysis of randomized controlled trials comparing first-line chemotherapy with supportive care alone was published in 2000 *(19)*. In total, seven trials and 614 patients were included. Overall, chemotherapy significantly prolonged 1-year survival, with a risk ratio of 0.69. It should be noted that none of the trials included in this analysis used oxaliplatin-based or irinotecan-based regimens, now regarded as part of the standard of care, which compared to fluoropyrimidines alone have further improved outcomes for patients with advanced disease. In addition to survival endpoints, quality of life is also an important endpoint in the setting of metastatic disease. Four trials in the meta-analysis included quality of life measures, demonstrating either maintenance of, or improvement in, quality of life scores in the chemotherapy arms compared to those receiving best supportive care.

Second-line chemotherapy (chemotherapy given at the time of disease progression after first-line chemotherapy) has also been demonstrated to improve survival outcomes. In 1993, Cunningham et al published a randomized phase III study of 189 patients who, after prior 5FU, received either single agent irinotecan plus best supportive care or best supportive care alone. This trial demonstrated a significantly better overall survival in the patients who received irinotecan (1-year survival 36.2% vs. 13.8%) *(20)*. Notably, quality of life parameters were also in favor of the irinotecan arm.

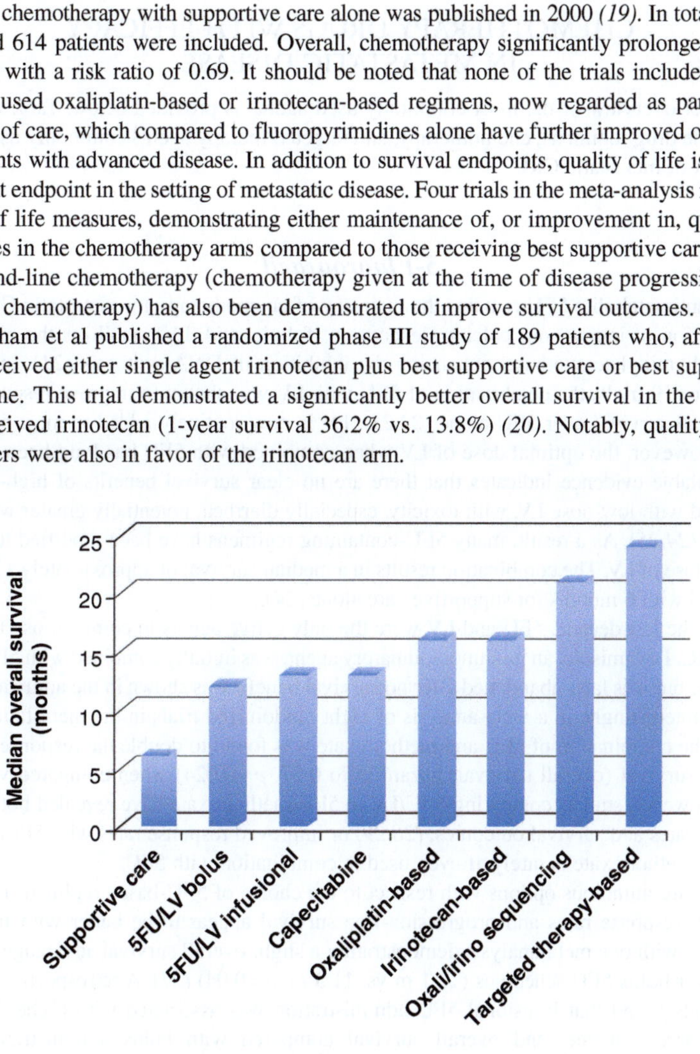

Fig. 1. Metastatic colorectal cancer: median survival estimates based on treatment received.

There have been significant improvements in the management options available for patients with metastatic rectal cancer, when considering that little over a decade ago, 5FU was the only chemotherapy drug available for patients with this disease. While fluoropyrimidine therapy remains the backbone of most chemotherapy regimens, there are now at least four chemotherapeutic agents and three targeted therapies in routine use around the globe for the treatment of metastatic disease. Increasing complexity regarding the options for using 5FU (bolus vs. short infusions vs. continuous 5FU) has resulted in numerous options with respect to treatment choices, particularly as newer drugs have become available. Furthermore, the survival gains obtained from this effort have been significant (Fig. 1).

CHEMOTHERAPY DRUGS WITH EFFICACY IN METASTATIC DISEASE

A brief overview of the most commonly used agents is provided below. Tables 2 and 3 outline the drug regimens, chemotherapy, and targeted therapy agents commonly used in the treatment of metastatic CRC.

5-Fluorouracil

The antimetabolite 5FU remains the mainstay of chemotherapy for metastatic CRC *(15)*. The addition of intravenous calcium leucovorin (folinic acid, LV) stabilizes the binding of 5FU to thymidylate synthase, enhancing the inhibition of DNA synthesis *(21)*. In a meta-analysis of 19 trials, the combination of 5FU with LV was shown to improve response rates and overall survival over 5FU alone *(22,23)*. LV is now routinely added to most 5FU regimens. However, the optimal dose of LV when combined with 5FU has long been debated. The available evidence indicates that there are no clear survival benefits of high-dose LV compared with low-dose LV, with toxicity, especially diarrhea, potentially greater with high-dose LV *(24,25)*. As a result, many 5FU-containing regimens have been modified to include a lower dose of LV. The combination results in a median survival of approximately 12 months compared with 6 months for supportive care alone *(24)*.

Until the last decade, 5FU and LV were the only active agents in common use for metastatic CRC. Levamisole, an immunomodulatory agent, was initially combined with 5FU-based regimens, but was later abandoned after no survival benefit was shown in the adjuvant setting *(26,27)*. Interestingly, in a meta-analysis of eight randomized trials in the metastatic disease setting, the combination of 5FU and methotrexate was found to double the response rate and improve survival (overall survival: hazard ratio 0.87, $p=0.024$) when compared with 5FU alone. However, studies comparing 5FU/LV to 5FU/methotrexate have revealed both similar response rates and survival outcomes, *(28,29)* or improved response rates with 5FU/LV *(30)*. As such, methotrexate is rarely, if ever, used in combination with 5FU.

There are numerous options with respect to the choice of 5FU-based regimens (Table 2). However, response rates and progression-free survival appear to be better with infusional schedules, with one meta-analysis demonstrating a slight overall survival advantage for infusional over bolus 5FU schedules (12.1 m vs. 11.3 m, $p=0.04$) *(31)*. A retrospective analysis of 22 trials found that infusional 5FU administration was associated with higher response rates, progression-free, and overall survival compared with bolus administration *(32)*. However, the various schedules result in differing side effect profiles: infusional 5FU causes more diarrhea and palmar-plantar fasciitis (hand-foot syndrome) while bolus 5FU carries a

Table 2
Common chemotherapy regimens for metastatic colorectal cancer

Regimen	*Description*	*Cycle length*
5FU Mayo *(170,171)*	5FU 425 mg/m²/day bolus days 1–5 LV 20 mg/m²/day, days 1–5	4 weeks
5FU Roswell Park *(27)*	5FU 500 mg/m²/day bolus weekly × 6 LV 500 mg/m²/day weekly × 6	8 weeks
LVFU2 *(172)* (de Gramont)	5FU 400 mg/m² bolus D1 and D2 LV 200 mg/m² D1 and D2 5FU 600 mg/m² CIVI 22 h D1 and D2	2 weeks
LV5FU2 (AIO) *(173)*	LV 500 mg/m² D1 weekly × 6 5FU 2,300–2,600 mg/m² CIVI 24 h D1 weekly × 6	8 weeks
Capecitabine *(35)*	1,250 mg/m² BD, D1–14	3 weeks
FOLFOX4 *(47)*	Oxaliplatin 85 mg/m² D1 LV 200 mg/m² D1 and D2 5FU 400 mg/m² D1 and D2 5FU 600 mg/m² CIVI 22 h D1 and D2	2 weeks
FOLFOX6 *(174)*	Oxaliplatin 100 mg/m² D1 LV 400 mg/m² D1 5FU 400 mg/m² D1 5FU 2,400–3,000 mg/m² CIVI 46 h (D1, D2)	2 weeks
FOLFOX7 *(82)*	Oxaliplatin 130 mg/m² D1 LV 400 mg/m² D1 5FU 2,400 mg/m² CIVI 46 h (D1, 2)	2 weeks
bFOL *(175)*	Oxaliplatin 85 mg/m² D1, D15 LV 20 mg/m² D1, D8, D15 5FU 500 mg/m² D1, D8, D15	4 weeks
FUFOX *(176)*	Oxaliplatin 85 mg/m² D1, 15, 29; LV 20 mg/m² D1, 8, 15, 22, 29; 5FU 500 mg/m² D1, 8, 15, 22, 29	8 weeks
FLOX *(177)*	Oxaliplatin 85 mg/m² D1 week 1, 3, 5 5FU 500 mg/m² bolus weekly weeks 1–6 LV 500 mg/m² bolus weekly weeks 1–6	8 weeks
FOLFIRI *(56)*	Irinotecan 180 mg/m² D1 LV 200 mg/m² D1 and D2 5FU 400 mg/m² bolus D1 and D2 5FU 600 mg/m² CIVI 22h D1 and D2	2 weeks
FOLFIRI3 *(83,84)*	Irinotecan 100 mg/m² D1 LV 400 mg/m² D1 5FU 2,400 mg/m² CIVI 46 h (D1,2) Irinotecan 100 mg/m² D3	2 weeks
IFL *(55)*	Irinotecan 100–125 mg/m² weekly × 4 weeks LV 20 mg/m² weekly × 4 weeks, 5FU 400–500 mg/m² bolus weekly × 4 weeks	6 weeks
XELOX *(48,178)*	Oxaliplatin 130 mg/m² D1 Capecitabine 1 g/m² BD D1–14	3 weeks

(continued)

Table 2
(continued)

Regimen	*Description*	*Cycle length*
CAPOX *(179)*	Capecitabine 1 g/m^2 BD D1–14 Oxaliplatin 70 mg/m^2 D1, D8 Numerous variations to regimen[a], *(49)*	3 weeks
XELIRI *(180)*	Irinotecan 200–250 mg/m^2 D1 Capecitabine 1 g/m^2 BD D1–14	3 weeks
CAPIRI *(57,181)*	Capecitabine 1 g/m^2 BD D1–14 Irinotecan 100 mg/m^2 D1, D8	3 weeks
FOLFOXIRI *(99,100)*	Irinotecan 125–175 mg/m^2 D1 Oxaliplatin 85–100 mg/m^2 D1 LV 200 mg/m^2 D1 5FU 400 mg/m^2 bolus D1 5FU 3,200 mg/m^2 CIVI 48 h	2 weeks

CIVI continuous intravenous infusion

[a]Regimens may also be 'modified', e.g., the leucovorin (LV) dose may be 'modified' to 50 mg, or LV5FU2 may be 'modified' or 'simplified' by omitting the Day 2 bolus and adjusting the infusional 5FU dose to compensate. Recommended capecitabine doses may vary depending on the geographic location

higher incidence of hematological toxicity. Presently, 5FU/LV is used alone in patients who are intolerant or have contra-indications to more complex regimens (see below).

Oral Fluoropyrimidines

Capecitabine has been available for use in metastatic CRC since the late 1990s. This oral prodrug is converted to 5FU in three enzymatic steps including the final activation by thymidine phosphorylase, a tumor-associated angiogenic factor, theoretically resulting in increased concentration of 5FU within the tumor cell *(33)*. Capecitabine is at least equivalent in efficacy to bolus 5FU in metastatic CRC *(34–36)* as well as in the adjuvant therapy setting *(37,38)*. The toxicity profile is similar to infusional 5FU with diarrhea and hand-foot syndrome occurring in some degree in up to 50–60% of patients, *(39)* not infrequently requiring a dose reduction. Although many patients prefer the use of an oral form of chemotherapy rather than hospital-based intravenous 5FU-based chemotherapy, compliance must be assured when such therapy is used. In the setting of disease refractory to intravenous 5FU, single-agent capecitabine appears to have minimal effect *(40–42)*.

Aside from capecitabine, other oral 5FU prodrugs have been developed, including *tegafur,* which has been demonstrated to be equivalent in survival outcomes to bolus 5FU in a phase III setting, *(43)* and *S*–1, which has been studied extensively in Asian countries in the management of both upper and lower gastro-intestinal cancers *(44)*.

Oxaliplatin

This platinum-based agent works by forming platinum-DNA adducts, thus blocking DNA replication *(45)*. Although it has minimal single-agent activity and hence should not be used as monotherapy, it is synergistic with 5FU in the treatment of metastatic CRC *(46)*. A phase

Table 3
Commonly used chemotherapy and targeted therapies used in metastatic rectal cancer

Drug name	*Drug class*	*Mechanism of action*	*Side effect profile*	*Single agent use*
5FU	Fluoropyrimidine	Pyrimidine analog (antimetabolite)	Diarrhea Mucositis Myelosuppression	Y
Capecitabine	Fluoropyrimidine	Oral prodrug, converted enzymatically to 5FU	Hand-foot syndrome Diarrhea Mucositis	Y
Oxaliplatin	Platinum agent	Forms platinum-DNA adducts	Neuropathy Myelosuppression	N
Irinotecan	Topoisomerase I inhibitor	Causes double stranded DNA breaks	Diarrhea Alopecia Myelosuppression	Y
Bevacizumab	Targeted therapy/Biologic agent Monoclonal antibody	Vascular endothelial growth factor (VEGF) antagonist	Hypertension Proteinuria Delayed wound healing GI perforation (rare)	N
Cetuximab	Targeted therapy/Biologic agent Monoclonal antibody	Epidermal growth factor receptor inhibitor	Acneiform rash Hypersensitivity reactions	Y
Panitumumab	Targeted therapy/Biologic agent Monoclonal antibody	Epidermal growth factor receptor inhibitor	Acneiform rash Hypomagnesaemia	Y (monotherapy only)

III trial of 420 patients (de Gramont et al) compared FOLFOX4 (Table 2) to infusional 5FU and demonstrated an improved response rate (50.7% vs. 22.3%, $p=0.0001$) and progression-free survival (9.0 months vs. 6.2 months, $p=0.0003$) in patients receiving FOLFOX4. Overall survival, while similarly improved (16.2 months vs. 14.7 months), was not statistically significantly different between the two arms ($p=0.12$) *(47)*, possibly attributable to patients in the control arm later receiving oxaliplatin, thus obscuring any survival benefit. Newer trials have combined capecitabine (rather than more complex 5FU schedules) with oxaliplatin (CAPOX or XELOX). A phase III study comparing first-line XELOX with FOLFOX4 met the primary endpoint of noninferiority for progression-free survival as well as overall survival (19.8 months vs. 19.6 months, hazard ratio 0.99) *(48)*. A meta-analysis of six randomized phase II and III trials comparing CAPOX with FOLFOX demonstrated similar progression-free and overall survival rates for both approaches, although response rate was slightly higher for the infusional 5FU-based regimens *(49)*.

The main toxicity of oxaliplatin is sensory peripheral neuropathy of which two types have been described – an acute, temporary cold-related dysesthesia, and a chronic cumulative persistent sensory neuropathy, which is dose-limiting but generally, although not invariably, reversible *(50)*. Up to 90% of patients experience some form of acute neurotoxicity *(51)* and 10–15% chronic neuropathy *(52)*. While most fully recover after a median time of 13 weeks *(53)*, in the MOSAIC study (a pivotal international study of adjuvant FOLFOX4), 29% of patients still had some degree of neurotoxicity 12 months following cessation of therapy *(50)*.

Irinotecan (CPT11)

Irinotecan, a camptothecin derivative, inhibits topoisomerase I, impeding DNA uncoiling and causing double-stranded DNA breaks *(54)*. It is used as monotherapy or in combination with a fluoropyrimidine. Saltz et al reported a phase III trial of 683 previously untreated patients with metastatic CRC who received either IFL (Table 2) vs. single agent irinotecan vs. bolus 5FU/LV (Mayo regimen, Table 2). Response rate, progression-free survival, and median overall survival (14.8 months vs. 12.6 months, $p=0.04$) were all significantly improved in patients receiving IFL *(55)*. A second phase III trial (Douillard et al) randomized a similar cohort of 387 patients to infusional and bolus 5FU combined with irinotecan (FOLFIRI) vs. the same 5FU schedule without irinotecan (LV5FU2, Table 2). This trial also demonstrated a higher overall survival (median 17.4 months vs. 14.1 months, $p=0.031$) in patients receiving irinotecan *(56)*. The IFL regimen is not generally used now due to concerns about toxicity and the improved tolerability of the FOLFIRI regimen.

Irinotecan has also been combined with capecitabine (CAPIRI or XELIRI) although results from a recent three-arm first-line phase III study comparing FOLFIRI to IFL or CAPIRI demonstrated significantly better progression-free survival for patients receiving FOLFIRI over the other two regimens (7.6 months, 5.9 months, and 5.8 months, respectively). Overall survival was also improved, although this was not statistically significant (FOLFIRI 23.1 months compared with IFL 17.6 months or CAPIRI 18.9 months) *(57)*.

The main dose-limiting side effect is of irinotecan is diarrhea, experienced by over 50% of patients in these studies. In rare circumstances and if not managed adequately, diarrhea can be life-threatening. Severe neutropenia can also occur, more commonly in patients with particular UGT1A1 (UDP-glucuronyltransferase 1A1) polymorphisms (UGT1A1 being a key enzyme involved in glucuronidation and inactivation of the drug) *(58)*. Gilbert's syndrome, a relatively common inherited disorder of metabolism whereby a mutation in the

UGT1A1 gene reduces its glucuronidation activity, is thus a pharmacogenetic risk factor for irinotecan toxicity *(59)*. At least partial alopecia occurs in up to 60% (unlike other drugs used in metastatic CRC where alopecia is rare). Irinotecan dose reductions are indicated in patients with liver impairment, and the drug should be used with extreme caution, if at all, in patients with an elevated bilirubin *(60)*, a situation which is relatively common in the setting of liver metastases. Some degree of hepatic steatosis and steatohepatitis is seen in up to 50% of specimens after resection of liver metastatic disease following irinotecan administration *(61,62)*.

Mitomycin C

This antineoplastic antibiotic is activated to become an alkylating agent in vivo, cross-linking and inhibiting DNA synthesis and function *(63)*. It demonstrates single-agent activity in metastatic CRC *(64,65)* but is accompanied by a significant risk of neutropenia and a small risk of hemolytic-uremic syndrome *(66)*. Although some earlier studies have shown efficacy in the first, second, and third-line disease settings *(67–71)*, its role has to a degree been superseded by irinotecan, oxaliplatin, and the biologics, and at present, mitomycin C is not one of the recommended drugs in the United States National Comprehensive Cancer Network (NCCN) Practice Guidelines in Oncology *(72)*.

Regional Chemotherapy: Hepatic Arterial Infusion Chemotherapy

Hepatic Arterial Infusion Chemotherapy (HAI) relies on the preferential blood supply of metastases from the hepatic artery and the dual blood supply of the liver from the portal vein *(73)*. Higher drug levels are delivered at sites of metastatic disease. The most common agent used in HAI is the 5FU analog floxuridine (FUDR). The most serious side effects of HAI include biliary sclerosis and catheter-related complications, both of which can be fatal *(74)*.

Until recently, trials comparing HAI to systemic chemotherapy in patients with liver metastases had demonstrated improved response rates although survival benefits were less clear cut *(74–76)*. A 2004 Cochrane review of HAI chemotherapy following resection or ablation of liver metastases secondary to CRC found no significant overall survival advantage for HAI *(77)*. However, a Phase III trial involving 135 patients receiving HAI (FUDR, leucovorin and dexamethasone) or systemic chemotherapy (5FU and leucovorin) showed an improvement in median overall survival favoring HAI (24.4 months vs. 20 months, $p=0.0034$). Conversely, time to extrahepatic progression was 7.7 months vs. 14.8 months with systemic chemotherapy ($p=0.029$) *(78)*. As more efficacious agents (oxaliplatin, irinotecan) are now used in the treatment of metastatic CRC, it is unclear as to whether the superiority of HAI in such patients will be maintained when using these agents as comparators, as this has not been tested to date in a randomized setting. Recently, House et al presented a retrospective comparison of 125 patients with CRC who underwent resection of liver-only metastases plus adjuvant HAI and concurrent FOLFOX or FOLFIRI, with 125 patients who received FOLFOX or FOLFIRI alone after liver resection. They demonstrated significantly improved liver recurrence-free survival (hazard ratio 0.39) and disease-specific survival (hazard ratio 0.5) for patients receiving both HAI and systemic chemotherapy *(79)*. Thus, it seems appropriate that a randomized study would be appropriate to prospectively evaluate the benefit of adding HAI to modern systemic chemotherapy in the setting of resected metastatic disease.

APPROACH TO CHEMOTHERAPY SCHEDULING (TABLE 4, FIG. 2)

Decisions as to the best choice of therapy are based on performance status, comorbidities, specific toxicities, and the preferences of the individual patient. When considering chemotherapy for metastatic CRC, initial chemotherapy options generally fall into three broad groups: 5FU/leucovorin or capecitabine alone; oxaliplatin-based regimens; and irinotecan-based regimens. The NCCN practice guidelines describe a wide range of appropriate first-line and second-line options for metastatic CRC and stratify choices based on the patient's ability to tolerate intensive therapy *(72)*. Numerous trials in the last decade have studied a broad array of regimens, leading to considerable variations in practice world-wide, albeit associated with some uncertainty as to what constitutes the optimal approach. Studies that have directly compared oxaliplatin-based and irinotecan-based regimens have suggested the overall efficacy and rate of severe toxicity is similar, although toxicity profiles themselves differ. In many cases, therefore, the choice of regimen is based on performance status, the likelihood of hepatic surgery, specific toxicities, comorbidities, and patient or physician preferences.

In addition to issues about the choice of initial regimen, unresolved questions about dose and schedule remain. One key question concerns the optimal 5FU regimen to use with oxaliplatin, as FOLFOX4, FOLFOX6, and FOLFOX7 utilize different doses and schedules of the same chemotherapy drugs, and have all been selected as standard regimens in recent trials *(80–82)*. Similarly, irinotecan may be used as a single agent, with varying doses and in different schedules; alternatively, irinotecan can be used in combination with bolus or infusional 5FU (commonly termed as the FOLFIRI regimen). As with the FOLFOX regimens, there have also been different modifications to the FOLFIRI regimen, with FOLFIRI3 (involving bifractionated irinotecan) providing improved clinical benefit in recent studies, even in patients previously exposed to irinotecan *(83)*. Similarly, this regimen has significantly improved progression-free survival in the second-line setting compared to other irinotecan-based regimens (including the commonly used FOLFIRI) *(84)*.

Table 4
Differing strategies for chemotherapy administration in metastatic rectal cancer

Method	*Example/trial*	*References*
Sequential	Tournigand/GERCOR group	*(80)*
Combination	FOLFOXIRI (HORG, GONO groups)	*(99,100)*
Sequential vs. combination	CAIRO	*(91)*
	FOCUS	*(90)*
Stop-and-go	OPTIMOX-1	*(82)*
	OPTIMOX-2	*(101)*
	CONcePT	*(104)*
Watch and wait (asymptomatic patients)	Nordic study	*(119)*
	Ackland 2-trial analysis	*(120)*
All three drugs at some stage in treatment	Grothey 7-trial analysis	*(93,94)*

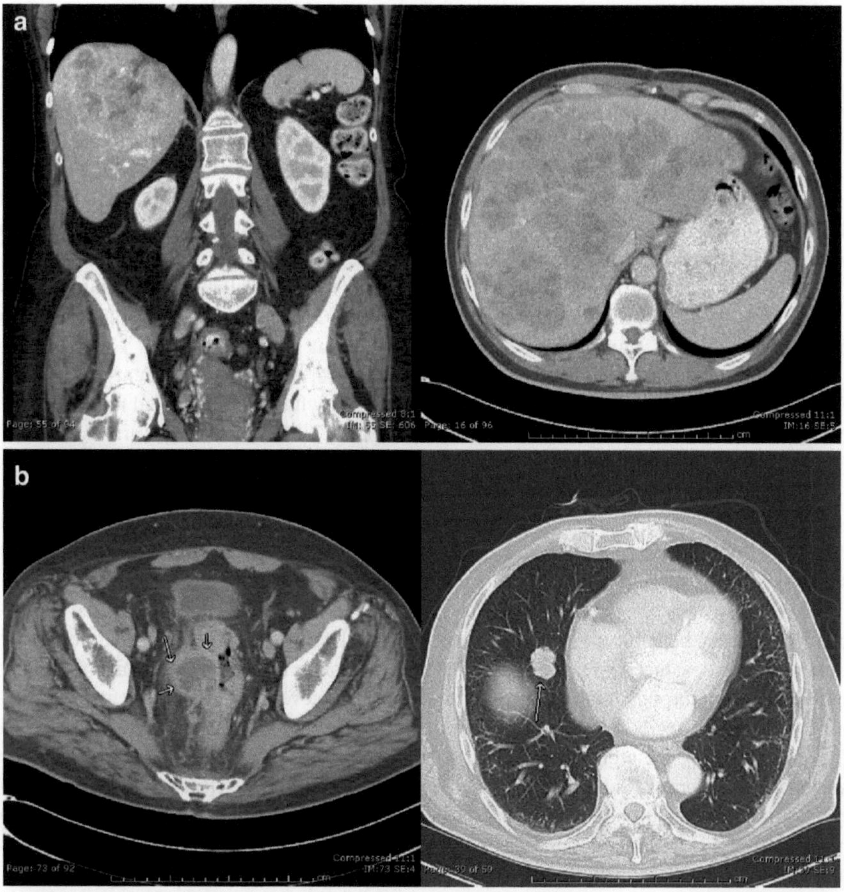

Fig. 2. Examples of different management strategies in metastatic rectal cancer depending on mode of presentation. *Example A*: Primary rectal cancer (asymptomatic) with large symptomatic liver metastases. Commenced palliative chemotherapy (FOLFOX) with good radiologic and symptomatic response. *Example B*: Primary rectal cancer (symptomatic, with bleeding and diarrhea) with small asymptomatic lung metastases. Commenced palliative chemoradiation therapy with infusional 5FU and good symptomatic response.

FOLFOX vs. FOLFIRI

There are three key trials that explore this issue. The first was a European study reported by Tournigand et al *(80)*. This randomized study of 220 patients receiving FOLFIRI followed by FOLFOX6 at progression vs. the reverse sequence demonstrated equivalent time to first progression (8.5 months vs. 8.0 months $p=0.26$) and median overall survival (21.5 months vs. 20.6 months, $p=0.99$) *(80)*. One statistically significant difference between the two arms was that 9% ($n=10$) of patients receiving FOLFIRI first-line had secondary surgery to remove liver metastases, compared with 22% ($n=24$) of those receiving FOLFOX first-line. However, as these types of comparisons represent posthoc analyses, they are of questionable value. In any case, this did not have any impact on overall survival. The authors' conclusions were that these sequencing strategies were equivalent in efficacy; and the main difference was the toxicity profile of the respective regimens.

The second trial was the N9741 Phase III study reported by Goldberg et al *(85)*. This trial of 795 patients was a three-arm study comparing FOLFOX4 with IFL and IROX (irinotecan and oxaliplatin). The IROX arm was later dropped. All outcome measures were better for the FOLFOX4 regimen compared to IFL with a 38% vs. 29% response rate and a 1-year survival of 71% vs. 58%. Median survival was 19.5 months (vs. 15 months for IFL, $p=0.0001$ and 17.4 months for IROX, $p=0.09$) *(85)*. The difference in overall survival may have been accentuated by differential access to second-line treatment for those in the two irinotecan-containing arms of the trial (at the time, irinotecan was readily available in the United States but oxaliplatin was not). Additionally, only the FOLFOX4 arm used infusional 5FU (as opposed to bolus 5FU), which may have contributed to its advantage.

The third trial was an Italian phase III study (Colucci et al) of 360 patients comparing FOLFIRI and FOLFOX4 (both using infusional 5FU), which demonstrated no difference in response rate (31% vs. 34%), time to progression (7 months for both arms), and OS (14 months vs. 15 months) between the two arms *(81)*.

Whether an oxaliplatin- or irinotecan-based regimen should be used initially given these data is unclear. The pivotal first-line phase III trial of oxaliplatin in metastatic disease resulting in its registration (de Gramont *(47)*), in fact did not demonstrate a statistically significant overall survival benefit. On the other hand, the two key first-line phase III trials comparing irinotecan-based regimens with 5FU/leucovorin (Saltz *(55)* and Douillard *(56)*) both demonstrated statistically significant benefits in overall survival. Potential factors influencing choice of initial treatment include concerns regarding toxicity of irinotecan in earlier trials in which the safety of irinotecan was brought under intense scruitiny *(86)*. However, the dosing strategy of irinotecan has since changed, and IFL in particular is no longer commonly used. Another potential factor determining the preference for initial treatment with oxaliplatin-based regimens is the somewhat unexpected finding that although FOLFOX has proven efficacy in reducing recurrence in the adjuvant disease setting for colon cancer (rectal cancer was not included in the two reported trials) *(50,87)*, the same has not been seen for irinotecan-based regimens used as adjuvant treatment in locally advanced disease *(88,89)*.

Sequential vs. Combination Therapy

Two pivotal studies have addressed the question of the optimal strategy for sequencing the various chemotherapy regimens in patients with incurable metastatic disease – the FOCUS and CAIRO studies, both published in the same edition of *The Lancet* in 2007 *(90,91)*. A third, the French FFCD-2005, has been presented but not yet published in full manuscript at this time *(92)*. These trials challenge the more commonly used aggressive approach using combination therapy (either FOLFOX or FOLFIRI) as initial therapy. The lack of benefit for less intense therapy but shorter overall survivals in each of these two studies (compared to trials that use more aggressive up-front therapy) is attributed by some to patient selection, and by others to the validity of the underlying hypothesis that both approaches are equally effective.

The FOCUS study conducted in the United Kingdom by the Medical Research Council (MRC) *(90)* was a randomized trial assessing three different strategies of sequential and combination chemotherapy for 2,135 patients with noncurative, metastatic CRC. Patients randomized to Arm A ('control') received infusional 5FU/leucovorin given until progression, then single-agent irinotecan; Arm B received infusional 5FU/leucovorin until progression, then either FOLFOX or FOLFIRI (randomly assigned); Arm C received FOLFOX or FOLFIRI initially (also randomly assigned). Treatment in both arms B and C was associated with a higher overall survival than Arm A; however, only Arm C with 'up-front' FOLFIRI was associated with a statistically significantly improvement in OS compared to the control arm. The authors concluded that combination chemotherapy up-front did not result in inferior outcomes and that initial monotherapy with (infusional) 5FU did not compromise survival. Notably, one-third of patients who were allocated to staged strategies did not receive second-line therapy, and only 19% received all three agents. This is a potential concern for some clinicians, in the potential to deny patients the opportunity to receive combination therapy, given the data that suggests that outcomes in metastatic CRC directly relate to the number of active agents patients have received during the course of their illness. Along these lines, Grothey et al published an analysis of seven phase III trials in metastatic CRC, which demonstrated that median overall survival significantly correlated with the percentage of patients who received all three drugs (5FU, irinotecan, and oxaliplatin) during the course of their disease, but not with the percentage of patients who received any therapy *(93,94)*.

The Dutch CAIRO study randomized 820 patients to either 'sequential' (first-line capecitabine, second-line irinotecan, third-line CAPOX) or 'combination' (first-line CAPIRI, second-line CAPOX) treatment. Combination treatment did not offer a significant overall survival advantage over the sequential approach (median survival 17.4 months vs. 16.3 months, hazard ratio 0.92, $p=0.3281$). This was despite the expected finding that combination therapy as first-line treatment resulted in a higher response rate and longer progression-free survival compared with monotherapy. Once again, only 36% of patients received all three agents. The toxicity profile was similar with the exception of higher grade 3 hand-foot syndrome in the sequential treatment arm *(91)*.

The optimal sequencing of chemotherapy remains the subject of ongoing debate in the literature *(95–98)*. What can be learned from these studies is that there are a number of strategies available for treating patients with incurable metastatic CRC, and no single strategy is necessarily superior to another, depending on the particular circumstances affecting individual patients. Together, these data have led to the paradigm that it is imperative to try to expose patients with metastatic disease, assuming they are willing and well enough, to all three active agents at some point in the treatment of their illness, rather than be concerned about the order in which these regimens are administered. It should be noted that this conclusion is subject to an inherent bias in that patients who are well enough to receive all three agents are those who are more likely to live longer. In their analysis, Grothey et al found that patients receiving combination vs. monotherapy as their initial treatment had an improved median survival, and were more likely to receive all three drugs in the course of their treatment. The data once again reflects a selection bias as this strategy favors patients with potentially curable disease being more likely to receive initial combination therapy. However, this does not detract from the findings of the FOCUS and CAIRO studies, which were prospectively designed to specifically examine the effect of different sequencing strategies.

This question leads to discussion as to the role of strategies combining all three drugs together as initial therapy (a regimen known most commonly as FOLFOXIRI). This strategy may be particularly important in patients for whom rapid control of disease is necessary - for example, in a younger patient with a large tumor volume for whom a failure to respond to first-line therapy may render the patient too unwell to tolerate therapy. There are some data that suggest a role for FOLFOXIRI (a combination of all three active agents) in such circumstances.

The Hellenic Oncology Research Group (HORG) reported a multicentre study in 283 patients receiving first-line chemotherapy, randomizing them to FOLFOXIRI or FOLFIRI *(99)*. There was no difference in overall survival (21.5 months vs. 19.5 months, $p=0.337$), response rates, or time to progression between the two arms, although toxicities (alopecia, diarrhea and neuropathy) were significantly higher with FOLFOXIRI. The rates of R0 resection (complete resection with negative margins) for metastatic disease was higher for the FOLFOXIRI arm (10% vs. 4%). This difference approached statistical significance ($p=0.08$). Notably, 70% of patients treated with FOLFIRI received second-line treatment (mainly oxaliplatin-based), and thus were exposed to all three active drugs *(99)*. A more recent phase III trial reported by the Italian Gruppo Oncologico Nord Ovest (GONO) group *(100)* compared FOLFOXIRI (both the regimen and scheduling were different from that used in the HORG study) with FOLFIRI in 244 patients and found a statistically significant median overall survival advantage of 22.6 months vs. 16.7 months ($p=0.032$) for the triplet arm, albeit with increased but manageable toxicities (mainly neutropenia and neurotoxicity). The response rate for FOLFOXIRI was reported at 70.4%; progression free survival (9.8 months vs. 6.9 months) and R0 resection rate (15% vs. 6%) were also significantly increased in the FOLFOXIRI arm. In the GONO study, 73% of those receiving FOLFIRI received second-line treatment (the majority receiving FOLFOX). The difference in outcomes between these two studies is likely to be multifactorial: a different study population (the HORG study recruited patients who were older and with a worse performance status) and lower drug doses and scheduling being at least two other potential factors.

Duration of Chemotherapy

Given the toxicities associated with chemotherapy, another important question is the optimal duration of therapy (assuming progression has not occurred and drug-related toxicities manageable). Again, to a degree, this decision is clinician and patient-dependent. This can be a difficult choice: continuing chemotherapy in the face of stable disease subjects the patient to potential drug toxicity and the burden of frequent hospital visits; on the other hand, ceasing chemotherapy carries with it the risk of disease progression, with the concern being that reintroduction of chemotherapy may not be as effective as maintaining continual disease control. Recent evidence suggests that rather than a drug holiday (stopping an active regimen with the plan to start again after progression or simply after a ‘break’ from chemotherapy), continued administration of a fluoropyrimidine is associated with improved survival.

The OPTIMOX1 trial was a European study *(82)* which assessed the efficacy of a stop-and-go approach to oxaliplatin in one of the treatment arms. In total, 620 patients were randomized to either FOLFOX4 until progression, or FOLFOX7 (Table 2) for six cycles, then maintenance fluoropyrimidine (LV5FU2) for 12 cycles, then routine reintroduction of FOLFOX7 for another six cycles. Both arms were equivalent as measured by progression-free (9 months vs. 8.7 months) and overall survival (19.3 months vs. 21.2 months, $p=\mathrm{NS}$). In addition, fewer patients experienced grade 3 or 4 toxicity in the stop-and-go arm. Essentially, efficacy was maintained while cumulative toxicity was reduced. Notably, only 40% of the patients in the stop-and-go arm actually went on to have reintroduction of FOLFOX, and in those who did, reintroduction was frequently delayed.

Given the equivalence in the two arms of OPTIMOX1, the OPTIMOX2 trial was designed to evaluate the complete cessation of chemotherapy instead of maintenance fluoropyrimidines *(101)*. The control arm was similar to arm B of OPTIMOX1 (FOLFOX7 for six cycles, then LV5FU2 till progression, then reintroduction of FOLFOX7 at progression; the investigation arm was the same as described above but without the ‘maintenance’ LV5FU2. Median overall survival was shorter in the investigation arm (24.6 m vs. 18.9 m, $p=0.05$), as was progression-free survival (8.3 m vs. 6.7 m, $p=0.04$). Thus, it appears that maintenance fluoropyrimidines prolong progression-free and overall survival.

However, not all trials have demonstrated that a drug "holiday" is inferior to maintenance chemotherapy. A multicenter randomized trial of 354 patients from the United Kingdom compared continuous treatment until progression with intermittent chemotherapy, and found no clear evidence of an overall survival benefit with the continuous approach *(102)*. Only 37% of patients assigned to intermittent treatment actually restarted chemotherapy. Chemotherapy in this trial (published in 2003) was either infusional 5FU or bolus ralitrexed (a drug no longer in routine use). More recently, Labianca et al reported a randomized study of continuous FOLFIRI (using a two weekly schedule) vs. intermittent FOLFIRI (the same schedule for 2 months on and 2 months off) *(103)*. In total, 336 patients were randomized; the median progression-free (8.8 m vs. 7.3 m) and overall survivals (16.9 m vs. 17.6 m) were similar across the two arms.

One of the potential benefits of intermittent chemotherapy is the avoidance of cumulative toxicities from repeated doses of chemotherapy. The CONcePT trial reported by Grothey et al was designed to evaluate the intermittent use of oxaliplatin with the aim to minimize toxicities (in particular the cumulative neuropathy associated with oxaliplatin) and hence reduce the incidence of chemotherapy cessation for neurotoxicity *(104)*. The trial randomized patients to receive FOLFOX7 (plus bevacizumab) with either continuous or intermittent (2 months on, 2 months off) oxaliplatin. Unfortunately, the trial was discontinued early due to an unplanned interim analysis which suggested there were lower response rates in patients receiving intravenous calcium and magnesium (a second randomization on the study). This was later refuted; however, only 139 patients were assessable. Nevertheless, time to treatment failure was found to be significantly longer in patients receiving intermittent oxaliplatin (5.6 months vs. 4.2 months, HR 0.58, $p=0.0025$). The incidence of severe neurotoxicity was also significantly reduced (10% vs. 24%, $p=0.048$).

CHEMOTHERAPY IN POTENTIALLY RESECTABLE METASTATIC DISEASE

In a select but increasing number of patients diagnosed with metastatic disease to the liver or lung, surgical resection of metastases can result in long-term cure. Treatment with curative intent is feasible in up to 15–20% of patients with liver metastases *(105)* and the 5-year survival may be over 30% *(106)* approaching 60% in some series of carefully selected patients *(107–109)*. Surgical techniques and considerations have been discussed in a separate chapter in this text. When a patient is considered potentially curable, a multidisciplinary approach is paramount and discussion in a multidisciplinary team setting to map out the treatment plan is essential (Fig. 3). Close liaison between the colorectal and hepatobiliary (or thoracic) surgeons and the medical oncologist, as well as the patient him/herself, is crucial. For rectal cancer in particular, the radiation oncologist is a critical member of the multidisciplinary team with respect to reducing the risk of local recurrence from the primary tumor in some presentations of synchronous metastatic disease, notably if the management plan has a curative intent.

Neoadjuvant chemotherapy for metastatic disease may downsize tumors to make surgery feasible and more successful and may also aid in the control of micrometastatic disease elsewhere in the body. There have been large studies demonstrating successful resection after neoadjuvant chemotherapy for liver metastases previously deemed unresectable *(110,111)*. Disease progression during chemotherapy is indicative of a very poor prognosis regardless of resection *(112)* (Table 5). Although complete disappearance of metastases on imaging may occur, without surgery, recurrence is the rule. Thus, current practice is to administer 2–3 months of neoadjuvant combination chemotherapy with repeat imaging to assess response, followed by surgery if appropriate.

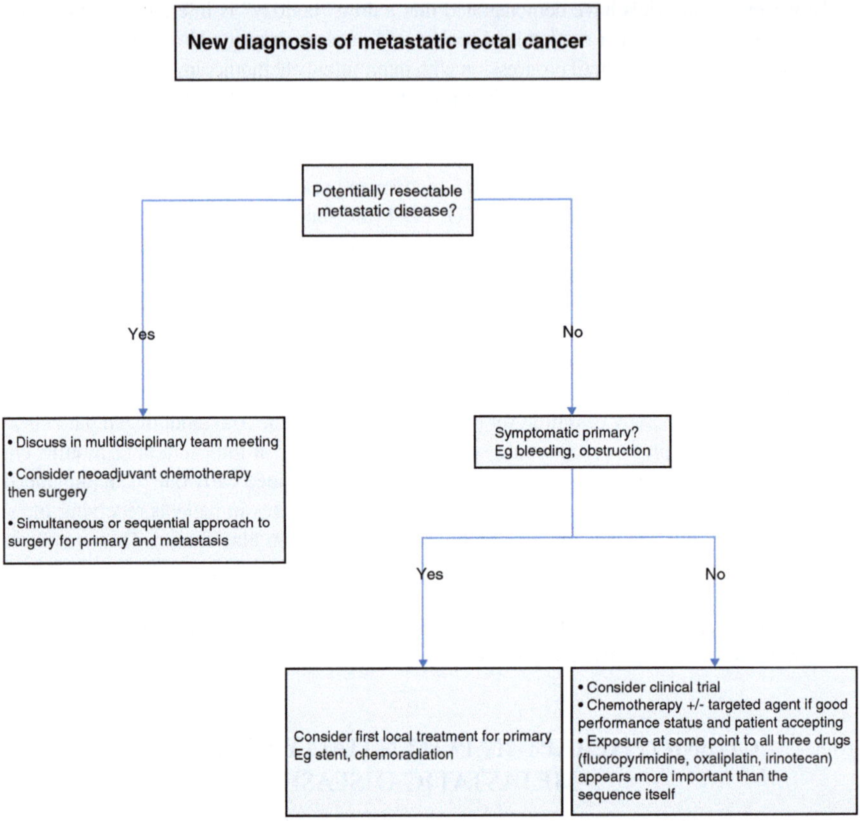

Fig. 3. Flow diagram of treatment options at initial presentation of metastatic rectal cancer.

Table 5
Neoadjuvant chemotherapy for potentially resectable metastatic disease: advantages and disadvantages

Advantages	*Disadvantages*
May convert initially unresectable lesions to resectable	May miss 'window of opportunity' for curative resection
Earlier treatment of micrometastatic disease	Potential hepatotoxicity of chemotherapy
Helps to determine response to chemotherapy	Complete response can make subsequent resection technically difficult
Helps to avoid morbidity of surgery if progress early	

Any chemotherapy regimen commonly used for CRC, if used for long periods of time, can induce varying degrees of hepatic dysfunction. 5FU is associated with fatty change; oxaliplatin with sinusoidal dilatation and obstruction; and irinotecan with steatosis and steatohepatitis *(61,62,113,114)*. However, rather than the choice of regimen itself, the more pertinent point may be a strategy of minimizing the number of cycles of chemotherapy administered before the resection of metastases, in order to avoid cumulative hepatotoxicity from chemotherapy, potentially rendering liver surgery more difficult and increasing postoperative morbidity from liver dysfunction.

Oxaliplatin-containing regimens are more commonly used as part of peri-operative (neoadjuvant or adjuvant) treatment in resectable disease. This is for a number of reasons. Firstly, both the Tournigand and N9741 studies (discussed in Section "FOLFOX vs. FOLFIRI"), when comparing oxaliplatin- and irinotecan-containing regimens, found that more patients on the oxaliplatin arms were rendered resectable. In the Tournigand study, 22% vs. 9% underwent an R0 resection *(80)*. Patients who underwent liver resection after participating in the Intergroup 9741 study (comparing IFL, FOLFOX and IROX) were followed up and results were published in 2005 *(110)*. Of the 795 patients, 24 (3.3%) underwent curative resection of metastatic disease – 92% of those patients ($n=22$) had received an oxaliplatin-based regimen. The median overall survival of resected patients was 42.4 months. The second reason underlying the choice of oxaliplatin-based regimens in this context relate to the incidence of chemotherapy-related hepatotoxicity, particularly steatohepatitis which is more commonly related to irinotecan and more likely to increase the risk of surgery *(113)*. Thirdly, a randomized phase III trial comparing 5FU/leucovorin vs. FOLFIRI as adjuvant treatment after complete resection of liver metastases *(115)* demonstrated no overall advantage in disease-free survival for the irinotecan arm, raising doubts as to the relative efficacy of this regimen – at least in this setting.

An analysis of patients who had participated in the Italian GONO group's phase II and III studies of FOLFOXIRI, and subsequently underwent R0 resection of metastatic disease, was recently published *(116)*. Of 196 patients in total participating in these trials, 37 who were initially unresectable eventually underwent R0 resection after a median of 5.5 months of FOLFOXIRI (longer than is conventionally used in the neoadjuvant setting). The 5-year and 8-year survival of these patients was 42% and 33%. Notably, steatohepatitis was seen in only 5% of the patients at surgery. While this was not a preplanned study of neoadjuvant therapy - a problem with most of these analyses of resection rates following chemotherapy - it nevertheless provides some insight into the benefits of aggressive neoadjuvant chemotherapy prior to resection.

With respect to whether the optimal approach for potentially resectable metastatic disease is neoadjuvant and/or adjuvant therapy, randomized clinical trials have been carried out, but to date do not provide all the necessary answers. A randomized EORTC Intergroup trial comparing preoperative chemotherapy with FOLFOX4 prior to surgery with surgery alone for resectable liver metastases was published in 2008 *(117)*. This international trial assessed 364 patients who had up to four liver metastases and received either six cycles of FOLFOX4 both before and after surgery, or surgery alone (without any chemotherapy). In the intention-to-treat analysis, the progression-free survival was 28.1% in the surgery-alone arm and 35.4% in the chemotherapy arm, the difference not quite statistically significant (hazard ratio 0.79, $p=0.058$). Overall survival is still being monitored at this time. Of note, the postoperative complication rate was significantly increased in patients who received neoadjuvant chemotherapy. In 2008, Mitry et al published a pooled analysis of two randomized trials (278 patients in total) assessing adjuvant therapy after potentially curative resection of CRC metastases (liver or lung), vs. surgery alone *(118)*. Both trials had closed prematurely due to slow accrual, so lacked statistical power; and both used bolus 5FU/leucovorin without oxaliplatin or irinotecan. Median progression-free survival was marginally higher in the adjuvant chemotherapy arms (27.9 months vs. 18.8 months, $p=0.058$). Median overall survival was higher, but not statistically significantly so (62.2 months vs. 47.3 months, $p=0.095$).

At present, we still do not have the answer to the question of whether preoperative (neoadjuvant) or postoperative (adjuvant) therapy, or both together (perioperative), are the most important aspects of chemotherapy treatment for resectable metastatic disease, and trials are planned which address further these questions. Our recommended current practice if metastatic disease is immediately resectable and the tumor burden is small is to operate first, then administer postoperative 'adjuvant metastatic' chemotherapy. If disease is borderline resectable or there is large volume disease, or there is strong likelihood of micrometastatic disease being present (e.g., due to high-risk nodal disease and/or short disease-free interval), then neoadjuvant combination chemotherapy with the aim to downsize is given, with close multidisciplinary evaluation (approximately every 6–8 weeks), in order to avoid toxicities (in particular hepatotoxicity) from chemotherapy. Generally, further postoperative chemotherapy should be given, even for an R0 (complete) resection and certainly for an incomplete or R1–R2 resection (microscopic or macroscopic residual disease). However, management strategies differ around the globe, *(106)* and ultimately results from further trials comparing neoadjuvant with adjuvant therapies are awaited.

WHEN SHOULD CHEMOTHERAPY BE GIVEN TO ASYMPTOMATIC PATIENTS?

Although cancer can cause a range of symptoms – both local (bleeding, obstruction, pain) and systemic (cachexia, fevers, pain) – it is not infrequent to encounter patients with metastatic disease who are relatively asymptomatic at the time of diagnosis. The decision whether to treat such patients up-front, or adapt a 'watch-and-wait' or expectant approach, reserving treatment for when a patient may become symptomatic or develop clear radiological or clinical progression, may be difficult.

Two publications in particular have addressed this question. The Nordic Gastrointestinal Tumor Adjuvant Therapy Group in 1992 published results from a randomized trial of 183 patients, using methotrexate (no longer used) and 5FU/leucovorin *(119)*. Overall survival was found to be better in the immediate chemotherapy group with a difference in median survival of around 5 months. Notably, 43% of patients randomized to the expectant arm did not end up receiving any chemotherapy. A more recent Australian meta-analysis of two randomized trials of early vs. delayed chemotherapy was published in 2005 *(120)*. This was prospectively planned and combined two trials from Australasia and Canada. The chemotherapy given was 5FU/leucovorin (not irinotecan or oxaliplatin), either up-front or at the time that defined clinical criteria were met. In total, 168 patients were assessed. Median survival was not significantly increased with immediate vs. delayed treatment (13 months vs. 11 months, hazard ratio 1.15, $p=0.49$), and there were no differences in quality of life between the two arms at any time point. In this study 30% of patients in the expectant arm did not receive any chemotherapy. The conclusion from this small meta-analysis was that withholding treatment until symptoms occurred is a reasonable strategy.

In helping a patient to make a decision regarding treatment of asymptomatic but incurable metastatic disease, the art of medicine comes into play, balancing the risk of toxicity and relative loss of freedom that regular chemotherapy administration entails, with the risk that untreated disease may ultimately shorten lifespan and the patient may deteriorate rapidly to the point that chemotherapy is unfeasible. Discussion about when to treat should always involve the patient in the decision-making process.

TARGETED THERAPIES IN CURRENT CLINICAL USE

Translational Research in Action

CRC provides an excellent example of the benefits of translational research, by which discoveries involving the molecular make-up of a cancer cell as well as factors other than DNA which promote replication, can be used as drug targets. In theory, these 'switches' or pathways are more active in cancer cells or the cancer microenvironment compared with normal cells or host tissues. While significant progress has already been made, intense research continues into targets and biomarkers which can be used to optimize therapy. Significant changes in management have occurred based on recent discoveries, which will be overviewed below.

Two particular targets that have led to the routine clinical use of targeted agents in metastatic CRC are vascular endothelial growth factor (VEGF) (and its receptor complex) and the epidermal growth factor receptor complex (EGFR). VEGF is an angiogenic factor overexpressed in approximately 50% of CRCs *(121)*. The binding of VEGF to receptors triggers a series of events in normal endothelial cells and potentially tumor cells involving cell proliferation, angiogenesis, and cell survival via intracellular tyrosine kinase pathways *(122)*. The EGFR gene is overexpressed or upregulated in 60–80% of CRCs *(123)*. Blocking the EGFR can lead to cell cycle arrest in the G1 phase and cell death via apoptosis *(124,125)*.

However, to be effective, inhibitors of the EGFR require a particular molecular genotype involving downstream signaling pathways – most specifically *k-ras*. This is an intracellular proto-oncogene, and part of the downstream pathway from EGFR. It is mutated in approximately 40% of colon cancers *(126,127)*, but less frequently in rectal cancers, between 15 and 30% *(128,129)*. Mutations can lead to constitutive activation of the intracellular pathway and render more proximal EGFR blockade ineffective. K-ras mutant tumors generally do not respond to therapy targeting the EGFR. This was not appreciated at the time of many of the earlier trials of anti-EGFR therapy and only became apparent in late 2007. Thus, prior trials have now been reassessed with a view to compare responses to therapy in patients with tumors that contain nonmutated k-ras (wild-type) vs. mutated versions of k-ras (k-ras mutant tumors). All subsequent studies using anti-EGFR therapies now exclude patients with k-ras mutant tumors. The use of biomarkers to help select patients for therapy has thus become a reality in this disease, and this is likely to continue to increase as more molecular targets are described.

Drugs in Routine Clinical Use

Bevacizumab

Bevacizumab is a humanized monoclonal antibody targeting VEGF; bevacizumab in combination with chemotherapy is now regarded as appropriate first-line therapy for metastatic CRC and is regarded as part of the standard of care in many countries. After a small phase II study suggested that bevacizumab had efficacy in combination with 5FU/LV in metastatic CRC *(130)*, a phase III trial in 813 previously untreated patients with metastatic CRC randomized to IFL +/– bevacizumab demonstrated a significant median overall survival advantage favoring the experimental arm (20.3 months vs. 15.6 months, $p<0.001$) *(131)*. An analysis of three trials using 5FU/LV +/– bevacizumab demonstrated a 17.9 months vs. 14.6 months ($p=0.008$) median overall survival advantage with the combination compared with 5FU-based treatment alone *(132)*. In the three arm ECOG 3200 study, FOLFOX4 +/– bevacizumab was compared with bevacizumab alone in 822 patients with previously treated metastatic CRC *(133)*. The bevacizumab-alone arm was discontinued due to inferiority at an interim analysis. An improvement in median survival (12.9 months vs. 10.8 months, $p=0.0024$) as well as a significant increased response rate and improved progression-free survival were seen in the FOLFOX4 plus bevacizumab arm. The TREE-2 study added bevacizumab to three different oxaliplatin-containing regimens in first-line therapy and found improved response rates and time to progression when compared to chemotherapy alone *(134)*. An additional large randomized study assessing FOLFOX4 or XELOX with or without bevacizumab enrolled 1,401 patients and demonstrated significant improvement in progression-free survival with the addition of bevacizumab (9.4 months vs. 8 months, $p=0.0023$) but the median overall survival benefit did not reach statistical significance (21.3 months vs. 19.9 months, $p=0.077$) *(135)*. Response rates were similar in the two arms. The authors postulated that the benefit of bevacizumab may have been diminished by the fact that only 29% of patients receiving bevacizumab actually continued the drug until progression. Kabbinavar et al combined data from three randomized clinical studies of first-line therapy comparing 5FU/LV with or without bevacizumab and demonstrated a significant survival improvement (17.9 months vs. 14.6 months, $p=0.008$) *(132)*. These trials all demonstrate that bevacizumab has activity when combined with a variety of chemotherapy regimens, and in both the first and second-line disease settings.

The toxicities of bevacizumab when added to chemotherapy may include hypertension, bleeding, arterial thrombotic events, proteinuria (mostly mild), and rarely, gastro-intestinal perforation *(131)*. The BRiTE and First BEAT registries were established to evaluate the safety profile of bevacizumab in a population outside that of clinical trials, using bevacizumab in combination with a range of chemotherapy regimens. The First BEAT registry enrolled approximately 2,000 patients from 41 countries *(136)*. No new safety issues were reported. The BRiTE registry conducted in the United States also enrolled around 2,000 patients *(137)*. Again, toxicities were similar to that reported in prior clinical trials. Given these toxicities, the use of bevacizumab in the perioperative setting has been closely examined. Bevacizumab is reported to be associated with wound healing complications *(138)*, and it is generally recommended that approximately 4–6 weeks elapse before or after surgery if bevacizumab has been or is to be administered. Early data suggest that this is a safe strategy *(139)*, and trials in the perioperative setting are ongoing.

Whether bevacizumab should be continued beyond disease progression, or used as maintenance therapy, remains subject to ongoing clinical trials. Data from the BRiTE registry seems to suggest a benefit. Of 1,445 patients who had developed disease progression on first-line therapy, physicians chose to continue bevacizumab in 642 of these patients, and these patients appeared to have a significantly improved survival compared to those who received chemotherapy without bevacizumab or received no chemotherapy (HR 0.48, $p<0.001$) *(137)*. However, this result is subject to potential bias as it is likely that patients who were more fit and had a better performance status were selected to receive ongoing bevacizumab.

Cetuximab

This chimeric monoclonal antibody, targeting the extracellular domain of the EGFR or HER-1, has demonstrated activity in metastatic CRC. The response to cetuximab in CRC appears to be independent of EGFR expression as measured by immunohistochemistry *(140,141)*, but is dependent on tumors demonstrating wild-type k-ras. Cetuximab is ineffective in K-ras mutant tumors. Thus, trials which were conducted and reported prior to the understanding of the importance of this biomarker have subsequently been reanalyzed where possible to look at outcomes for patients with k-ras wild-type vs. k-ras mutant tumors. In the main, striking results have been seen.

Unlike bevacizumab, cetuximab has single-agent activity as well as demonstrating activity in combination with chemotherapy. In the BOND-1 study of 329 participants refractory to oxaliplatin and irinotecan, randomized to cetuximab plus irinotecan or cetuximab alone, a significantly higher response rate and median time to progression for the combination was seen, although overall survival was no different *(141)*. A multinational study (CO.17) of 572 patients exposed to prior fluoropyrimidine, irinotecan, and oxaliplatin compared cetuximab monotherapy with best supportive care *(142)*. Cetuximab was associated with a significant improvement in overall survival (median survival 6.1 months vs. 4.6 months; hazard ratio 0.77, $p=0.005$) and progression-free survival (hazard ratio 0.68, $p<0.001$). Importantly, quality of life was also better preserved in the cetuximab group. These findings were observed in the total study population, including those patients whose tumors contained k-ras mutations. As information regarding the significance of k-ras became available, this trial was reanalyzed: of the 572 patients who participated, tumor samples were available for 394 patients and 42.3% had at least one mutation *(143)*. For k-ras wild-type tumors, the median survival seen in the group randomized to cetuximab was 9.5 months vs. 4.8 months (hazard ratio 0.55, $p<0.001$) in the control arm. Patients with tumors harboring mutated k-ras derived no clinical benefit with cetuximab (hazard ratio for death 0.98). In this study, for patients receiving supportive care alone, the mutation status of the k-ras gene was not significantly associated with overall survival (implying that k-ras mutational status is a predictive but not a prognostic factor).

Key studies of cetuximab in combination with chemotherapy are the CRYSTAL and OPUS studies. The CRYSTAL study randomized 1,198 patients to FOLFIRI with or without cetuximab in the first-line setting and demonstrated significant improvements in progression-free survival and overall response for the combination *(144)* When reanalyzed, looking specifically at k-ras status, tumor samples were evaluable for 540 of the patients; 35.6% had tumors with mutated k-ras. Similarly to the CO.17 analysis, the addition of cetuximab to chemotherapy benefitted patients with k-ras wild-type tumors but not k-ras mutant tumors *(144)*. An improvement in median survival by 3.9 months (24.9 months vs. 21 months) was seen for patients whose tumors were k-ras wild-type but the difference was not statistically significant ($p=0.22$), perhaps because of cross-over to cetuximab on progression in patients in the control arm of this study. Interestingly of those receiving FOLFIRI alone, median overall survival was 21 months for k-ras wild-type and 17.7 months for k-ras mutant tumors. The OPUS study was a randomized phase II trial comparing first-line FOLFOX with FOLFOX plus cetuximab *(145)*. It did not demonstrate significant improvements in overall response or progression-free survival for the combination arm. However, when analyzed by k-ras mutational status (tumor samples were available for 233 of the 337 original patients), response rates (61% vs. 37%) and progression free survival (7.7 months vs. 7.2 months) were significantly improved in patients whose tumors were k-ras wild-type with the addition of cetuximab.

The main side effect of cetuximab is an acneiform skin rash, occurring in up to 89% of patients *(146)*; the degree of skin reaction correlates with response rate which may relate to the relative expression of the EGFR in normal tissues relative to tumors *(140,147)*. The EVEREST trial further demonstrated that in patients with tumors that were wild-type k-ras, the efficacy of cetuximab could be improved by escalating the dose of cetuximab in patients with grade 0 or 1 skin reactions *(148)*.

Panitumumab

This antibody also targets the EGFR but in contrast to cetuximab, it is derived from a transgenic mouse which produces fully human antibodies *(149)*. It is generally used as monotherapy. There is currently no evidence to suggest that panitumumab is effective after progression on cetuximab, and vice-versa, and the NCCN does not recommend use of one after failure on the other *(150)*. Similar to cetuximab, k-ras mutational status is predictive of response to panitumumab. A phase III trial comparing panitumumab with best supportive care in 463 patients with metastatic CRC after progression on irinotecan and oxaliplatin, showed that panitumumab significantly prolonged progression-free survival; although the median difference was small (8 weeks vs. 7.3 weeks, $p<0.0001$), the hazard ratio was significantly different (HR 0.54), and the response rate 10% vs. 0% *(151)*. There was no difference in overall survival (but crossover was permitted, so the majority of patients assigned to best supportive care received panitumumab on disease progression). The trial was reanalyzed after the importance of k-ras became known: 427 of the 463 patients entered were able to have k-ras status tested *(126)*. Progression-free survival for patients with k-ras wild-type tumors was significantly better (12.3 weeks vs. 7.3 weeks, HR 0.45, $p<0.0001$) while there was no difference in outcome for patients whose tumors were k-ras mutant. Thus, the clinical benefit of panitumumab was seen entirely in k-ras wild-type tumors. In this study, wild-type k-ras status was a predictor for overall survival in both the panitumumab and best supportive care arms. This is contrary to the finding from the CO.17 study where k-ras status had no effect on the survival outcomes of patients in the best supportive care arm and again raises the possibility of k-ras being a prognostic as well as a predictive factor.

Rash of some degree occurred in over 90% of patients (although prophylactic or early intervention strategies may ameliorate the rash in the majority of patients *(152,153)*), and hypomagnesaemia occurred in 38% of patients in this trial, although in general allergic reactions appear less frequent than is the case with cetuximab.

Combining Targeted Therapies: Lessons Learned

Similarly to chemotherapy approaches which combine all active agents (e.g., FOLFOXIRI), studies examining the effectiveness of combining multiple targeted agents together have also been conducted. The theory behind this approach, while plausible (attacking multiple growth pathways in cancer cells at once may be more effective at killing cells and reducing resistance than doing so sequentially), has not proved fruitful. Despite preclinical studies suggesting benefits from the combination of combined anti-VEGF and anti-EGFR therapy, results have been disappointing.

While encouraging results were initially seen – the BOND-2 randomized phase II study demonstrated efficacy in treating patients with irinotecan-refractory CRC with cetuximab and bevacizumab *(154)* – this could not be proven in much larger phase III studies (specifically, the CAIRO-2 and PACCE trials – see below). In the BOND-2 trial, 83 patients were randomized to receive cetuximab and bevacizumab, with or without irinotecan. Toxicities were similar to that expected from each agent alone. Patients in the three-drug arm had better outcomes: time to progression 7.3 months vs. 4.9 months, response rate 37% vs. 20%, and median survival 14.5 months vs. 11.4 months *(154)*.

The CAIRO-2 study was a Dutch trial involving 775 patients randomized to receive CAPOX plus bevacizumab, with or without cetuximab, as first-line therapy *(155)*. K-ras mutation status was evaluated in all patients. Unexpectedly, progression-free survival was worse in the cetuximab arm (9.4 months vs. 10.7 months, $p=0.01$). Quality of life was also worse for the combination arm. Overall survival and response rates did not differ significantly. Patients with k-ras mutations treated with cetuximab had a significantly worse progression-free survival, not just compared with wild-type tumors treated with cetuximab, but also compared to patients with a similar genotype treated without cetuximab. Similar adverse outcomes were also seen in the PACCE study, a study conducted in patients with previously untreated metastatic CRC : 823 patients received either FOLFOX or FOLFIRI (at the treating doctor's discretion) and bevacizumab, with or without panitumumab (randomized) *(156)*. Median progression-free survival was worse in the panitumumab arm (10.0 months vs. 11.4 months) as was the median survival (19.4 months vs. 24.5 months). Adverse outcomes for the panitumumab arm were seen in both k-ras wild-type and mutant groups. There was also an excess of serious toxicity including skin toxicity, diarrhea, and infections. The reasons for these inferior outcomes when combining bevacizumab and cetuximab or panitumumab remain puzzling. A phamacokinetic or pharmacodynamic interaction between the two monoclonal antibodies is possible.

Despite such setbacks along the way, targeted therapies have brought significant benefits to patients with metastatic CRC. A large meta-analysis by Golfinopoulos et al *(157)* reviewed 242 randomized trials (56,677 patients) from 1967 to 2007 comparing systemic treatment regimens in advanced CRC. The sheer number of trials alone exemplifies the work that has been carried out over these four decades in the treatment of this disease. Thirty-seven of the trials were used in a multiple-treatment meta-analysis, which found that compared with 5FU/leucovorin alone, the risk of death was most decreased with the addition of irinotecan plus bevacizumab (hazard ratio 0.6) and significant benefits were seen with the addition of irinotecan plus oxaliplatin (FOLFOXIRI) (HR 0.72), oxaliplatin plus bevacizumab (HR 0.72), bevacizumab alone (HR 0.78), and oxaliplatin alone (HR 0.87). The absolute survival benefit for the use of irinotecan plus bevacizumab is estimated at 8 months (compared with 5FU/leucovorin alone). Since this study, considerably more trials have been published, particularly in the context of improved selection of patients given the role of k-ras as a biomarker, so whether these findings would improve further is likely but speculative at this point.

MOLECULAR DIFFERENCES BETWEEN COLON AND RECTAL CANCER

With the increased understanding of the importance of molecular subtypes of tumors using biomarkers which may be used as prognostic and/or predictive markers, an appreciation of the differences between colon and rectal cancers has been emerging in recent years. It is well-known that microsatellite instability (MSI) is more commonly associated with proximal tumors and is seldom seen in rectal tumors *(158,159)*; however, it appears that multiple biological differences exist between colon and rectal cancers. The hope is that this knowledge will translate into trials specifically designed to target the biology of a particular tumor, rather than the more conventional approach which has been to group colon and rectal cancers together. While there are similarities, more recent research suggests that it may be more accurate to regard colon and rectal cancer as two distinct entities.

Frattini et al in a molecular study of sporadic CRC described two distinct pathways in CRC development: k-ras dependent (more commonly in colon cancers) and k-ras independent (more commonly in rectal cancers) *(129)* and found significant differences in combinations of genetic alterations (including the APC, TP53, and k-ras genes as well as in chromosome 18q) between colon and rectal cancers. Other researchers have also demonstrated significant differences in gene mutations and other biomarkers in rectal vs. colon cancers *(160,161)*, supporting the theory that the mechanisms of oncogenesis may be different in rectal cancers from colon cancers.

One of the next generation of biomarkers likely to be of considerable interest in CRC is b-raf. This gene encodes a tyrosine kinase, which plays an important role in the ras-raf-MEK-ERK signaling pathway and is thought to be associated with the MSI pathway of colorectal tumorigenesis. B-raf and k-ras mutations are mutually exclusive *(162)*. B-raf mutations also appear to confer resistance to anti-EGFR monoclonal antibody therapy *(163)*. B-raf inhibitors are undergoing early phase clinical trials in a number of malignancies including CRC. However, the important point that colon and rectal cancer are not the same disease is exemplified by the fact that b-raf mutations are seen almost exclusively in colon cancer and rarely in rectal cancer *(164,165)*. It seems likely that in the future, clinical trials may need to distinguish rectal cancers from colon cancers, a step which to date has not happened in the treatment of metastatic disease.

WHAT LIES AHEAD?

Progress in the management of metastatic CRC over the last decade has been significant. We are now starting to be able to tailor therapy based on particular tumor characteristics, as exemplified by the k-ras story. It seems likely that in the future, as the significance of other biomarkers becomes apparent, that other tailoring strategies based on tumor phenotype or genotype will be feasible. The ultimate goal is personalized therapy, for which the characteristics of an individual patient and their tumor are taken into consideration when choosing therapy, recognizing and understanding the influence of each on response to treatment and likely outcomes (Fig. 4). Gene expression signatures may be used in the future to predict response to particular anticancer agents *(166)* as more prognostic and predictive factors continue to emerge for both CRC and other malignancies.

The evolution of targeted therapies and their integration into routine practice is likely to expand. In particular, the role of 'maintenance' targeted agents is being explored in studies such as the DREAM (OPTIMOX3) trial, which is assessing the role of maintenance bevacizumab and erlotinib (an oral EGFR tyrosine kinase inhibitor) *(167)*. The efficacy of continuing bevacizumab beyond disease progression into the second-line setting will also be evaluated prospectively.

There are many ongoing trials in metastatic CRC. A systematic review of actively enrolling metastatic CRC trials from the databases of the National Cancer Institute and Investigative Drug Branch was published in 2008, finding over 100 trials were currently enrolling at the time *(168)*. A concern was raised that only 13% of trials were investigating novel agents not yet FDA-approved for any oncology indication, and that only 3% of patients were enrolled onto trials centered on tumor characteristics hypothesized to improve clinical benefit. This is likely to change as the recognition of specific tumor characteristics as biomarkers and prognostic or predictive markers expands. An international collaborative approach is necessary to conduct trials using biomarkers, which will by definition reduce the number of patients suitable for a particular study – as a result, the 'gold standard' randomized study is likely to be less feasible when investigating therapies based on specific tumor or patient characteristics. Different approaches to clinical trial design have been suggested, such as a multiarm, multistage strategies in which intermediate outcomes are measured and experimental arms discontinued early if they do not show promise *(169)*. There are multiple ongoing studies evaluating the role of novel agents such as angiogenesis inhibitors and growth factor inhibitors in metastatic CRC. As more is understood about the molecular pathways that help to drive cancer, it seems likely that more and more novel agents will be developed; however, patients will need to be carefully selected for participation in trials depending on their tumor phenotype and genotype.

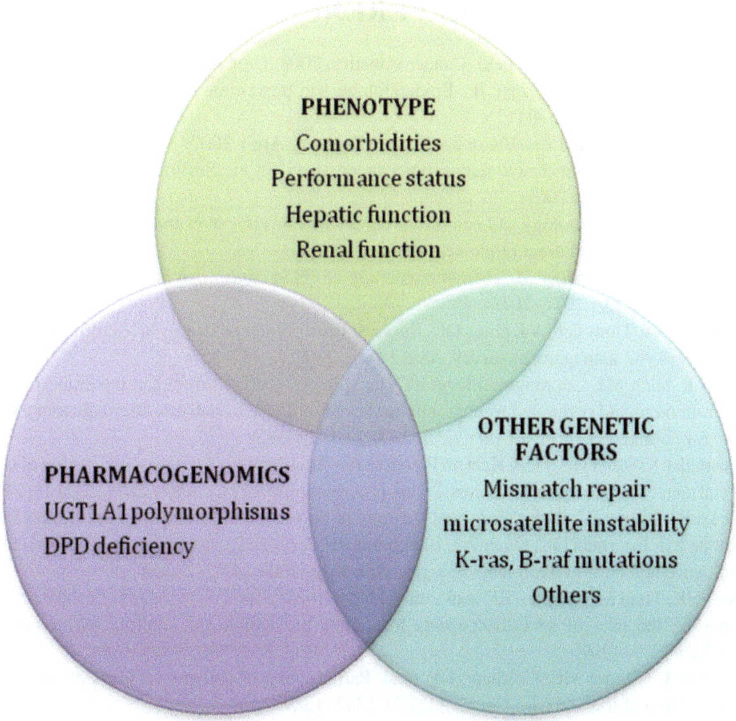

Fig. 4. Interactions between phenotype and genotype which may help to guide personalized therapy.

CONCLUSION

The management of metastatic CRC in the twenty-first century is becoming increasingly complex, with the development of innovative new therapies and further scope for combinations of active agents. In addition, there have been significant advances in surgical and other ablative and local techniques. It seems certain that targeted therapies will become a major component of the management of early as well as advanced CRC in the future. Multidisciplinary input into the management of this disease remains critical as significant advances based on translational research and the further understanding of tumor biology emerge. In ideal circumstances, at the time of diagnosis, the genetic and biological profile of a tumor and the normal host tissues of a patient would be assessed, prognostic and predictive markers analyzed in the former and risk factors for treatment toxicities in the latter, and a treatment regimen developed for an individual patient based on these factors. The likelihood of such individualized therapy is on our doorstep but relies on the continuing liaison between scientists and clinicians to bring these strategies from the bench to the bedside and the bedside to the bench.

Overall, the significant gains made in the last decade are beginning to significantly impact the survival and the quality of life for people affected with this devastating disease, leading to much hope that terminal metastatic CRC may one day become a rarity.

REFERENCES

1. Jemal A, Siegel R, Ward E, et al. Cancer statistics, 2008. *CA Cancer J Clin.* 2008;58:71–96.
2. Hawk ET, Limburg PJ, Viner JL. Epidemiology and prevention of colorectal cancer. *Surg Clin North Am.* 2002;82:905–941.
3. Cancer survival, Victoria. Victorian Cancer Registry, April 2007. http://www.cancervic.org.au/downloads/about_our_research/canstats/cancer_survival_vic/Survival_2007_Full_Report.pdf; 2007. Accessed June 2009.
4. Surveillance epidemiology and end results cancer fact sheets: colon and rectum. http://seer.cancer.gov/statfacts/html/colorect.html; Accessed June 2009.
5. Cunningham D, Findlay M. The chemotherapy of colon cancer can no longer be ignored. *Eur J Cancer.* 1993;29A:2077–2079.
6. McLeish JA, Thursfield VJ, Giles GG. Survival from colorectal cancer in Victoria: 10-year follow up of the 1987 management survey. *ANZ J Surg.* 2002;72:352–356.
7. Chau I, Allen MJ, Cunningham D, et al. The value of routine serum carcino-embryonic antigen measurement and computed tomography in the surveillance of patients after adjuvant chemotherapy for colorectal cancer. *J Clin Oncol.* 2004;22:1420–1429.
8. Kosmider S, Stella DL, Field K, et al. Preoperative investigations for metastatic staging of colon and rectal cancer across multiple centres – what is current practice? *Colorectal Dis.* 2009;11:592–600.
9. Heald RJ, Moran BJ. Embryology and anatomy of the rectum. *Semin Surg Oncol.* 1998;15:66–71.
10. Koppe MJ, Boerman OC, Oyen WJ, Bleichrodt RP. Peritoneal carcinomatosis of colorectal origin: incidence and current treatment strategies. *Ann Surg.* 2006;243:212–222.
11. Weir HK, Thun MJ, Hankey BF, et al. Annual report to the nation on the status of cancer, 1975–2000, featuring the uses of surveillance data for cancer prevention and control. *J Natl Cancer Inst.* 2003;95:1276–1299.
12. Lewis JH, Kilgore ML, Goldman DP, et al. Participation of patients 65 years of age or older in cancer clinical trials. *J Clin Oncol.* 2003;21:1383–1389.
13. Hutchins LF, Unger JM, Crowley JJ, Coltman CA Jr, Albain KS. Underrepresentation of patients 65 years of age or older in cancer-treatment trials. *N Engl J Med.* 1999;341:2061–2067.
14. DeVita VT Jr, Chu E. A history of cancer chemotherapy. *Cancer Res.* 2008;68:8643–8653.
15. Heidelberger C, Chaudhuri NK, Danneberg P, et al. Fluorinated pyrimidines, a new class of tumour-inhibitory compounds. *Nature.* 1957;179:663–666.
16. Moertel CG. Gastrointestinal cancer. Treatment with fluorouracil-nitrosourea combinations. *JAMA.* 1976;235:2135–2136.
17. Moertel CG. Chemotherapy of gastrointestinal cancer. *N Engl J Med.* 1978;299:1049–1052.
18. Moertel CG. Colorectal cancer: chemotherapy as surgical adjuvant treatment. *Bull Cancer.* 1983;70:329–338.
19. Jonker DJ, Maroun JA, Kocha W. Survival benefit of chemotherapy in metastatic colorectal cancer: a meta-analysis of randomized controlled trials. *Br J Cancer.* 2000;82:1789–1794.
20. Cunningham D, Pyrhonen S, James RD, et al. Randomised trial of irinotecan plus supportive care versus supportive care alone after fluorouracil failure for patients with metastatic colorectal cancer. *Lancet.* 1998;352:1413–1418.
21. Petrelli N, Douglass HO Jr, Herrera L, et al. The modulation of fluorouracil with leucovorin in metastatic colorectal carcinoma: a prospective randomized phase III trial. Gastrointestinal Tumor Study Group. *J Clin Oncol.* 1989;7:1419–1426.
22. Advanced Colorectal Cancer Meta-Analysis Project. Modulation of fluorouracil by leucovorin in patients with advanced colorectal cancer: evidence in terms of response rate. *J Clin Oncol.* 1992;10:896–903.
23. Zhang ZG, Harstrick A, Rustum YM. Modulation of fluoropyrimidines: role of dose and schedule of leucovorin administration. *Semin Oncol.* 1992;19:10–15.
24. Ychou M, Fabbro-Peray P, Perney P, et al. A prospective randomized study comparing high- and low-dose leucovorin combined with same-dose 5-fluorouracil in advanced colorectal cancer. *Am J Clin Oncol.* 1998;21:233–236.

25. Jager E, Heike M, Bernhard H, et al. Weekly high-dose leucovorin versus low-dose leucovorin combined with fluorouracil in advanced colorectal cancer: results of a randomized multicenter trial. Study Group for Palliative Treatment of Metastatic Colorectal Cancer Study Protocol 1. *J Clin Oncol.* 1996;14:2274–2279.
26. Dencausse Y, Hartung G, Sturm J, et al. Adjuvant chemotherapy in stage III colon cancer with 5-fluorouracil and levamisole versus 5-fluorouracil and leucovorin. *Onkologie.* 2002;25:426–430.
27. Haller DG, Catalano PJ, Macdonald JS, et al. Phase III study of fluorouracil, leucovorin, and levamisole in high-risk stage II and III colon cancer: final report of Intergroup 0089. *J Clin Oncol.* 2005;23:8671–8678.
28. Valone FH, Friedman MA, Wittlinger PS, et al. Treatment of patients with advanced colorectal carcinomas with fluorouracil alone, high-dose leucovorin plus fluorouracil, or sequential methotrexate, fluorouracil, and leucovorin: a randomized trial of the Northern California Oncology Group. *J Clin Oncol.* 1989;7:1427–1436.
29. Petrelli N, Herrera L, Rustum Y, et al. A prospective randomized trial of 5-fluorouracil versus 5-fluorouracil and high-dose leucovorin versus 5-fluorouracil and methotrexate in previously untreated patients with advanced colorectal carcinoma. *J Clin Oncol.* 1987;5:1559–1565.
30. Poon MA, O'Connell MJ, Moertel CG, et al. Biochemical modulation of fluorouracil: evidence of significant improvement of survival and quality of life in patients with advanced colorectal carcinoma. *J Clin Oncol.* 1989;7:1407–1418.
31. Meta-analysis Group In Cancer. Efficacy of intravenous continuous infusion of fluorouracil compared with bolus administration in advanced colorectal cancer. *J Clin Oncol.* 1998;16:301–308.
32. Folprecht G, Cunningham D, Ross P, et al. Efficacy of 5-fluorouracil-based chemotherapy in elderly patients with metastatic colorectal cancer: a pooled analysis of clinical trials. *Ann Oncol.* 2004;15:1330–1338.
33. Papamichael D. The use of thymidylate synthase inhibitors in the treatment of advanced colorectal cancer: current status. *Oncologist.* 1999;4:478–487.
34. Hoff PM, Ansari R, Batist G, et al. Comparison of oral capecitabine versus intravenous fluorouracil plus leucovorin as first-line treatment in 605 patients with metastatic colorectal cancer: results of a randomized phase III study. *J Clin Oncol.* 2001;19:2282–2292.
35. Van Cutsem E, Hoff PM, Harper P, et al. Oral capecitabine vs intravenous 5-fluorouracil and leucovorin: integrated efficacy data and novel analyses from two large, randomised, phase III trials. *Br J Cancer.* 2004;90:1190–1197.
36. Van Cutsem E, Twelves C, Cassidy J, et al. Oral capecitabine compared with intravenous fluorouracil plus leucovorin in patients with metastatic colorectal cancer: results of a large phase III study. *J Clin Oncol.* 2001;19:4097–4106.
37. Twelves C, Wong A, Nowacki MP, et al. Capecitabine as adjuvant treatment for stage III colon cancer. *N Engl J Med.* 2005;352:2696–2704.
38. Glen H, Cassidy J. Redefining adjuvant chemotherapy in patients with stage III colon cancer: X-ACT trial. *Expert Rev Anticancer Ther.* 2008;8:547–551.
39. Hoff PM, Cassidy J, Schmoll HJ. The evolution of fluoropyrimidine therapy: from intravenous to oral. *Oncologist.* 2001;6(suppl 4):3–11.
40. Hoff PM, Pazdur R, Lassere Y, et al. Phase II study of capecitabine in patients with fluorouracil-resistant metastatic colorectal carcinoma. *J Clin Oncol.* 2004;22:2078–2083.
41. Lee JJ, Kim TM, Yu SJ, et al. Single-agent capecitabine in patients with metastatic colorectal cancer refractory to 5-fluorouracil/leucovorin chemotherapy. *Jpn J Clin Oncol.* 2004;34:400–404.
42. Gubanski M, Naucler G, Almerud A, Lidestahl A, Lind PA. Capecitabine as third line therapy in patients with advanced colorectal cancer. *Acta Oncol.* 2005;44:236–239.
43. Douillard JY, Hoff PM, Skillings JR, et al. Multicenter phase III study of uracil/tegafur and oral leucovorin versus fluorouracil and leucovorin in patients with previously untreated metastatic colorectal cancer. *J Clin Oncol.* 2002;20:3605–3616.
44. Saif MW, Syrigos KN, Katirtzoglou NA. S-1: a promising new oral fluoropyrimidine derivative. *Expert Opin Investig Drugs.* 2009;18:335–348.

45. Raymond E, Buquet-Fagot C, Djelloul S, et al. Antitumor activity of oxaliplatin in combination with 5-fluorouracil and the thymidylate synthase inhibitor AG337 in human colon, breast and ovarian cancers. *Anticancer Drugs*. 1997;8:876–885.
46. Rothenberg ML, Oza AM, Bigelow RH, et al. Superiority of oxaliplatin and fluorouracil-leucovorin compared with either therapy alone in patients with progressive colorectal cancer after irinotecan and fluorouracil-leucovorin: interim results of a phase III trial. *J Clin Oncol*. 2003;21:2059–2069.
47. de Gramont A, Figer A, Seymour M, et al. Leucovorin and fluorouracil with or without oxaliplatin as first-line treatment in advanced colorectal cancer. *J Clin Oncol*. 2000;18:2938–2947.
48. Cassidy J, Clarke S, Diaz-Rubio E, et al. Randomized phase III study of capecitabine plus oxaliplatin compared with fluorouracil/folinic acid plus oxaliplatin as first-line therapy for metastatic colorectal cancer. *J Clin Oncol*. 2008;26:2006–2012.
49. Arkenau HT, Arnold D, Cassidy J, et al. Efficacy of oxaliplatin plus capecitabine or infusional fluorouracil/leucovorin in patients with metastatic colorectal cancer: a pooled analysis of randomized trials. *J Clin Oncol*. 2008;26:5910–5917.
50. Andre T, Boni C, Mounedji-Boudiaf L, et al. Oxaliplatin, fluorouracil, and leucovorin as adjuvant treatment for colon cancer. *N Engl J Med*. 2004;350:2343–2351.
51. Cersosimo RJ. Oxaliplatin-associated neuropathy: a review. *Ann Pharmacother*. 2005;39:128–135.
52. Gamelin E, Gamelin L, Bossi L, Quasthoff S. Clinical aspects and molecular basis of oxaliplatin neurotoxicity: current management and development of preventive measures. *Semin Oncol*. 2002;29:21–33.
53. Cassidy J, Misset JL. Oxaliplatin-related side effects: characteristics and management. *Semin Oncol*. 2002;29:11–20.
54. Hsiang YH, Liu LF. Identification of mammalian DNA topoisomerase I as an intracellular target of the anticancer drug camptothecin. *Cancer Res*. 1988;48:1722–1726.
55. Saltz LB, Cox JV, Blanke C, et al. Irinotecan plus fluorouracil and leucovorin for metastatic colorectal cancer. Irinotecan Study Group. *N Engl J Med*. 2000;343:905–914.
56. Douillard JY, Cunningham D, Roth AD, et al. Irinotecan combined with fluorouracil compared with fluorouracil alone as first-line treatment for metastatic colorectal cancer: a multicentre randomised trial. *Lancet*. 2000;355:1041–1047.
57. Fuchs CS, Marshall J, Mitchell E, et al. Randomized, controlled trial of irinotecan plus infusional, bolus, or oral fluoropyrimidines in first-line treatment of metastatic colorectal cancer: results from the BICC-C Study. *J Clin Oncol*. 2007;25:4779–4786.
58. Toffoli G, Cecchin E, Corona G, et al. The role of UGT1A1*28 polymorphism in the pharmacodynamics and pharmacokinetics of irinotecan in patients with metastatic colorectal cancer. *J Clin Oncol*. 2006;24:3061–3068.
59. Lankisch TO, Schulz C, Zwingers T, et al. Gilbert's Syndrome and irinotecan toxicity: combination with UDP-glucuronosyltransferase 1A7 variants increases risk. *Cancer Epidemiol Biomarkers Prev*. 2008;17:695–701.
60. Field KM, Michael M. Part II: Liver function in oncology: towards safer chemotherapy use. *Lancet Oncol*. 2008;9:1181–1190.
61. Morris-Stiff G, Tan YM, Vauthey JN. Hepatic complications following preoperative chemotherapy with oxaliplatin or irinotecan for hepatic colorectal metastases. *Eur J Surg Oncol*. 2008;34:609–614.
62. Fernandez FG, Ritter J, Goodwin JW, Linehan DC, Hawkins WG, Strasberg SM. Effect of steatohepatitis associated with irinotecan or oxaliplatin pretreatment on resectability of hepatic colorectal metastases. *J Am Coll Surg*. 2005;200:845–853.
63. Haskell CM. *Cancer Treatment*. 3rd ed. Philadelphia: WB Saunders Co; 1990.
64. Hartmann JT, Kanz L, Bokemeyer C. Phase II study of continuous 120-hour-infusion of mitomycin C as salvage chemotherapy in patients with progressive or rapidly recurrent gastrointestinal adenocarcinoma. *Anticancer Res*. 2000;20:1177–1182.
65. Anderson N, Lokich J, Moore C, Bern M, Coco F. A dose-escalation phase II clinical trial of infusional mitomycin C for 7 days in patients with advanced measurable colorectal cancer refractory or resistant to 5-fluorouracil. *Cancer Invest*. 1999;17:586–593.
66. Zakarija A, Bennett C. Drug-induced thrombotic microangiopathy. *Semin Thromb Hemost*. 2005;31:681–690.

67. Ross P, Norman A, Cunningham D, et al. A prospective randomised trial of protracted venous infusion 5-fluorouracil with or without mitomycin C in advanced colorectal cancer. *Ann Oncol.* 1997;8:995–1001.
68. Yamada Y, Shirao K, Hyodo I, et al. Phase II study of biweekly irinotecan and mitomycin C combination therapy in patients with fluoropyrimidine-resistant advanced colorectal cancer. *Cancer Chemother Pharmacol.* 2003;52:125–130.
69. Rao S, Cunningham D, Price T, et al. Phase II study of capecitabine and mitomycin C as first-line treatment in patients with advanced colorectal cancer. *Br J Cancer.* 2004;91:839–843.
70. Chong G, Dickson JL, Cunningham D, et al. Capecitabine and mitomycin C as third-line therapy for patients with metastatic colorectal cancer resistant to fluorouracil and irinotecan. *Br J Cancer.* 2005;93:510–514.
71. Lim DH, Park YS, Park BB, et al. Mitomycin-C and capecitabine as third-line chemotherapy in patients with advanced colorectal cancer: a phase II study. *Cancer Chemother Pharmacol.* 2005;56:10–14.
72. National Comprehensive Cancer Network Clinical Practice Guidelines in Oncology: Rectal Cancer. Version 2, 2009. Accessed June 2009.
73. Breedis C, Young G. The blood supply of neoplasms in the liver. *Am J Pathol.* 1954;30:969–977.
74. Lorenz M, Muller HH. Randomized, multicenter trial of fluorouracil plus leucovorin administered either via hepatic arterial or intravenous infusion versus fluorodeoxyuridine administered via hepatic arterial infusion in patients with nonresectable liver metastases from colorectal carcinoma. *J Clin Oncol.* 2000;18:243–254.
75. Allen-Mersh TG, Earlam S, Fordy C, Abrams K, Houghton J. Quality of life and survival with continuous hepatic-artery floxuridine infusion for colorectal liver metastases. *Lancet.* 1994;344:1255–1260.
76. Rougier P, Laplanche A, Huguier M, et al. Hepatic arterial infusion of floxuridine in patients with liver metastases from colorectal carcinoma: long-term results of a prospective randomized trial. *J Clin Oncol.* 1992;10:1112–1118.
77. Nelson RL, Freels S. A systematic review of hepatic artery chemotherapy after hepatic resection of colorectal cancer metastatic to the liver. *Dis Colon Rectum.* 2004;47:739–745.
78. Kemeny NE, Niedzwiecki D, Hollis DR, et al. Hepatic arterial infusion versus systemic therapy for hepatic metastases from colorectal cancer: a randomized trial of efficacy, quality of life, and molecular markers (CALGB 9481). *J Clin Oncol.* 2006;24:1395–1403.
79. House M, Kemeny N, Jarnagin W, et al. Comparison of adjuvant systemic chemotherapy with or without hepatic arterial infusional chemotherapy after hepatic resection for metastatic colorectal cancer. In: *Proceedings of the American Society of Clinical Oncology – Gastrointestinal Cancers Symposium*; San Francisco, January 2009, Abstract 383.
80. Tournigand C, Andre T, Achille E, et al. FOLFIRI followed by FOLFOX6 or the reverse sequence in advanced colorectal cancer: a randomized GERCOR study. *J Clin Oncol.* 2004;22:229–237.
81. Colucci G, Gebbia V, Paoletti G, et al. Phase III randomized trial of FOLFIRI versus FOLFOX4 in the treatment of advanced colorectal cancer: a multicenter study of the Gruppo Oncologico Dell'Italia Meridionale. *J Clin Oncol.* 2005;23:4866–4875.
82. Tournigand C, Cervantes A, Figer A, et al. OPTIMOX1: a randomized study of FOLFOX4 or FOLFOX7 with oxaliplatin in a stop-and-Go fashion in advanced colorectal cancer–a GERCOR study. *J Clin Oncol.* 2006;24:394–400.
83. Viel E, Demarchi MF, Chaigneau L, et al. A retrospective study of bifractionated CPT-11 with LF5FU infusion (FOLFIRI-3) in colorectal cancer patients pretreated with oxaliplatin and CPT-11 containing chemotherapies. *Am J Clin Oncol.* 2008;31:89–94.
84. Bidard FC, Tournigand C, Andre T, et al. Efficacy of FOLFIRI-3 (irinotecan D1, D3 combined with LV5-FU) or other irinotecan-based regimens in oxaliplatin-pretreated metastatic colorectal cancer in the GERCOR OPTIMOX1 study. *Ann Oncol.* 2009;20(6):1042–1047.
85. Goldberg RM, Sargent DJ, Morton RF, et al. A randomized controlled trial of fluorouracil plus leucovorin, irinotecan, and oxaliplatin combinations in patients with previously untreated metastatic colorectal cancer. *J Clin Oncol.* 2004;22:23–30.

86. Rothenberg ML, Meropol NJ, Poplin EA, Van Cutsem E, Wadler S. Mortality associated with irinotecan plus bolus fluorouracil/leucovorin: summary findings of an independent panel. *J Clin Oncol.* 2001;19:3801–3807.
87. Kuebler JP, Wieand HS, O'Connell MJ, et al. Oxaliplatin combined with weekly bolus fluorouracil and leucovorin as surgical adjuvant chemotherapy for stage II and III colon cancer: results from NSABP C-07. *J Clin Oncol.* 2007;25:2198–2204.
88. Saltz L, Niedzwiecki D, Hollis D, et al. Irinotecan plus fluorouracil/leucovorin (IFL) versus fluorouracil/leucovorin alone (FL) in stage III colon cancer (intergroup trial CALGB C89803). *J Clin Oncol.* 2004;22(14S (July 15 Supplement)):3500. 2004 ASCO Annual Meeting Proceedings (Post-Meeting Edition).
89. Van Cutsem E, Labianca R, Hossfeld D, et al. Randomized phase III trial comparing infused irinotecan/5-fluorouracil (5-FU)/folinic acid (IF) versus 5-FU/FA (F) in stage III colon cancer patients (pts) (PETACC 3). *J Clin Oncol.* 2005;23(16S (June 1 Supplement)):LBA8. 2005 ASCO Annual Meeting Proceedings.
90. Seymour MT, Maughan TS, Ledermann JA, et al. Different strategies of sequential and combination chemotherapy for patients with poor prognosis advanced colorectal cancer (MRC FOCUS): a randomised controlled trial. *Lancet.* 2007;370:143–152.
91. Koopman M, Antonini NF, Douma J, et al. Sequential versus combination chemotherapy with capecitabine, irinotecan, and oxaliplatin in advanced colorectal cancer (CAIRO): a phase III randomised controlled trial. *Lancet.* 2007;370:135–142.
92. Bouche O, Castaing M, Etienne P, et al. Randomized strategical trial of chemotherapy in metastatic colorectal cancer (FFCD 2000–05): preliminary results. *J Clin Oncol.* 2007;25(18S):4069. 2007 ASCO Annual Meeting Proceedings Part I.
93. Grothey A, Sargent D, Goldberg RM, Schmoll HJ. Survival of patients with advanced colorectal cancer improves with the availability of fluorouracil-leucovorin, irinotecan, and oxaliplatin in the course of treatment. *J Clin Oncol.* 2004;22:1209–1214.
94. Grothey A, Sargent D. Overall survival of patients with advanced colorectal cancer correlates with availability of fluorouracil, irinotecan, and oxaliplatin regardless of whether doublet or single-agent therapy is used first line. *J Clin Oncol.* 2005;23:9441–9442.
95. Schmoll HJ, Sargent D. Single agent fluorouracil for first-line treatment of advanced colorectal cancer as standard? *Lancet.* 2007;370:105–107.
96. Seymour MT, Punt CJ. Cairo and focus. *Lancet.* 2007;370:1904–1905. author reply 5.
97. Schmoll HJ, Sargent D. CAIRO and FOCUS – authors' reply. *Lancet.* 2007;370:1905.
98. Fricker J. No end in sight for chemotherapy debate. *Lancet Oncol.* 2008;9:204.
99. Souglakos J, Androulakis N, Syrigos K, et al. FOLFOXIRI (folinic acid, 5-fluorouracil, oxaliplatin and irinotecan) vs FOLFIRI (folinic acid, 5-fluorouracil and irinotecan) as first-line treatment in metastatic colorectal cancer (MCC): a multicentre randomised phase III trial from the Hellenic Oncology Research Group (HORG). *Br J Cancer.* 2006;94:798–805.
100. Falcone A, Ricci S, Brunetti I, et al. Phase III trial of infusional fluorouracil, leucovorin, oxaliplatin, and irinotecan (FOLFOXIRI) compared with infusional fluorouracil, leucovorin, and irinotecan (FOLFIRI) as first-line treatment for metastatic colorectal cancer: the Gruppo Oncologico Nord Ovest. *J Clin Oncol.* 2007;25:1670–1676.
101. Maindrault-Goebel F, Lledo G, Chibaudel B, et al. Final results of OPTIMOX2, a large randomized phase II study of maintenance therapy or chemotherapy-free intervals (CFI) after FOLFOX in patients with metastatic colorectal cancer (MRC): a GERCOR study. *J Clin Oncol.* 2007;25(18S):4013. 2007 ASCO Annual Meeting Proceedings Part I.
102. Maughan TS, James RD, Kerr DJ, Ledermann JA, Seymour MT, Topham C, McArdle C, Cain D, Stephens RJ and on behalf of the Medical Research Council Colorectal Cancer Group. Comparison of intermittent and continuous palliative chemotherapy for advanced colorectal cancer: a multicentre randomised trial. *The Lancet.* 2003;361(9356):457–464.
103. Labianca R, Floriani I, Cortesi E, et al. Alternating versus continuous "FOLFIRI" in advanced colorectal cancer (ACC): a randomized "GISCAD" trial. *J Clin Oncol.* 2006;24(18S):3505. 2006 ASCO Annual Meeting Proceedings Part I.

104. Grothey A, Hart L, Rowland K, et al. Intermittent oxaliplatin (oxali) administration and time-to-treatment-failure (TTF) in metastatic colorectal cancer (mCRC): final results of the phase III CONcePT trial. *J Clin Oncol.* 2008;26:4010.
105. Sharma S, Camci C, Jabbour N. Management of hepatic metastasis from colorectal cancers: an update. *J Hepatobiliary Pancreat Surg.* 2008;15:570–580.
106. Petrelli NJ. Perioperative or adjuvant therapy for resectable colorectal hepatic metastases. *J Clin Oncol.* 2008;26:4862–4863.
107. Fernandez FG, Drebin JA, Linehan DC, Dehdashti F, Siegel BA, Strasberg SM. Five-year survival after resection of hepatic metastases from colorectal cancer in patients screened by positron emission tomography with F-18 fluorodeoxyglucose (FDG-PET). *Ann Surg.* 2004;240:438–447.
108. Choti MA, Sitzmann JV, Tiburi MF, et al. Trends in long-term survival following liver resection for hepatic colorectal metastases. *Ann Surg.* 2002;235:759–766.
109. Pawlik TM, Scoggins CR, Zorzi D, et al. Effect of surgical margin status on survival and site of recurrence after hepatic resection for colorectal metastases. *Ann Surg.* 2005;241:715–722.
110. Delaunoit T, Alberts SR, Sargent DJ, et al. Chemotherapy permits resection of metastatic colorectal cancer: experience from Intergroup N9741. *Ann Oncol.* 2005;16:425–429.
111. Adam R, Vibert E, Pitombo M. Induction chemotherapy and surgery of colorectal liver metastases. *Bull Cancer.* 2006;93(suppl 1):S45-S49.
112. Adam R, Pascal G, Castaing D, et al. Tumor progression while on chemotherapy: a contraindication to liver resection for multiple colorectal metastases? *Ann Surg.* 2004;240:1052–1061. discussion 1061–1064.
113. Zorzi D, Laurent A, Pawlik TM, Lauwers GY, Vauthey JN, Abdalla EK. Chemotherapy-associated hepatotoxicity and surgery for colorectal liver metastases. *Br J Surg.* 2007;94:274–286.
114. Rubbia-Brandt L, Audard V, Sartoretti P, et al. Severe hepatic sinusoidal obstruction associated with oxaliplatin-based chemotherapy in patients with metastatic colorectal cancer. *Ann Oncol.* 2004;15:460–466.
115. Ychou M, Hohenberger W, Thezenas S, et al. Randomized phase III trial comparing infused 5-fluorouracil/folinic acid (LV5FU) versus LV5FU+irinotecan (LV5FU+IRI) as adjuvant treatment after complete resection of liver metastases from colorectal cancer (LMCRC). (CPT-GMA-301). *J Clin Oncol.* 2008;26:LBA4013.
116. Masi G, Loupakis F, Pollina L, et al. Long-term outcome of initially unresectable metastatic colorectal cancer patients treated with 5-fluorouracil/leucovorin, oxaliplatin, and irinotecan (FOLFOXIRI) followed by radical surgery of metastases. *Ann Surg.* 2009;249:420-425.
117. Nordlinger B, Sorbye H, Glimelius B, et al. Perioperative chemotherapy with FOLFOX4 and surgery versus surgery alone for resectable liver metastases from colorectal cancer (EORTC Intergroup trial 40983): a randomised controlled trial. *Lancet.* 2008;371:1007–1016.
118. Mitry E, Fields AL, Bleiberg H, et al. Adjuvant chemotherapy after potentially curative resection of metastases from colorectal cancer: a pooled analysis of two randomized trials. *J Clin Oncol.* 2008;26:4906–4911.
119. Nordic Gastrointestinal Tumor Adjuvant Therapy Group. Expectancy or primary chemotherapy in patients with advanced asymptomatic colorectal cancer: a randomized trial. *J Clin Oncol.* 1992;10:904–911.
120. Ackland SP, Jones M, Tu D, et al. A meta-analysis of two randomised trials of early chemotherapy in asymptomatic metastatic colorectal cancer. *Br J Cancer.* 2005;93:1236–1243.
121. Lee JC, Chow NH, Wang ST, Huang SM. Prognostic value of vascular endothelial growth factor expression in colorectal cancer patients. *Eur J Cancer.* 2000;36:748–753.
122. Mulcahy MF, Benson AB 3rd. Bevacizumab in the treatment of colorectal cancer. *Expert Opin Biol Ther.* 2005;5:997–1005.
123. Porebska I, Harlozinska A, Bojarowski T. Expression of the tyrosine kinase activity growth factor receptors (EGFR, ERB B2, ERB B3) in colorectal adenocarcinomas and adenomas. *Tumour Biol.* 2000;21:105–115.
124. Chou JL, Fan Z, DeBlasio T, Koff A, Rosen N, Mendelsohn J. Constitutive overexpression of cyclin D1 in human breast epithelial cells does not prevent G1 arrest induced by deprivation of epidermal growth factor. *Breast Cancer Res Treat.* 1999;55:267–283.

125. Wu X, Fan Z, Masui H, Rosen N, Mendelsohn J. Apoptosis induced by an anti-epidermal growth factor receptor monoclonal antibody in a human colorectal carcinoma cell line and its delay by insulin. *J Clin Invest.* 1995;95:1897–1905.
126. Amado RG, Wolf M, Peeters M, et al. Wild-type KRAS is required for panitumumab efficacy in patients with metastatic colorectal cancer. *J Clin Oncol.* 2008;26:1626–1634.
127. Freeman DJ, Juan T, Reiner M, et al. Association of K-ras mutational status and clinical outcomes in patients with metastatic colorectal cancer receiving panitumumab alone. *Clin Colorectal Cancer.* 2008;7:184–190.
128. Servomaa K, Kiuru A, Kosma VM, Hirvikoski P, Rytomaa T. p53 and K-ras gene mutations in carcinoma of the rectum among Finnish women. *Mol Pathol.* 2000;53:24–30.
129. Frattini M, Balestra D, Suardi S, et al. Different genetic features associated with colon and rectal carcinogenesis. *Clin Cancer Res.* 2004;10:4015–4021.
130. Kabbinavar F, Hurwitz HI, Fehrenbacher L, et al. Phase II, randomized trial comparing bevacizumab plus fluorouracil (FU)/leucovorin (LV) with FU/LV alone in patients with metastatic colorectal cancer. *J Clin Oncol.* 2003;21:60–65.
131. Hurwitz H, Fehrenbacher L, Novotny W, et al. Bevacizumab plus irinotecan, fluorouracil, and leucovorin for metastatic colorectal cancer. *N Engl J Med.* 2004;350:2335–2342.
132. Kabbinavar FF, Hambleton J, Mass RD, Hurwitz HI, Bergsland E, Sarkar S. Combined analysis of efficacy: the addition of bevacizumab to fluorouracil/leucovorin improves survival for patients with metastatic colorectal cancer. *J Clin Oncol.* 2005;23:3706–3712.
133. Giantonio BJ, Catalano PJ, Meropol NJ, et al. Bevacizumab in combination with oxaliplatin, fluorouracil, and leucovorin (FOLFOX4) for previously treated metastatic colorectal cancer: results from the Eastern Cooperative Oncology Group Study E3200. *J Clin Oncol.* 2007;25:1539–1544.
134. Hochster HS, Hart LL, Ramanathan RK, et al. Safety and efficacy of oxaliplatin and fluoropyrimidine regimens with or without bevacizumab as first-line treatment of metastatic colorectal cancer: results of the TREE Study. *J Clin Oncol.* 2008;26:3523–3529.
135. Saltz LB, Clarke S, Diaz-Rubio E, et al. Bevacizumab in combination with oxaliplatin-based chemotherapy as first-line therapy in metastatic colorectal cancer: a randomized phase III study. *J Clin Oncol.* 2008;26:2013–2019.
136. Van Cutsem E, Rivera F, Berry S, et al. Safety and efficacy of first-line bevacizumab with FOLFOX, XELOX, FOLFIRI and fluoropyrimidines in metastatic colorectal cancer: the BEAT study. *Ann Oncol.* 2009;20(11):1842–1847.
137. Grothey A, Sugrue MM, Purdie DM, et al. Bevacizumab beyond first progression is associated with prolonged overall survival in metastatic colorectal cancer: results from a large observational cohort study (BRiTE). *J Clin Oncol.* 2008;26:5326–5334.
138. Scappaticci FA, Fehrenbacher L, Cartwright T, et al. Surgical wound healing complications in metastatic colorectal cancer patients treated with bevacizumab. *J Surg Oncol.* 2005;91:173–180.
139. Gruenberger B, Tamandl D, Schueller J, et al. Bevacizumab, capecitabine, and oxaliplatin as neoadjuvant therapy for patients with potentially curable metastatic colorectal cancer. *J Clin Oncol.* 2008;26:1830–1835.
140. Saltz LB, Meropol NJ, Loehrer PJ Sr, Needle MN, Kopit J, Mayer RJ. Phase II trial of cetuximab in patients with refractory colorectal cancer that expresses the epidermal growth factor receptor. *J Clin Oncol.* 2004;22:1201–1208.
141. Cunningham D, Humblet Y, Siena S, et al. Cetuximab monotherapy and cetuximab plus irinotecan in irinotecan-refractory metastatic colorectal cancer. *N Engl J Med.* 2004;351:337–345.
142. Jonker DJ, O'Callaghan CJ, Karapetis CS, et al. Cetuximab for the treatment of colorectal cancer. *N Engl J Med.* 2007;357:2040–2048.
143. Karapetis CS, Khambata-Ford S, Jonker DJ, et al. K-ras mutations and benefit from cetuximab in advanced colorectal cancer. *N Engl J Med.* 2008;359:1757–1765.
144. Van Cutsem E, Kohne CH, Hitre E, et al. Cetuximab and chemotherapy as initial treatment for metastatic colorectal cancer. *N Engl J Med.* 2009;360:1408–1417.
145. Bokemeyer C, Bondarenko I, Hartmann J, et al. KRAS status and efficacy of first-line treatment of patients with metastatic colorectal cancer (mCRC) with FOLFOX with or without cetuximab: the OPUS experience. *J Clin Oncol.* 2008;26, Abstract 4000.

146. Vincenzi B, Santini D, Russo A, et al. Angiogenesis modifications related with cetuximab plus irinotecan as anticancer treatment in advanced colorectal cancer patients. *Ann Oncol.* 2006;17:835–841.
147. Chong G, Cunningham D. The role of cetuximab in the therapy of previously treated advanced colorectal cancer. *Semin Oncol.* 2005;32:S55-S58.
148. Van Cutsem E, Humblet Y, Gelderblom H, et al. Cetuximab dose-escalation study in patients with metastatic colorectal cancer (mCRC) with no or slight skin reactions on cetuximab standard dose treatment (EVEREST): pharmacokinetic and efficacy data of a randomized study. In: *Proceedings of the American Society of Clinical Oncology – Gastrointestinal Cancers Symposium*; 2007, Abstract 237.
149. Green LL. Antibody engineering via genetic engineering of the mouse: XenoMouse strains are a vehicle for the facile generation of therapeutic human monoclonal antibodies. *J Immunol Methods.* 1999;231:11–23.
150. National Comprehensive Cancer Network Clinical Practice Guidelines in Oncology: Colon Cancer. Version 2. http://www.nccn.org/; 2009. Accessed June 2009.
151. Van Cutsem E, Peeters M, Siena S, et al. Open-label phase III trial of panitumumab plus best supportive care compared with best supportive care alone in patients with chemotherapy-refractory metastatic colorectal cancer. *J Clin Oncol.* 2007;25:1658–1664.
152. Melosky B, Burkes R, Rayson D, Alcindor T, Shear N, Lacouture M. Management of skin rash during egfr-targeted monoclonal antibody treatment for gastrointestinal malignancies: Canadian recommendations. *Curr Oncol.* 2009;16:16–26.
153. Lacouture M, Mitchell E, Shearer H, et al. Impact of pre-emptive skin toxicity (ST) treatment (tx) on panitumumab (pmab)-related skin toxicities and quality of life (QOL) in patients (pts) with metastatic colorectal cancer (mCRC): results from STEPP. In: *Proceedings of the American Society of Clinical Oncology – Gastrointestinal Cancers Symposium*; 2009, Abstract 291.
154. Saltz LB, Lenz HJ, Kindler HL, et al. Randomized phase II trial of cetuximab, bevacizumab, and irinotecan compared with cetuximab and bevacizumab alone in irinotecan-refractory colorectal cancer: the BOND-2 study. *J Clin Oncol.* 2007;25:4557–4561.
155. Tol J, Koopman M, Cats A, et al. Chemotherapy, bevacizumab, and cetuximab in metastatic colorectal cancer. *N Engl J Med.* 2009;360:563–572.
156. Hecht JR, Mitchell E, Chidiac T, et al. A randomized phase IIIB trial of chemotherapy, bevacizumab, and panitumumab compared with chemotherapy and bevacizumab alone for metastatic colorectal cancer. *J Clin Oncol.* 2009;27:672–680.
157. Golfinopoulos V, Salanti G, Pavlidis N, Ioannidis JP. Survival and disease-progression benefits with treatment regimens for advanced colorectal cancer: a meta-analysis. *Lancet Oncol.* 2007;8:898–911.
158. Thibodeau SN, Bren G, Schaid D. Microsatellite instability in cancer of the proximal colon. *Science.* 1993;260:816–819.
159. Chen WS, Chen JY, Liu JM, et al. Microsatellite instability in sporadic-colon-cancer patients with and without liver metastases. *Int J Cancer.* 1997;74:470–474.
160. Gervaz P, Bouzourene H, Cerottini JP, et al. Dukes B colorectal cancer: distinct genetic categories and clinical outcome based on proximal or distal tumor location. *Dis Colon Rectum.* 2001;44:364–372.
161. Kapiteijn E, Liefers GJ, Los LC, et al. Mechanisms of oncogenesis in colon versus rectal cancer. *J Pathol.* 2001;195:171–178.
162. Velho S, Moutinho C, Cirnes L, et al. BRAF, KRAS and PIK3CA mutations in colorectal serrated polyps and cancer: primary or secondary genetic events in colorectal carcinogenesis? *BMC Cancer.* 2008;8:255.
163. Di Nicolantonio F, Martini M, Molinari F, et al. Wild-type BRAF is required for response to panitumumab or cetuximab in metastatic colorectal cancer. *J Clin Oncol.* 2008;26:5705–5712.
164. Fransen K, Klintenas M, Osterstrom A, Dimberg J, Monstein HJ, Soderkvist P. Mutation analysis of the BRAF, ARAF and RAF-1 genes in human colorectal adenocarcinomas. *Carcinogenesis.* 2004;25:527–533.
165. Tie J, Sieber OM, Gibbs P, et al. Selecting subjects for a therapeutic target in colorectal cancer (CRC): using a clinical database to enrich for patients harboring the BRAFV600E mutation. *J Clin Oncol.* 2009;27:15s. suppl; abstr 11003.

166. Del Rio M, Molina F, Bascoul-Mollevi C, et al. Gene expression signature in advanced colorectal cancer patients select drugs and response for the use of leucovorin, fluorouracil, and irinotecan. *J Clin Oncol*. 2007;25:773–780.
167. Tournigand C, Lledo G, Delord JP, et al. Modified (m)Folfox7/bevacizumab (B) or modified (m) Xelox/bevacizumab with or without erlotinib (E) in first-line metastatic colorectal cancer (MCRC): results of the feasibility phase of the DREAM-OPTIMOX3 study (GERCOR). *J Clin Oncol*. 2007;25(18S):4097. 2007 ASCO Annual Meeting Proceedings Part I.
168. Kopetz S, Overman M, Chang DZ, et al. Systematic survey of therapeutic trials for metastatic colorectal cancer: room for improvement in the critical pathway. *J Clin Oncol*. 2008;26:2000–2005.
169. Parmar MK, Barthel FM, Sydes M, et al. Speeding up the evaluation of new agents in cancer. *J Natl Cancer Inst*. 2008;100:1204–1214.
170. O'Connell MJ. A phase III trial of 5-fluorouracil and leucovorin in the treatment of advanced colorectal cancer. A Mayo Clinic/North Central Cancer Treatment Group study. *Cancer*. 1989;63:1026–1030.
171. O'Connell MJ, Mailliard JA, Kahn MJ, et al. Controlled trial of fluorouracil and low-dose leucovorin given for 6 months as postoperative adjuvant therapy for colon cancer. *J Clin Oncol*. 1997;15:246–250.
172. de Gramont A, Louvet C, Andre T, et al. Modulation of 5-fluorouracil with folinic acid in advanced colorectal cancers. Groupe d'etude et de recherche sur les cancers de l'ovaire et digestifs (GERCOD). *Rev Med Interne*. 1997;18(suppl 4):372s-378s.
173. Ychou M, Duffour J, Pinguet F, et al. Individual 5FU-dose adaptation schedule using bimonthly pharmacokinetically modulated LV5FU2 regimen: a feasibility study in patients with advanced colorectal cancer. *Anticancer Res*. 1999;19:2229–2235.
174. Maindrault-Goebel F, Louvet C, Andre T, et al. Oxaliplatin added to the simplified bimonthly leucovorin and 5-fluorouracil regimen as second-line therapy for metastatic colorectal cancer (FOLFOX6). GERCOR. *Eur J Cancer*. 1999;35:1338–1342.
175. Hochster H, Chachoua A, Speyer J, Escalon J, Zeleniuch-Jacquotte A, Muggia F. Oxaliplatin with weekly bolus fluorouracil and low-dose leucovorin as first-line therapy for patients with colorectal cancer. *J Clin Oncol*. 2003;21:2703–2707.
176. Moehler M, Hoffmann T, Hildner K, Siebler J, Galle PR, Heike M. Weekly oxaliplatin, high-dose folinic acid and 24h-5-fluorouracil (FUFOX) as salvage therapy in metastatic colorectal cancer patients pretreated with irinotecan and folinic acid/5-fluorouracil regimens. *Z Gastroenterol*. 2002;40:957–964.
177. Sorbye H, Dahl O. Nordic 5-fluorouracil/leucovorin bolus schedule combined with oxaliplatin (Nordic FLOX) as first-line treatment of metastatic colorectal cancer. *Acta Oncol*. 2003;42:827–831.
178. Cassidy J, Tabernero J, Twelves C, et al. XELOX (capecitabine plus oxaliplatin): active first-line therapy for patients with metastatic colorectal cancer. *J Clin Oncol*. 2004;22:2084–2091.
179. Chang DZ, Abbruzzese JL. Capecitabine plus oxaliplatin vs infusional 5-fluorouracil plus oxaliplatin in the treatment of colorectal cancer. Pro: the CapeOx regimen is preferred over FOLFOX. *Clin Adv Hematol Oncol*. 2005;3:400–404.
180. Delord JP, Pierga JY, Dieras V, et al. A phase I clinical and pharmacokinetic study of capecitabine (Xeloda) and irinotecan combination therapy (XELIRI) in patients with metastatic gastrointestinal tumours. *Br J Cancer*. 2005;92:820–826.
181. Kim TW, Kang WK, Chang HM, et al. Multicenter phase II study of oral capecitabine plus irinotecan as first-line chemotherapy in advanced colorectal cancer: a Korean Cancer Study Group trial. *Acta Oncol*. 2005;44:230–235.

13 Radiation Therapy: Adjuvant vs. Neoadjuvant Therapy

Rolf Sauer and Claus Rödel

INTRODUCTION

The rationale for using combinations of radiation and systemic chemotherapy as a component of (neo)adjuvant treatment in rectal cancer is based on the risk of relapse following surgery alone and the evidence of radio- and drug-responsiveness derived from both laboratory studies and clinical trials. The last four decades have witnessed the development of a variety of preoperative and postoperative radiotherapy (RT) and radiochemotherapy (RCT) schedules designed to optimize the sequence of treatment modalities and the most appropriate scheduling of irradiation and 5-fluorouracil-based chemotherapy.

RANDOMIZED TRIALS OF POSTOPERATIVE RCT

Historically, the combination of postoperative RT and 5-FU-based chemotherapy has been shown in several randomized trials to reduce local recurrence rates and to improve overall survival compared with (non-TME) surgery alone or surgery plus postoperative RT (Table 1). In the early GITSG 7175 trial, the best local control was achieved with combined RCT (local relapse rate of 11% vs. 20% with RT alone), while no impact on local control was seen with chemotherapy as single adjuvant treatment (local relapse rate of 27% vs. 24% with surgery alone) *(1)*. Although rates of distant metastases were slightly lower in the two arms that contained chemotherapy, no single arm had a significant impact on distant failure rates. Thus, the survival advantage achieved with combined RCT appeared to relate primarily to the marked reduction in local relapse rates. These results were later confirmed by a trial conducted by the Norwegian Adjuvant Rectal Cancer Project Group *(2)*. Again, the local relapse rate was significantly decreased from 30 to 12% by combined postoperative RCT compared with surgery alone, an effect which also translated into an improvement in 5-year survival, though no significant impact on distant metastases was achieved. The more recent NSABP R-02 also showed that combined RCT resulted in a

From: *Current Clinical Oncology: Rectal Cancer*,
Edited by: B.G. Czito and C.G. Willett, DOI: 10.1007/978-1-60761-567-5_13,

Table 1
Randomized trials of postoperative radiation (RT), chemotherapy (CT), or combined radiochemotherapy (RCT) for locally advanced rectal cancer (UICC II and III)

Series	*Treatment*	*Local failure*		*Distant failure*		*5-year survival*	
GITSG 7175 *(1)*	Surgery	24%	$p=0.08$	34%		45%	$p<0.05$
	Surgery + RT	20%		30%		52%	
	Surgery + 5-FU/MeCCNU	27%		27%		56%	
	Surgery + RT + 5-FU/MeCCNU	11%		26%		59%	
NCCTG/Mayo 794751 *(5)*	Surgery + RT	25%	$p=0.04$	46%	$p=0.01$	48%	$p=0.025$
	Surgery + RT + 5-FU/MeCCNU	13.5%		29%		58%	
Norway trial *(2)*	Surgery	30%	$p=0.01$	39%		50%	$p=0.05$
	Surgery + RT + 5-FU	12%		33%		64%	
NSABP R-02 *(3)*	Surgery + CT[a]	13%	$p=0.02$	29%		64%	
	Surgery + RCT	8%		31%		64%	
Italy trial *(4)*	Surgery + RT	20%		38%		59%	
	Surgery + 5-FU/LEV + RT + 5-FU/LEV (RT and CT applied sequentially)	22%		27%		43%	

[a]Male patients received MOF (MeCCNU, Vincristine, 5-FU) or 5-FU/LV; female patients only 5-FU/LV

significantly reduced local failure rate compared with chemotherapy alone (8% vs. 13%); however, this rather small absolute reduction did not translate into a difference in overall survival *(3)*. In all these trials, the effect of concomitant 5-FU chemotherapy appeared to be primarily mediated through its radiosensitizing properties rather than through its own systemic efficacy. This conclusion is further strengthened by a recent Italian study that showed no significant effect on local control and survival when postoperative RT and chemotherapy were delivered sequentially rather than concomitantly *(4)*.

The NCCTG 794751 trial was the first study to integrate a course of full-dose chemotherapy preceding as well as following combined RCT in an attempt to exploit both the radiosensitizing properties of 5-FU and its potential to reduce the incidence of distant metastases *(5)*. Indeed, this was also the first trial in which both local relapse and distant metastasis rates were significantly reduced in the experimental arm. The NCI Consensus Conference concluded in 1990 that combined RCT was the standard adjuvant treatment for patients with TNM stages II and III rectal cancer *(6)*.

RANDOMIZED TRIALS TO OPTIMIZE 5-FU-BASED POSTOPERATIVE RCT

Further trials by the GITSG (7180) and NCCTG (864751) investigated the need for methyl-CCNU in the chemotherapy regimen and concluded that it added no benefit to the 5-FU regimen (Table 2) *(7,8)*. Thus, methyl-CCNU is no longer used for adjuvant RCT in rectal cancer. NCCTG (864751) also evaluated the optimal method of administering 5-FU during RT: Bolus 5-FU (500 mg/m^2 for 3 days during weeks 1 and 5 of radiation therapy) was compared with continuous infusion (225 mg/m^2 during the entire course of RT). A 10% disease-free and overall survival advantage was achieved with continuous infusion 5-FU during RT (Table 2). The INT 0144 trial compared infusion 5-FU vs. bolus 5-FU before and after RCT (or modulation of 5-FU through the addition of leucovorin and levamisole) and whether further increases tumor control could be achieved (Table 2) *(9)*. There was no significant difference in local control or survival. Results of a four-arm Intergroup trial, INT 0114, also showed no significant differences in local control and survival among patients receiving either bolus 5-FU, bolus 5-FU + folinic acid, bolus 5-FU + levamisole, or bolus 5-FU + folinic acid + levamisole *(10)*. However, gastrointestinal toxicity was higher in folinic acid-containing regimens.

Given all these results, the standard design of postoperative RCT is to deliver six cycles of 5-FU chemotherapy with concurrent radiation therapy during cycles 3 and 4. During RT, continuous infusion 5-FU regimens [e.g., 225 mg/m^2/day during the entire course of radiation, or 1,000 mg/m^2/day as 120-h continuous infusion during weeks 1 and 5 of radiation, as delivered in the German CAO/ARO/AIO-95-study (see below)] are recommended. A recent randomized Korean trial (Table 2) suggests that radiation should start with cycle 1 rather than cycle 3, supporting the radiobiological paradigm that subclinical disease in the pelvis is best controlled if RT is applied as soon as possible after surgical resection to account for any regrowth of residual tumor cells *(11)*.

The main advantage with a postoperative approach is improved patient selection based on operative and pathologic staging. The primary disadvantages include an increased rates of acute and chronic toxicity related to the increased amount of small bowel in the radiation field, a potentially more radio-resistant hypoxic postsurgical bed and, if the patient has undergone an APR, the radiation field has to be extended to include the perineal scar.

Table 2
Randomized trials of postoperative combined radiochemotherapy (RCT) in locally advanced rectal cancer

Series	*Postoperative treatment*	*DFS*	*OS*
GITSG 7180 *(7)*	RCT bolus 5-FU+bolus 5-FU (6 cycles, escalating 5-FU) RCT bolus 5-FU+bolus 5-FU/ MeCCNU (12 months treatment)	68% (3y) 54% (3y) p=0.20	75% (3y) 66% (3y) p=0.58
NCCTG 864751 *(8)*	2 Cycles of bolus 5-FU (±MeCCNU)+RCT bolus 5-FU+2 cycles of bolus 5-FU (±MeCCNU) 2 Cycles of bolus 5-FU (±MeCCNU)+RCT PVI 5-FU+2 cycles of bolus 5-FU (±MeCCNU)	53% (4y) 63% (4y) p=0.01	60% (4y) 70% (4y) p=0.005
INT 0114 *(10)*	2 Cycles bolus 5-FU+bolus 5-FU+2 cycles bolus 5-FU 2 Cycles bolus 5-FU/LV+RCT bolus 5-FU/LV+2 cycles bolus 5-FU/LV 2 Cycles bolus 5-FU/LEV+RCT bolus 5-FU+2 cycles bolus 5-FU/LEV 2 Cycles bolus 5-FU/LV/LEV+RCT bolus 5-FU/LV+2 cycles bolus 5-FU/LV/LEV	54% (all) No significant difference	64% (all) No significant difference
INT 0144 *(9)*	2 Cycles bolus 5-FU+RCT PVI 5-FU+2 cycles bolus 5-FU PVI 5-FU+RCT PVI 5-FU+PVI 5-FU 2 Cycles bolus 5-FU/LV/LEV+RCT bolus 5-FU/LV+2 cycles bolus 5-FU/LV/LEV	68–69% (3y) No significant difference	81–83% (3y) No significant difference
Korean Trial *(11)*	RCT bolus FU/LV+6 cycles bolus 5-FU/LV 2 Cycles bolus 5-FU/LV+RCT bolus FU/LV+4 cycles bolus 5-FU/LV	81% (4y) 70% (4y) p=0.04	84% (4y) 82% (4y) p=0.39

PREOPERATIVE RADIATION

Potential advantages of a preoperative approach include decreased tumor seeding at resection, less acute and chronic toxicity, increased radiosensitivity due to more oxygenated cells, and the potential for improved rates of sphincter preservation. The primary disadvantage is potential overtreatment of patients with early stage (pT1-2N0) or undetected metastatic disease. However, this disadvantage becomes less important with contemporary imaging modalities (endorectal ultrasound and high-resolution phased-array magnetic resonance imaging), which allow more accurate preoperative staging and predicting of a negative circumferential margins *(12)*.

There are more than 15 randomized trials of preoperative RT without concurrent chemotherapy for clinically resectable rectal cancer. All used low-to-moderate doses of RT and most showed a decrease in local recurrence. The Swedish Rectal Cancer Trial is the only study (out of eight studies) with more than 500 patients that reported a survival advantage for the overall treatment group *(13)*. Two meta-analyzes evaluating RT alone have reported conflicting results.

While both revealed a decrease in local recurrence, the analysis by Camma et al., reported a survival advantage, whereas the Colorectal Cancer Collaborative Group did not *(14,15)*. The Swedish Council of Technology Assessment in Health Care performed a systematic review of RT trials *(16)*. They analyzed data from 42 randomized trials, 3 meta-analyzes, 36 prospective studies, 7 retrospective studies, and 17 other cohorts, for a total of 25,351 patients. The primary conclusion was that preoperative RT at biologically effective doses above 30 Gy decreases the relative risk of local failure by 50–70%, that postoperative RT decreases this risk by 30–40% through doses that are usually higher than those used preoperatively, and that survival is improved by about 10% using preoperative RT. Therefore, in recent years preoperative therapy has gained a large acceptance as standard therapy for rectal cancer.

RANDOMIZED TRIALS TO OPTIMIZE THE SEQUENCE

Until recently, the only randomized trial that directly compared preoperative to postoperative RT (both without chemotherapy) in rectal cancer was the Uppsala trial, which was conducted in Sweden between 1980 and 1985 *(17)*. In the preoperative arm, patients received intensive short-course radiation (five fractions of 5.1 Gy to a total dose of 25.5 Gy in 1 week). In the postoperative arm, conventional radiation therapy (2 Gy to a total of 60 Gy with a 2-week break after 40 Gy) was delivered. Preoperative RT significantly decreased local failure rates (13% vs. 22%, $p=0.02$); however, there was no significant difference in 5-year survival rates (42% vs. 38%).

Prospective randomized trials comparing the efficacy of preoperative with standard postoperative RCT in UICC-stage II and III rectal cancer were initiated in the United States both through the Radiation Therapy Oncology Group (RTOG 94-01) and the NSABP (R-03) as well as in Germany (Protocol CAO/ARO/AIO-94). Unfortunately, both US trials suffered from lack of accrual and were closed prematurely. The German study (CAO/ARO/AIO-94), however, completed accrual with more than 820 patients included. The design of this trial and the treatment schedule is depicted in Fig. 1. Five-year results were reported in 2004 (Table 3). Compared with postoperative RCT, the preoperative combined modality approach was superior in terms of local control, downstaging, acute and chronic toxicity, and sphincter preservation in those patients judged by the surgeon to require an APR *(18)*. Given these advantages, preoperative RCT is now the preferred therapeutic approach for patients with locally advanced rectal cancer. However, it should be emphasized that, with a median follow-up of 46 months, there was no difference in 5-year disease-free and overall survival rates between both treatment arms.

The United Kingdom Medical Research Council Trial MRC C07 randomized patients with clinical stage I–III rectal cancer to preoperative RT (5×5 Gy) and TME (total mesorectal excision) or to selective postoperative RCT, which was delivered only to patients with a histologic circumferential radial margin <1 mm. Preliminary results showed local recurrence rates at 5 years of 5 and 11%, significantly favoring the unselected preoperative treatment approach *(19)*.

CONCOMITANT CHEMOTHERAPY WITH PREOPERATIVE RADIATION THERAPY?

The concurrent use of chemotherapy as part of the preoperative regimen is another important point. For the treatment of primarily "unresectable," fixed, T4-rectal cancer, several institutions have applied preoperative radiation therapy and RCT. The goal is to convert ("downsize") the tumor, which is clinically not amenable to curative resection at presentation, to a resectable

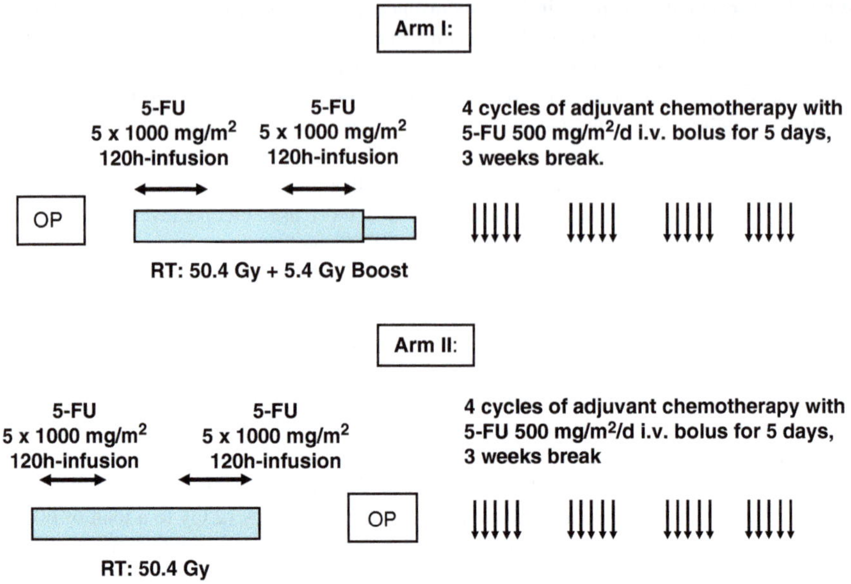

Fig. 1. Design of the German CAO/ARO/AIO-94 study comparing postoperative (arm I) with preoperative radiochemotherapy (arm II) in locally advanced rectal cancer.

Table 3
German Rectal Cancer Study Group randomized trial of preoperative compared with postoperative radiochemotherapy for rectal cancer *(18)*

5-year outcome	*Preoperative RCT(%)*	*Postoperative RCT(%)*	*p Value*
Locoregional recurrence rate	6	13	0.006
Distant recurrence rate	36	38	0.84
Disease-free survival	68	65	0.32
Overall survival	74	76	0.80
Any grade 3/4-acute toxicity	27	40	0.001
Any grade 3/4-late toxicity	14	24	0.01
Sphincter preservation rate[a]	39	19	0.004

[a]In patients deemed to require abdominal perineal resection by the surgeon before randomization

status. Minsky et al., compared preoperative RT (50.4 Gy) with or without 5-FU/folinic acid and showed that 90% of the patients with initially "unresectable" tumors were converted to resectable lesions by preoperative combined therapy as compared with only 64% of those who received radiation therapy alone *(20)*. Moreover, a complete pathologic response was found in 20% of patients receiving combined modality therapy as compared to 6% receiving RT alone, indicating an enhancement of radiation-induced "downstaging" with the use of concomitant 5-FU-based RCT. In a recent randomized phase III study comparing RT alone (n=109) with combined 5-FU-based RCT (n=98) for primarily "unresectable" T4-rectal cancer or locally recurrent disease, Braendengen et al., demonstrated that the addition of chemotherapy to RT significantly improved R0-resection rates, local control, time to treatment failure, and cancer-specific survival *(21)*.

A Polish randomized trial compared preoperative short-course irradiation (5×5 Gy) and immediate surgery with conventionally fractionated RCT (1.8 Gy–50.4 Gy) and delayed surgery in 316 patients with locally advanced (T3/T4) low rectal cancer. The primary endpoint of the trial was the rate of sphincter preserving surgery. Despite a significant increase in tumor response in the RCT group (pathologic complete remission 16% vs. 1%; mean largest tumor diameter on the operative specimen, 29 mm vs. 48 mm), the rate of sphincter preservation was 61% in the immediate surgery group and 58% in the delayed group, possibly indicating a strong commitment of the surgeons in this trial to maintain their surgical approach no matter what degree of tumor response was seen following neoadjuvant RCT *(22,23)*. The actuarial 4-year overall survival was 67% in the short-course group and 66% the chemoradiation group (p=NS); no significant differences were found in disease-free survival, incidence of local recurrence and severe late toxicity.

Two randomized trials have examined whether chemotherapy improves the results of preoperative radiation in patients with cT3 rectal cancer (Table 4). The EORTC 22921 is a four-arm randomized trial of preoperative radiation (45 Gy) with or without concurrent bolus 5FU/leucovorin followed by surgery, with or without four cycles of postoperative 5FU/ leucovorin. A significant decrease in local recurrence was observed in three chemotherapy groups: 8.8, 9.6, 8.0% with either preoperative RCT, postoperative CT and both, vs. 17.1% without (p=0.002) *(24)*. Five-year overall survival was not affected by chemotherapy at a median follow-up of 5.4 years: 66% vs. 65% (p=0.8) for preoperative RCT vs. preoperative RT; 67% vs. 63% (p=0.132) for postoperative CT vs. no chemotherapy. An increased rate of ypT0 responses (14% vs. 5%, p=0.0001) were observed with the addition of preoperative chemotherapy, although no difference in sphincter saving surgery (52.8% vs. 50.5%, p=0.47) was seen. Only 42.9% of patients received planned adjuvant CT. The authors stated that in view of the benefit of preoperative RCT and the poor compliance with postoperative CT, preoperative RCT should be preferred. The second trial (FFCD 9203) compared preoperative

Table 4
Preoperative conventionally fractionated radiotherapy with or without 5-FU/LV-based chemotherapy. Results of EORTC 22921 and FFCD 9203 randomized trials *(24,25)*

5-year outcome	*Preoperative RT*	*Preoperative RCT*	*p Value*
EORTC 22921 (n = 1011)			
pCR rate	5.3%	13.7%	<0.001
ypN0	60.5%	71.9%	<0.001
Tumor size (median)	30 mm	25 mm	<0.0001
Sphincter preserved	50.5%	52.8%	0.47
Local failure	17%	8%	0.002
Overall survival	64.8%	65.6%	0.79
FFCD 9203 (n = 762)			
pCR rate	3.7%	11.7%	<0.0001
Sphincter preserved	52.6%	51.7%	n.s.
Grade 3/4 toxicity	2.7%	14.6%	<0.0001
Local failure	8%	16.5%	n.g.
Overall survival	66%	67%	n.g.

RT (45 Gy) with or without bolus 5FU/leucovorin. All patients received postoperative chemotherapy. An improvement in the pCR rate (12% vs. 4%, $p=0.0001$) and local recurrence rate (8% vs. 16.5%, $p=0.004$) was seen in the preoperative RCT group *(25)*. Overall survival at 5 years was the same (67%).

There are insufficient data to make firm conclusions on the role of postoperative chemotherapy following preoperative treatment with RT or RCT. In the EORTC 22921 trial, the delivery of postoperative chemotherapy demonstrated a nonsignificant improvement in rates of local relapse, relapse-free, and overall survival. An exploratory subgroup analysis suggested that only good-prognosis patients with downstaging of cT3-4 tumors to ypT0-2 disease benefit from adjuvant CT *(26)*. In patients treated with preoperative radiation using a regimen of 5×5 Gy, the role of postoperative chemotherapy is currently being investigated in a randomized trial (the SCRIPT trial, Simply Capecitabine in Rectal cancer after Irradiation Plus TME).

INTEGRATING NOVEL CHEMOTHERAPEUTIC AGENTS INTO PREOPERATIVE COMBINED MODALITY TREATMENT

With optimized local treatment, including RT/RCT and TME surgery, distant metastasis development is by far the predominant pattern of tumor failure in rectal cancer presently. One future challenge is to integrate more effective systemic therapy into the multimodal approach of this disease. Novel chemotherapeutic agents such as capecitabine, UFT, tomudex, oxaliplatin, and irinotecan as well as targeted therapies, such as bevacizumab and cetuximab, have improved outcomes of patients treated in the adjuvant and metastatic setting of colorectal cancer, and have also been incorporated into phase I/II combined modality programs for rectal cancer as well *(27)*. Most suggest higher pathologic complete response (pCR) rates compared with 5-FU-based RCT alone. However, for some agents, this increased pCR rate is associated with an increase in acute toxicity. Clearly, phase III trials are needed to determine if these regimens offer an advantage compared with 5-FU-based combined modality regimens. These studies have been initiated in Europe and the USA (Table 5).

FUTURE CHALLENGES FOR COMBINED MODALITY RECTAL CANCER TREATMENT

As depicted in Fig. 2, there have been two major developments in rectal cancer treatment over the past two decades. The first has been to apply RT and CT as early as possible in the treatment course. Since 2004, preoperative RCT has been considered therapy, with more recent studies even incorporating neodjuvant chemotherapy prior to preoperative RCT *(28)*. As a consequence, surgery has been gradually postponed. Indeed, the need for radical surgery is now challenged by series of patients treated with definitive RCT that report excellent outcomes in patients achieving clinical complete response *(29)*. The second major development has been to integrate concurrent chemotherapy with preoperative RT. More recent series have used "triple combinations," including RT, combination chemotherapy, and targeted therapies *(30,31)*. Phase III trials are needed to determine if these novel combination regimen offer an advantage compared with 5-FU-based combined modality therapy.

Moreover, improved knowledge of microscopic lymphatic spread within the mesorectum has led to the use of total mesorectal excision for mid- and low rectal cancer. With this "optimized" surgery, local control rates have improved markedly and local failure rates greater than 10–15% are now no longer acceptable. Technical advances in RT, including

Table 5
Ongoing phase III trials with novel agents for rectal cancer patients

	Preoperative treatment	*Surgery*	*Postoperative treatment*
ACCORD 12	RT 45 Gy + Capecitabine vs.	TME	Per institutional policy
	RT 50 Gy + Capecitabine + Oxaliplatin	TME	Per institutional policy
STAR	RT 50.4 Gy + 5-FU PVI vs.	TME	5-FU-based CT
	RT 50.4 Gy + 5-FU + Oxaliplatin	TME	5-FU-based CT
NSABP R-04	RT 50.4 Gy + 5-FU vs.	TME	(Patients may enter ECOG-E5204)
	RT 50.4 Gy + 5-FU + Oxaliplatin vs.	TME	
		TME	
	RT 50.4 Gy + Capecitabine vs.	TME	
	RT 50.4 Gy + Capecitabine + Oxaliplatin		
ECOG-E5204	RT 40-55.8 Gy + Chemotherapy according to NSABP-04 or 5-FU PVI/ Capecitabine ± Oxaliplatin or 5-FU + Leucovorin	TME	Oxaliplatin + 5-FU/ Leucovorin vs.
		TME	Oxaliplatin + 5-FU/ Leucovorin + Bevacizumab
CAO/ARO/ AIO-04	RT 50.4 Gy + 5-FU vs.	TME	5-FU vs.
	RT 50.4 Gy + 5-FU + Oxaliplatin	TME	5-FU + Oxaliplatin
CHRONICLE	RT ≥ 45 Gy + 5-FU ± Leucovorin or Capecitabine	TME	Observation vs. Capecitabine + Oxaliplatin
PETACC 6	RT 45 Gy + Capecitabine vs.	TME	Capecitabine vs.
	RT 45 Gy + Capecitabine + Oxaliplatin	TME	Capecitabine + Oxaliplatin
SCRIPT	RT 25 Gy/1 week	TME	Observation vs.
		TME	Capecitabine

RT radiotherapy, *TME* total mesorectal excision, *CT* chemotherapy, *PVI* protracted venous infusion, *ACCORD* Actions Concertées dans les Cancers Colorectaux et Digestifs, *STAR* Studio nazionaleTerapia neoAdiuvante Retto, *NSABP* National Surgical Adjuvant Breast and Bowel Project, *SCRIPT* Simply Capecitabine in Rectal Cancer after Irradiation Plus TME, *CAO/ARO/AIO* Chirurgische Arbeitsgemeinschaft für Onkologie/ Arbeitsgemeinschaft Radiologische Onkologie/Arbeitsgemeinschaft Internistische Onkologie, *CHRONICLE* Chemotherapy or no chemotherapy in clear margins after neoadjuvant chemoradiotherapy in locally advanced rectal cancer, *ECOG* Eastern Cooperative Oncology Group, *PETACC* Pan-European Trials in Alimentary Tract Cancer

tumor- and radiobiologically optimized fractionation, 3D treatment planning and intensity-modulated radiation therapy will further allow more sophisticated treatment delivery resulting in reduced irradiation of normal tissue and increase in therapeutic index. Uniform treatment approaches, established by studies performed more than a decade ago, which apply the same schedule of preoperative or postoperative 5-FU-based RCT to all patients with TNM stage II/III rectal cancer or deliver preoperative, intensive short-course radiation for all patients with resectable rectal cancer, irrespective of tumor stage and treatment goal (e.g., sphincter preservation), need to be questioned. The inclusion of multimodal treatments into the traditional surgical oncological approach, adapted to the tumor location and stage and to individual patient's risk factors, is mandatory. Clearly, future developments will aim at identifying and

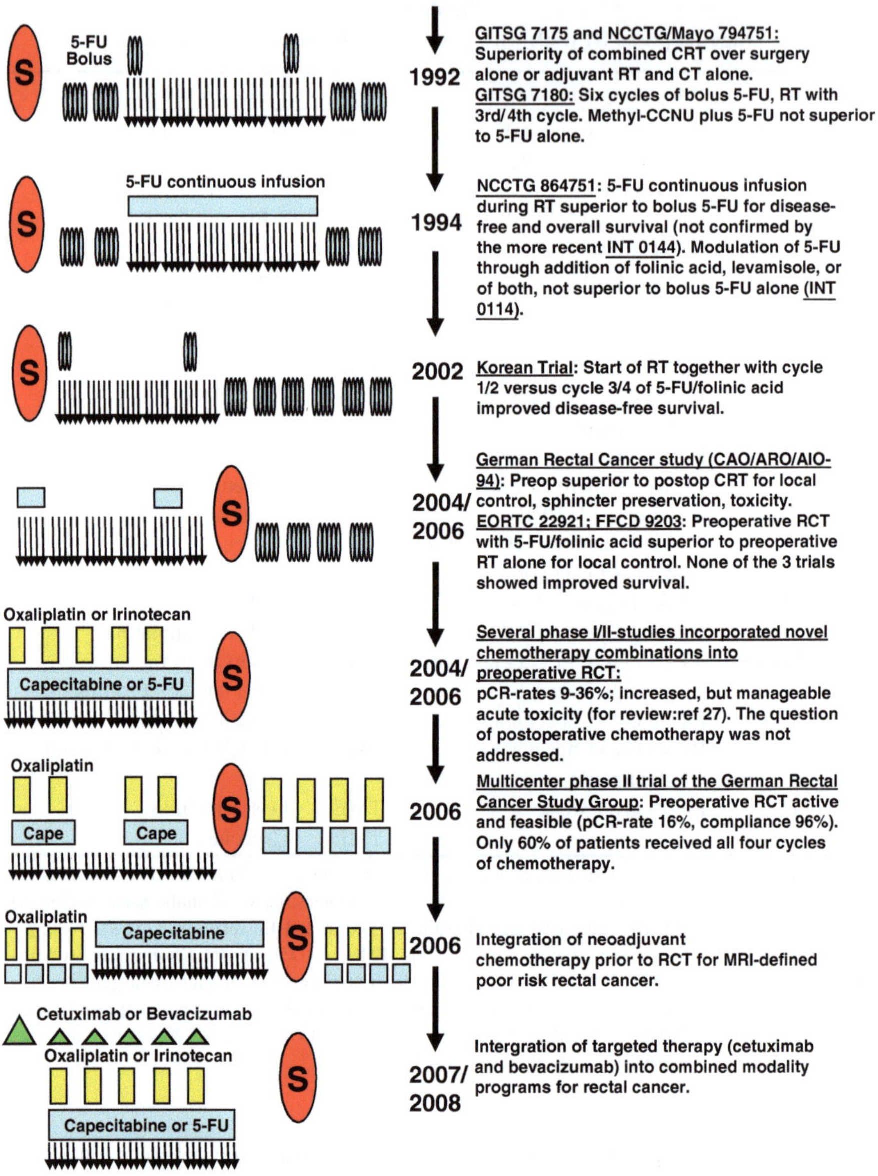

Fig. 2. Timeline of major advances in rectal cancer therapy. S= Surgery

selecting patients for optimal, individualized treatment approaches. Thus, clinicopathological and molecular features as well as accurate preoperative imaging and staging methods with endorectal ultrasound and magnetic resonance imaging will take an important and integrative place in the multimodality treatment of rectal cancer.

REFERENCES

1. Gastrointestinal Tumor Study Group. Prolongation of the disease-free interval in surgically treated rectal carcinoma. *N Engl J Med.* 1985;312(23):1465–1472.
2. Tveit KM, Guldvog I, Hagen S, et al. Randomized controlled trial of postoperative radiotherapy and short-term time-scheduled 5-fluorouracil against surgery alone in the treatment of Dukes B and C rectal cancer. Norwegian Adjuvant Rectal Cancer Project Group. *Br J Surg.* 1997;84(8):1130–1135.
3. Wolmark N, Wieand HS, Hyams DM, et al. Randomized trial of postoperative adjuvant chemotherapy with or without radiotherapy for carcinoma of the rectum: National Surgical Adjuvant Breast and Bowel Project Protocol R-02. *J Natl Cancer Inst.* 2000;92(5):388–396.
4. Cafiero F, Gipponi M, Lionetto R, P.A.R. Cooperative Study Group. Randomized clinical trial of adjuvant postoperative RT vs. sequential postoperative ER plus 5-FU and levamisole in patients with stage II-III resectable rectal cancer: a final report. *J Surg Oncol.* 2003;83(3):140–146.
5. Krook JE, Moertel CG, Gunderson LL, et al. Effective surgical adjuvant therapy for high-risk rectal carcinoma. *N Engl J Med.* 1991;324(11):709–715.
6. NIH consensus conference. Adjuvant therapy for patients with colon and rectal cancer. *JAMA.* 1990;264(11):1444–1450.
7. Gastrointestinal Tumor Study Group. Radiation therapy and fluorouracil with or without semustine for the treatment of patients with surgical adjuvant adenocarcinoma of the rectum. *J Clin Oncol.* 1992;10(4):549–557.
8. O'Connell MJ, Martenson JA, Wieand HS, et al. Improving adjuvant therapy for rectal cancer by combining protracted-infusion fluorouracil with radiation therapy after curative surgery. *N Engl J Med.* 1994;331(8):502–507.
9. Smalley SR, Benedetti JK, Williamson SK, et al. Phase III trial of fluorouracil-based chemotherapy regimens plus radiotherapy in postoperative adjuvant rectal cancer: GI INT 0144. *J Clin Oncol.* 2006;24(22):3542–3547.
10. Tepper JE, O'Connell M, Niedzwiecki D, et al. Adjuvant therapy in rectal cancer: analysis of stage, sex, and local control–final report of intergroup 0114. *J Clin Oncol.* 2002;20(7):1744–1750.
11. Lee JH, Lee JH, Ahn JH, et al. Randomized trial of postoperative adjuvant therapy in stage II and III rectal cancer to define the optimal sequence of chemotherapy and radiotherapy: a preliminary report. *J Clin Oncol.* 2002;20(7):1751–1758.
12. MERCURY Study Group. Diagnostic accuracy of preoperative magnetic resonance imaging in predicting curative resection of rectal cancer: prospective observational study. *BMJ.* 2006;333(7572):779.
13. Swedish Rectal Cancer Trial. Improved survival with preoperative radiotherapy in resectable rectal cancer. *N Engl J Med.* 1997;336(14):980–987.
14. Camma C, Giunta M, Fiorica F, Pagliaro L, Craxi A, Cottone M. Preoperative radiotherapy for resectable rectal cancer: a meta-analysis. *JAMA.* 2000;284(8):1008–1015.
15. Colorectal Cancer Collaborative Group. Adjuvant radiotherapy for rectal cancer: a systematic overview of 8507 patients from 22 randomised trials. *Lancet.* 2001;358(9290):1291–1304.
16. Glimelius B, Gronberg H, Jarhult J, Wallgren A, Cavallin-Stahl E. A systematic overview of radiation therapy effects in rectal cancer. *Acta Oncol.* 2003;42(5-6):476–492.
17. Frykholm GJ, Glimelius B, Pahlman L. Preoperative or postoperative irradiation in adenocarcinoma of the rectum: final treatment results of a randomized trial and an evaluation of late secondary effects. *Dis Colon Rectum.* 1993;36(6):564–572.
18. Sauer R, Becker H, Hohenberger W, et al. Preoperative versus postoperative chemoradiotherapy for rectal cancer. *N Engl J Med.* 2004;351(17):1731–1740.
19. Sebag-Montefiore D, Steele R, Quirke P, et al. Routine short course pre-op radiotherapy or selective post-op chemoradiotherapy for resectable rectal cancer? Preliminary results of the MRC CR07 randomised trial. *J Clin Oncol.* 2006;24:abstr 3511.
20. Minsky BD, Cohen AM, Kemeny N, et al. Enhancement of radiation-induced downstaging of rectal cancer by fluorouracil and high-dose leucovorin chemotherapy. *J Clin Oncol.* 1992;10(1):79–84.
21. Braendengen M, Tveit KM, Berglund A, et al. Randomized phase III study comparing preoperative radiotherapy with chemoradiotherapy in nonresectable rectal cancer. *J Clin Oncol.* 2008;26(22):3687–3694.

22. Bujko K, Nowacki MP, Nasierowska-Guttmejer A, et al. Sphincter preservation following preoperative radiotherapy for rectal cancer: report of a randomised trial comparing short-term radiotherapy vs. conventionally fractionated radiochemotherapy. *Radiother Oncol.* 2004;72(1):15–24.
23. Bujko K, Nowacki MP, Nasierowska-Guttmejer A, Michalski W, Bebenek M, Kryj M. Long-term results of a randomized trial comparing preoperative short-course radiotherapy with preoperative conventionally fractionated chemoradiation for rectal cancer. *Br J Surg.* 2006;93(10):1215–1223.
24. Bosset JF, Collette L, Calais G, et al. Chemotherapy with preoperative radiotherapy in rectal cancer. *N Engl J Med.* 2006;355(11):1114–1123.
25. Gerard JP, Conroy T, Bonnetain F, et al. Preoperative radiotherapy with or without concurrent fluorouracil and leucovorin in T3-4 rectal cancers: results of FFCD 9203. *J Clin Oncol.* 2006;24(28): 4620–4625.
26. Collette L, Bosset JF, den Dulk M, et al. Patients with curative resection of cT3-4 rectal cancer after preoperative radiotherapy or radiochemotherapy: does anybody benefit from adjuvant fluorouracil-based chemotherapy? A trial of the European Organisation for Research and Treatment of Cancer Radiation Oncology Group. *J Clin Oncol.* 2007;25(28):4379–4386.
27. Rodel C, Sauer R. Integration of novel agents into combined-modality treatment for rectal cancer patients. *Strahlenther Onkol.* 2007;183(5):227–235.
28. Chau I, Brown G, Cunningham D, et al. Neoadjuvant capecitabine and oxaliplatin followed by synchronous chemoradiation and total mesorectal excision in magnetic resonance imaging-defined poor-risk rectal cancer. *J Clin Oncol.* 2006;24(4):668–674.
29. Habr-Gama A, Perez RO, Proscurshim I, et al. Patterns of failure and survival for nonoperative treatment of stage c0 distal rectal cancer following neoadjuvant chemoradiation therapy. *J Gastrointest Surg.* 2006;10(10):1319–1329.
30. Willett CG, Boucher Y, di Tomaso E, et al. Direct evidence that the VEGF-specific antibody bevacizumab has antivascular effects in human rectal cancer. *Nat Med.* 2004;10(2):145–147.
31. Rodel C, Arnold D, Hipp M, et al. Phase I-II trial of cetuximab, capecitabine, oxaliplatin, and radiotherapy as preoperative treatment in rectal cancer. *Int J Radiat Oncol Biol Phys.* 2008;70(4): 1081–1086.

14 Radiation Therapy: Short Versus Long Course

Krzysztof Bujko and Magdalena Bujko

INTRODUCTION

Two randomized trials in rectal cancer have demonstrated that preoperative radiotherapy is superior to postoperative radiotherapy in its ability to decrease the risk of local recurrence *(1,2)*. In addition, the rates of early and late adverse effects have been shown to be lower with a preoperative approach. For those reasons, preoperative radiation therapy has become a standard treatment approach in patients with rectal cancer. When preoperative, conventionally fractionated irradiation has been used, the addition of simultaneous chemotherapy to radiation has produced benefit in terms of local control *(3–5)*. In Southern Europe and the USA, a protracted course of preoperative chemoradiation is most commonly used, whereas in the Northern Europe, a short course of radiation alone (5×5 Gy) given immediately prior to surgery is the most commonly used regimen for resectable rectal cancer, with preoperative chemoradiation reserved for unresectable lesions or when the surgical plane of resection (margins) is threatened *(3)*. The aim of this chapter is to provide a theoretical rationale for short-course radiation therapy, to present its efficacy, and to evaluate the advantages and limitations of its use in relation to a chemoradiotherapy regimen.

RATIONALE FOR USING SHORT-COURSE RADIATION THERAPY

Rectal cancer clonogens generally proliferate rapidly, which is reflected in the short mean potential doubling volume time of approximately 5 days *(6,7)*. This observation has led to the concept of shortening the overall irradiation time in efforts to limit the ability of cancer cells to repopulate. This concept was supported by animal model data as reported by Basha et al. *(8)*. In this study, tumors were irradiated with 5×5 Gy over 5 days, 10×3 Gy over 10 days, or 10×3 Gy (twice per day) over 5 days. A significantly higher degree of cancer

From: *Current Clinical Oncology: Rectal Cancer*,
Edited by: B.G. Czito and C.G. Willett, DOI: 10.1007/978-1-60761-567-5_14,

cell killing was observed following both schedules of radiation delivered over 5 days compared to that delivered over 10 days. As performed in the above experiment, the overall treatment time can be shortened by increasing the dose per fraction with total dose reduction (hypofractionation) or by delivering conventional doses per fraction two times per day (accelerated regimen). The advantages of hypofractionated regimens over accelerated regimens include convenience (savings in time for patients and departments) and lower cost. This advantage is especially evident in departments with long waiting lists. On the other hand, large doses per fraction lead to the concern of increasing the risk of late adverse effects. It should be noted, however, that the estimated, biologically equivalent dose of short-course radiation therapy for late damage is slightly less than that calculated for conventionally fractionated schedules (Table 1). This is because the total dose of short-course schedule is drastically reduced to 25 Gy. This lower total dose raises concerns of inadequate cancer cells killing effect, especially when one calculates an isoeffective dose using high α/β ratio of 10 Gy (Table 1). For many years, it was commonly believed that an α/β ratio of approximately 10 Gy is appropriate for most tumors. However, recent data has demonstrated that the α/β estimate is lower for prostate and breast adenocarcinomas *(9,10)* and is closer to that calculated for late adverse effects. Similarly, the α/β ratio for rectal adenocarcinoma has been suggested to be low (5 Gy) *(11)*. Table 1 demonstrates that the radiobiological isoeffective dose estimates of the short-course schedule compare favorably to that calculated for conventionally fractionated schedules in regard to tumor control when the time-corrected linear-quadratic model and low α/β ratio were used. However, in contrast to a chemoradiotherapy regimen, the disadvantage of the short-course radiation-alone schedule is that the synergistic effect of simultaneously delivered radiation and chemotherapy cannot be exploited. This is because the toxicity of the simultaneous delivery of 5×5 Gy and chemotherapy is believed to be prohibitive.

Table 1
Biologically equivalent doses to fractionation given at 2 Gy per fraction *(48)* in two commonly used schedules of preoperative radiotherapy for rectal cancer

	Biologically equivalent doses to fractionation given with 2-Gy fractions (Gy)[a]	
	25 Gy in 5 fractions of 5 Gy	*50.4 Gy in 28 fractions of 1.8 Gy*
Tumor control, $\alpha/\beta=5$ Gy, *(11)* time correction *(49)*[b]	35.7	30.4
Tumor control, $\alpha/\beta=10$ Gy, time correction	31.3	31.0
Late damage, $\alpha/\beta=3$ Gy	40.0	48.4

The following formulas were used:

[a]Biologically equivalent doses (2 Gy per fraction) = nd ($d+\alpha/\beta$/2 Gy + α/β); where n = number of fractions, d = dose (Gy) per fraction *(48)*

[b]Biologically equivalent doses (2 Gy per fraction) with time correction = biologically equivalent doses (2 Gy per fraction) − 0.6 Gy (T − 7); where T = overall treatment time in days. In this formula, it was assumed that 0.6 Gy is lost per day due to the tumor clonogens repopulation starting after 7 days from the beginning of radiation *(49)*

THE EVIDENCE OF LOCAL EFFICACY OF SHORT-COURSE RADIATION THERAPY

Table 2 summarizes randomized trials evaluating a preoperative 5×5 Gy radiation regimen. Three large Swedish randomized trials have compared the regimen of 5×5 Gy preoperatively delivered radiotherapy and immediate surgery vs. surgery alone: Stockholm I, Stockholm II, and the Swedish Rectal Cancer Trial *(12–14)*. The relative reduction of local recurrence incidence in the radiation arms ranged from 52 to 65%. In the largest study (1,168 patients), a statistically significant 8% absolute overall survival benefit at 13 years was reported ($p=0.008$) *(14)*. In the other two trials (Stockholm I and Stockholm II), a benefit in terms of disease-specific survival or in overall survival in the subgroup of curatively treated patients was demonstrated *(12,13)*.

One small randomized trial compared short-course preoperative radiotherapy with conventionally fractionated postoperative radiotherapy *(1)* (Table 2). Superior rates of local control and late complications were seen in the preoperative radiotherapy group although survival did not differ between the groups.

Admittedly, all of the aforementioned Swedish studies were conducted prior to the widespread implementation of modern surgical standard of total mesorectal excision (TME). Thus, local recurrence rates in those trials were higher than reported in more contemporary studies. The low incidence of local recurrence following TME has raised the question of whether preoperative radiation therapy is still needed. To address this question, two large randomized studies have been conducted: the Dutch TME trial *(15,16)* and MRC CR07 trial *(17)*. These studies compared 5×5 Gy preoperative radiotherapy and immediate surgery with the selective use of postoperative radiochemotherapy for patients deemed at high risk for local recurrence (Table 2). Both trials showed a statistically significant benefit in local control with use of short-course preoperative radiotherapy although the absolute benefit was only about 5%. Neither trial showed any overall survival benefit. In the Dutch TME trial, there was no difference in disease-free survival between the arms. In contrast, the MRC CR07 trial showed that disease-free survival was significantly improved in the preoperatively irradiated group. This, however, was initially reported as a 3-year actuarial figure, with many patients having follow-up time of less than 1 year. Thus, this data is not mature enough for definitive conclusions to be drawn.

EARLY ADVERSE EFFECTS AND COMPLIANCE OF SHORT-COURSE RADIATION THERAPY

When surgery is carried out within a week following radiation therapy, the main organ at risk for early toxicity (the rectum) is removed before adverse effects manifest. The symptoms of acute radiation toxicity including enteritis, cystitis, and dermatitis generally occur with a delay of at least 1 week following irradiation, thus within the early postoperative period *(18)*. For this reason, early toxicities of the short-course schedule are underreported, as it may not be distinguished from surgery-related complications.

The most accurate data on the acute toxicity of the 5×5 Gy regimen was presented by Marijnen et al., *(19)* based on results of the Dutch TME trial. Compliance to the irradiation schedule was 98%. Any occurrence of early adverse effects was reported in 26% of patients, and in 7% of those, these complications were recorded as severe (grade II or III). No deaths due to an acute toxicity were reported. Of these, gastrointestinal side effects were most frequently observed. Sacral pain, usually of short duration, was reported in 10% of patients;

Table 2
Randomized trials evaluating short-course (5×5 Gy) preoperative radiotherapy

Study name, reference	*Study design*	*Number of patients*	*Median follow-up, years*	*Main findings and remarks*
Stockholm I *(12)*	5×5 Gy with immediate surgery vs. surgery alone	849	4.5	No difference in overall survival. Improved disease-specific survival (RR=0.76, 95% CI 0.54–1.00, $p=0.05$) and local recurrence rates (11% vs. 23%, $p<0.01$) with radiotherapy but with higher postoperative mortality (8% vs. 2%, $p<0.01$)
Uppsala *(1,21)*	5×5.1 Gy with immediate surgery vs. postoperative radiotherapy 60 Gy, 2 Gy per fraction	471	Minimum 5	No difference in overall survival. Improved local recurrence rates (13% vs. 22%, $p=0.02$) and lower incidence of late small bowel obstruction (5% vs. 11%, $p<0.01$) with preoperative radiotherapy
Stockholm II *(13)*	5×5 Gy with immediate surgery vs. surgery alone	557	9	No difference in overall survival for all patients. Improved overall survival for curatively treated patients (46% vs. 39%, $p=0.03$), fewer local recurrences (12% vs. 25%, $p<0.001$) and more deaths of intercurrent disease within 6 months of surgery (5% vs. 1%, $p=0.02$) with radiotherapy
Swedish trial *(14,22, 25,27,28,50)*	5×5 Gy with immediate surgery vs. surgery alone	1,168	13	Improved overall survival at 13 years (38% vs. 30%, $p=0.008$) with fewer local recurrences (9% vs. 26%, $p<0.001$) with radiotherapy, without increase postoperative morbidity. No increased risk of late toxicity resulting in hospital admission with the exception of late small bowel obstruction. Radiation impaired anorectal function. More patients treated with radiotherapy developed secondary cancer; RR=1.85 (95% CI 1.23–2.78)
Dutch TME trial *(15,16,19,26, 29,30,40)*	5×5 Gy with immediate surgery vs. surgery alone (postoperative radiotherapy 50.4 Gy, 1.8 Gy per fraction for patients with positive CRM or tumor spill at surgery). Of patients allocated to the selective postop radiotherapy arm, 18% were CRM positive although only 11% received radiotherapy).	1,861	6	No difference in overall survival (64.2% in the preoperative radiation group and 63.5% at 5 years in the selective postoperative radiation group, $p=0.90$.) Fewer local recurrences (5.6% vs. 10.9% at 5 years, $p<0.001$) with preoperative radiotherapy. No downstaging in patients with an interval of <10 days between radiation initiation and TME. Radiation impaired anorectal and sexual function

MRC CR07 *(17)*	5×5 Gy with immediate surgery vs. selective postoperative chemoradiation for patients with positive CRM (of patients allocated to the selective postop chemoradiotherapy group, 11% were CRM positive although only 70% of them received chemoradiotherapy)	1,350	3	No difference in overall survival. At 3 years, significantly improved disease-free survival (80% vs. 75%) and local recurrence rates (5% vs. 11%) with preoperative radiotherapy (abstract only)
Polish trial *(20,33, 34,36,39)*	5×5 Gy with immediate surgery vs. chemoradiation (50.4 Gy, 1.8 Gy per fraction + 5-FU/LV) with delayed surgery	312	4	No difference in sphincter preservation (primary endpoint). Less acute adverse events with short-course radiotherapy (grade III–IV 3% vs. 18%, $p<0.001$) but slightly more postoperative complications (27% vs. 21%, $p=0.27$ for absolute patient rates, 31% vs. 22%, $p=0.06$ for number of events). No difference in the rate of patients with severe complications (10% vs. 11%, $p=0.85$). More favorable postoperative pathology with chemoradiotherapy with tumor, on average, 1.9 cm smaller ($p<0.001$); more pathological complete responses (16% vs. 1%, $p<0.001$), fewer positive radial margins (4% vs. 13%, $p=0.017$) and fewer stage III disease patients (32% vs. 48%, $p=0.007$) with chemoradiotherapy. At 4 years, no differences in overall survival, disease-free survival, incidence of local recurrences, late toxicity, anorectal and sexual function
TROG 0104 trial *(23)*	5×5 Gy with immediate surgery vs. chemoradiation (50.4 Gy, 1.8 Gy per fraction + 5-FU/LV) with delayed surgery	326	–	Less postradiotherapy acute toxicity with short-course radiotherapy (grade III–IV 1.9% vs. 28%, $p<0.001$). Similar rates of postoperative complications (51% in the short-course group vs. 49% in the chemoradiotherapy group) (abstract only)

CRM circumferential resection margin, *LV* leucovorin, *5-FU* 5-fluorouracil, *RR* relative risk, *CI* confidence interval the majority of these patients did not require any intervention. However, in 2.5% of patients, the pain was severe and required treatment interruption. Similar results have been reported in other randomized trials *(13,20–23)*.

POSTOPERATIVE COMPLICATIONS FOLLOWING SHORT-COURSE PREOPERATIVE RADIATION THERAPY

In the Stockholm I trial, *(12)* an increase in postoperative mortality was observed in patients receiving radiotherapy compared with those treated with surgery alone (8% vs. 2%, $p<0.01$). Combined analysis of Stockholm I and Stockholm II trials revealed that this increase in mortality was related to a two-portal radiotherapy technique delivered to a relatively large target volume and not observed in patients treated with a four-portal technique to a more limited target volume *(24)*. In trials in which modern radiotherapy techniques were used, no difference in postoperative mortality was seen between radiotherapy plus surgery groups compared to surgery-alone groups *(25,26)*.

Based on data from the Dutch TME trial, detailed information regarding postoperative complications with the use of modern radiotherapy and surgical techniques were reported by Marijnen et al. *(19)* They found no difference in median operation time and hospital stay between the 5×5 Gy preoperative radiotherapy group and the surgery-alone group. Operative blood loss was slightly increased in the radiotherapy group (100 ml). The overall postoperative complication rate was higher in the preoperative radiotherapy group (48% vs. 41%, $p=0.008$). This difference was mainly attributed to an increase in perineal wound complication rates (29% vs. 18%, $p=0.008$). Among irradiated patients, this complication was more frequently observed in those in whom the perineum was included in the radiation treatment volume. The rate of severe postoperative complications, including anastomotic leakage, did not differ between groups, although these results might be biased as temporary stomas were more frequently performed in the preoperative radiation group. The above data is similar to reports of other randomized trials *(12,21,22)*.

LATE ADVERSE EFFECTS OF SHORT-COURSE RADIATION THERAPY

Based on the Swedish Rectal Cancer Trial, Birgisson et al. *(27)* provided data regarding late adverse effects following short-course radiotherapy. In this report, minimal follow-up time was 11 years, and data were retrieved from the national register that included all hospital admissions. No difference in the risk for overall hospital admission was found between the irradiated group and surgery-alone group (relative risk (RR) = 1.07, 95% confidence interval (CI) 0.91–1.26). However, an increased risk for admission during the first 6 months following treatment was seen in irradiated patients (RR = 1.64, 95% CI 1.21–2.22). The primary reasons for this increase were gastrointestinal disorders and infection. Eight years following treatment, an increase in hospital admission for bowel obstruction, nausea, and unspecific abdominal pain were seen in irradiated patients. The cumulative incidence of small bowel obstruction at 14 years was 13.9% in the irradiated group compared to 5.5% in surgery-alone group ($p<0.001$) *(28)*. A trend toward higher rates of bowel obstruction was observed in patients irradiated with a two-field technique as compared to patients treated with multiple fields. Of note, the upper border of the radiation fields in this study was located at middle of the forth lumbar vertebra, which is higher than is generally accepted presently and would result in larger amounts of bowel being irradiated.

The results presented above indicate that there is no significant increase in the risk of severe, late adverse effects of such magnitude to warrant hospital admission following radiation therapy. This, however, does not rule out late toxicity that potentially impairs patients' quality of life. Peeters et al. *(29)* and Marijnen et al. *(30)* provided data regarding sexual function, bowel function, and quality of life following short-course preoperative radiotherapy compared to surgery alone, based on the Dutch TME trial. Increased rates of fecal incontinence (62% vs. 38%, $p<0.001$) and sexual disorders in males ($p=0.004$) and females ($p<0.001$) were reported in the irradiated group. Despite this increase, formally measured, health-related quality of life was similar in the irradiated and surgery-alone groups *(30)*.

One major concern about the use of short-course radiotherapy is the late development of chronic neurotoxicity. In a study from Uppsala, generally reversible sacral pain of long duration was reported in 7 out of 503 patients (1.4%) during a follow-up period ranging from 3 to 14 years. Three (0.6%) patients also developed other neurological symptoms including weakness, numbness, and paralysis of the lower extremities *(31)*. This neurotoxic effect, however, did not translate to detectable differences in formal questionnaire responses regarding neurologic function between the 5×5 Gy group and the surgery-alone group of Dutch TME trial *(29)*. Similarly, in the Swedish Rectal Cancer Trial, there was no difference between groups with regard to hospital admissions due to the neurological disorders *(27)*. In a combined analysis of the Stockholm I and Stockholm II trials, 5.3% of irradiated patients and 2.4% of unirradiated patients ($p=0.03$) were hospitalized because of femoral or pelvic fractures *(32)*. In contrast, no increase in femoral or pelvic fractures following a radiation regimen of 5×5 Gy was observed in other randomized trials *(27,29)*.

RANDOMIZED TRIALS COMPARING PREOPERATIVE SHORT-COURSE RADIATION THERAPY VERSUS PREOPERATIVE CHEMORADIATION THERAPY IN RESECTABLE RECTAL CANCER

The regimens of 5×5 Gy preoperative radiation therapy and conventionally fractionated preoperative chemoradiation therapy were compared in two randomized trials: in the Polish trial *(20,33)* and in the Australian TROG 0104 trial *(23)* (Table 2). The TROG trial was recently closed to accrual following accrual of 326 patients; thus, only acute adverse effects have been reported.

The Polish trial randomized 312 patients with a primary endpoint of evaluating whether the downstaging effect of preoperative chemoradiation therapy results in an improved rate of sphincter preservation when compared to preoperative short-course radiotherapy alone. Trial results showed that anterior resection rates did not differ between groups, accounting for 61% of anterior resections in the short-course group and 58% in the chemoradiation group ($p=0.57$). Similarly, two recent meta-analyses have shown no impact of preoperative radio(chemo)therapy on anterior resection rates *(34,35)*. Both Polish and Australian trials showed higher rates of early radiation toxicity in the chemoradiation group compared to the 5×5 Gy group (Table 2). This lower acute toxicity rate with short-course radiation therapy translated into improved compliance compared to the chemoradiation therapy protocol in the Polish trial (98% vs. 69%) *(20)*. Additionally, in the Polish study, two toxic deaths (1.5%) occurred in the chemoradiation group vs. none in the short-course group. However, the incidence of postoperative complications was slightly higher following short-course radiation therapy vs. chemoradiation therapy in the Polish study *(36)*. This, however, was not confirmed by the Australian trial (Table 2). In the Polish trial, there were no significant differences in survival and local control between both groups *(33)* with actuarial overall survival (at a median follow-up of 4 years) 67% in the short-course group vs. 66% in the chemoradiation group ($p=0.96$). Corresponding values for disease-free survival were 58% vs. 56% ($p=0.82$) and for crude incidence of local recurrence 9% vs. 14% ($p=0.17$). Limitations of this study include that it was underpowered to detect small differences in survival and local control outcomes, as it was designed to detect differences of ≥15% in sphincter preservation rates. It is interesting to note that despite the fact more favorable postoperative pathology was observed in the chemoradiation group compared to the short-course group (Table 2), long-term outcomes were similar. This may be due to the fact that cancer cells damaged after radiotherapy require time to develop necrosis *(37)* and for a period following irradiation, nonviable cancer cells may appear (morphologically) viable *(38)*.

No increase of late toxicity in the short-course irradiation group was observed compared to the chemoradiation group, although follow-up was too short (median 4 years) to draw any definitive conclusions. The crude overall incidence of late toxicity was 28% for patients in the short-course group and 27% in the chemoradiation group ($p=0.81$) *(33)*. The corresponding values of severe late toxicity were 10% vs. 7% ($p=0.36$). No significant differences were observed between the two groups with respect to quality of life, anorectal or sexual function *(39)*. These findings suggest that a preoperative regimen of 5×5 Gy and preoperative long-course chemoradiation therapy may be equivalent management options for patients with resectable rectal cancer. In some countries of Northern Europe, the short-course preoperative radiation regimen is preferred to a chemoradiation regimen due to lower acute toxicity rates, better compliance, and lower cost.

Recently, the short-course radiation regimen has been used in other clinical settings which are described below.

PREOPERATIVE SHORT-COURSE RADIATION THERAPY ALONE OR COMBINED WITH CONSOLIDATION CHEMOTHERAPY IN UNRESECTABLE RECTAL CANCER, WITH OR WITHOUT SYNCHRONOUS DISTANT METASTASES

As tumor shrinkage depends heavily on the interval duration between radiotherapy completion and surgery, *(20,37,40)* no downstaging and very limited downsizing is observed with a regimen of 5×5 Gy and immediate surgery *(40)*. For this reason, this approach is not used in patients with unresectable lesions or when the plane of surgical resection is threatened by tumor invasion on pelvic MRI. Instead, conventionally fractionated chemoradiotherapy is considered as a standard approach for those patients *(3,41)*. However, elderly patients with poor performance status and comorbidities are often unfit for chemotherapy. In addition, a prolonged 5- to 6-week hospital stay or transportation required to undergo conventionally fractionated radiation may be a significant burden for some patients. Due to these issues, short-course radiation therapy with a long interval to surgery (which is required to allow for possible tumor shrinkage) might be an alternative approach. Two retrospective reports have described results of such management. Radu et al. *(42)* reported a series of 24 patients unfit for chemotherapy (mean age 79 years) with unresectable T4NxM0 disease, treated with preoperative regimen of 5×5 Gy with median 7-week interval to surgery. The rate of margin-negative resection was 88% with a pathological complete response rate of 9%. During follow-up (range 7–54 months), local recurrence was detected in one patient. A report by Sebag-Montfiore et al. *(43)* reported on 43 patients unfit for chemotherapy (mean age 80 years) with either fixed tumor or with MRI evidence of tumor within 2 mm of the circumferential resection margin. Forty percent of patients did not proceed to resection for various reasons. The remaining 60% of patients underwent tumor resection at a median of 8 weeks following radiation completion. R0 resection was achieved in 84% of those patients, with pathological complete response seen in 7.5%. In patients undergoing resection, no local recurrences were observed at a median follow-up of 18 months. The results of both series show that short-course radiation therapy with delayed resection is a useful option for patients deemed unfit for chemotherapy with either unresectable disease or with threatened surgical margins.

During conventionally fractionated chemoradiation therapy, the conventional dose of chemotherapy must be reduced by approximately 20% to facilitate acceptable rates of acute toxicity. In patients with unresectable primary tumors with synchronous distant metastatic disease, short-course radiotherapy and chemotherapy delivered in close sequence enable intensification of both systemic treatment and radiation. Radu et al. *(42)* reported a series of 13 patients with unresectable primary tumor with synchronous metastatic disease treated with this approach. In some of these patients, the treatment goal was to make both primary and distant disease resectable. All patients received up-front chemotherapy, mainly a combination of 5-FU/leucovorin/oxaliplatin. Six patients received an additional one or two courses of chemotherapy during the interval between short-course radiotherapy and surgery. Nine patients underwent primary tumor resection. Of these, R0 resection was achieved in six patients and two of the surgical specimens demonstrated pathological complete response. Subsequent surgery for metastatic disease was carried out in two patients. In the entire cohort, ten patients died, and three were alive (all without local symptoms) at a median of 31-month follow-up. These results suggest that the integration of a regimen of 5×5 Gy and chemotherapy is a reasonable option for patients with unresectable primary tumors and distant metastases.

Widder et al. *(44)* reported on two patients with cT3N2 resectable tumors who received 5×5 Gy followed by three courses of oxaliplatin and capecitabine during the interval before surgery. Symptoms decreased rapidly following irradiation and early tolerance was acceptable. In both cases, pathological complete response was observed.

The above clinical reports suggest that the integration of a regimen of 5×5 Gy with sequential consolidating chemotherapy is feasible and promising. The other rationale for this approach is based on the results of the aforementioned Polish study showing similar local efficacy of a regimen of 5×5 Gy and long-course chemoradiation therapy. Thus, it might be expected that the addition consolidating chemotherapy to a 5×5 Gy regimen may produce higher antitumor activity (due to enhanced tumor cytotoxicity) than traditional long-course chemoradiation therapy regimens. Further support for this concept is provided by radiobiological parameters shown in Table 1. In addition, there is the potential to deliver a higher chemotherapy dose intensity compared to the traditional chemoradiation approach. It should be emphasized that at least a 1-week interval between completion of the 5×5 Gy regimen and chemotherapy initiation should be maintained to avoid overlap of early adverse treatment effects (for detailed data about early toxicity of short-course radiation therapy, see prior sections of this chapter). For patients fit for chemotherapy presenting with unresectable cancer, a regimen of 5×5 Gy integrated with consolidating chemotherapy during a prolonged interval to surgery may result in higher rates of curative resection compared to traditional chemoradiation regimens. To test this hypothesis, a phase III study has been launched in Poland.

SHORT-COURSE RADIATION THERAPY PRIOR TO FULL-THICKNESS LOCAL EXCISION

Full-thickness local excision is an attractive treatment for a variety of reasons. It prevents a permanent stoma in patients who would otherwise require abdominoperineal resection. In addition, when compared with transabdominal surgery, the risk of postoperative morbidity is lower.

In this context, it is also worth pointing out that a recent European population-based study showed a 6-month mortality rate as high as 16% following transabdominal rectal cancer surgery in patients older than 75 years compared to 3.9% in younger patients *(45)*. In addition, local excision may be the only surgical option for elderly patients with comorbidities precluding transabdominal resection. Also, improved anorectal function has been observed following local excision compared to low anterior resection. Lastly, local excision does not impair sexual and urinary function. Unfortunately, apart from selected T1 lesions, local excision is associated with high rates of local failure, even when combined with postoperative radio(chemo)therapy *(46)*. However, preoperative radiation therapy may be more effective in preventing local relapse compared to postoperative radiation therapy *(1,2)*. Furthermore, preoperative radiation therapy may expand the use of local excision for T2–3, radiosensitive tumors.

To explore the value of preoperative radiotherapy prior to local excision in a systematic fashion, a prospective, multicenter study was launched. The rationale for designing this trial and early results have been described in detail elsewhere *(18,47)*. Briefly, two series of selection criteria were used to determine patient eligibility in this trial. The first selection was based on tumor size: disease had to be no larger than 3–4 cm and clinically staged as T1, T2, or "borderline" T2–T3. The second selection depended on response to radiation therapy, due to the potential relationship between tumor radiosensitivity and decreased rectal cancer aggressiveness as well as a potentially strong correlation between primary tumor radioresponsiveness and radioresponsiveness of mesorectal nodal disease (which are usually left intact following local excision). If pathological complete response of the primary tumor or downstaging to ypT1 disease with clear surgical margins was achieved following radiation, local excision was considered definitive therapy. For patients with more radioresistant cancer (i.e., in whom the risk of residual mesorectal nodal disease may be higher), immediate conversion to radical resection was planned. Prior to radiotherapy, the mucosa at the tumor edges was tattooed to allow excision of the pretreatment tumor volume in cases of complete or substantial regression. Patients were treated with either 5×5 Gy plus a 4-Gy boost following a 1-week interval (N=31) or with chemoradiotherapy (50.4 Gy plus 5.4 Gy boost at 1.8 Gy per fraction with concurrent 5-fluorouracil and leucovorin) (N=13). Thirteen patients in the short-course radiation group were deemed unfit for chemotherapy. Grade I–II acute radiation toxicity was observed in 11 patients (33%) who were treated with short-course radiotherapy. Of note, in those patients, the onset of early radiation side effects (usually abdominal pain and cramps, fecal urgency and increased stool frequency) was delayed by 3–7 days following 5×5 Gy, i.e., during the 1-week interval between 5×5 Gy and the 4 Gy boost. In all but one patient, these symptoms resolved within 1 week. In five patients, the boost was delayed by a few days beyond that mandated by the protocol (1 week), due to acute toxicity. There was no grade III toxicity in this group. The interval from radiation completion to full-thickness local excision was 6 weeks. Study results showed that pathological complete response was achieved in 35% of patients in the short-course group and 54% of patients in the chemoradiotherapy group. The incidence of patients who were deemed to require conversion to a transabdominal surgery were 39% and 23%, respectively. However, among these, only 53% actually underwent radical resection as the remaining 47% refused or were deemed unfit. During the 14-month median follow-up, local recurrence was detected in 7% of patients and all underwent salvage surgery.

In conclusion, this study suggests that short-course radiation therapy prior to local excision is a viable treatment option for patients unfit for chemotherapy and transabdominal surgery. Additional patients and longer follow-up are required to further evaluate the ultimate efficacy of this treatment.

REFERENCES

1. Frykholm GJ, Glimelius B, Pahlman L. Preoperative or postoperative irradiation in adenocarcinoma of the rectum: final treatment results of a randomized trial and evaluation of late secondary effects. *Dis Colon Rectum.* 1993;36:564–572.
2. Sauer R, Becker H, Hohenberger W, et al. Preoperative versus postoperative chemoradiotherapy for rectal cancer. *N Engl J Med.* 2004;351:1731–1740.
3. Braendengen M, Tveit KM, Berglund A, et al. Randomized phase III study comparing preoperative radiotherapy with chemoradiotherapy in nonresectable rectal cancer. *J Clin Oncol.* 2008;26:3687–3694.
4. Bosset JF, Collette L, Calais G, et al. Chemotherapy with preoperative radiotherapy in rectal cancer. *N Engl J Med.* 2006;355:1114–1123.
5. Gérard JP, Conroy T, Bonnetain F, et al. Preoperative radiotherapy with or without concurrent fluorouracil and leucovorin in T3-4 rectal cancers: results of FFCD 9203. *J Clin Oncol.* 2006;24:4620–4625.
6. Rew DA, Wilson GD, Taylor I, Weaver PC. Proliferation characteristics of human colorectal carcinomas measured in vivo. *Br J Surg.* 1991;78:60–66.
7. Suwinski R, Taylor JM, Withers HR. Rapid growth of microscopic rectal cancer as a determinant of response to preoperative radiation therapy. *Int J Radiat Oncol Biol Phys.* 1998;42:943–951.
8. Basha G, Landuyt W, Fowler J, et al. An experimental evaluation of three preoperative radiation regimens for resectable rectal cancer. *Ann Surg Oncol.* 2002;9:292–297.
9. Brenner DJ, Martinez AA, Edmundson GK, Mitchell C, Thames HD, Armour EP. Direct evidence that prostate tumors show high sensitivity to fractionation (low alpha/beta ratio), similar to late-responding normal tissue. *Int J Radiat Oncol Biol Phys.* 2002;52:6–13.
10. START Trialists' Group, Bentzen SM, Agrawal RK, Aird EG, et al. The UK Standardisation of Breast Radiotherapy (START) Trial A of radiotherapy hypofractionation for treatment of early breast cancer: a randomised trial. *Lancet Oncol.* 2008;9:331–341.
11. Suwinski R, Wzietek I, Tarnawski R, et al. Moderately low alpha/beta ratio for rectal cancer may best explain the outcome of three fractionation schedules of preoperative radiotherapy. *Int J Radiat Oncol Biol Phys.* 2007;69:793–799.
12. Stockholm Colorectal Cancer Study Group. Preoperative short-term radiation therapy in operable rectal carcinoma. A prospective randomized trial. *Cancer.* 1990;66:49–55.
13. Martling AL, Holm T, Johansson H, Rutqvist LE, Cedermark B. The Stockholm II trial on preoperative radiotherapy in rectal carcinoma: long-term follow-up of a population-based study. *Cancer.* 2001;92:896–902.
14. Folkesson J, Birgisson H, Pahlman L, Cedermark B, Glimelius B, Gunnarsson U. Swedish Rectal Cancer Trial: long lasting benefits from radiotherapy on survival and local recurrence rate. *J Clin Oncol.* 2005;23:5644–5650.
15. Marijnen CA, Nagtegaal ID, Kapiteijn E, et al. Radiotherapy does not compensate for positive resection margins in rectal cancer patients: report of a multicenter randomized trial. *Int J Radiat Oncol Biol Phys.* 2003;55:1311–1320.
16. Peeters KC, Marijnen CA, Nagtegaal ID, et al. The TME trial after a median follow-up of 6 years: increased local control but no survival benefit in irradiated patients with resectable rectal carcinoma. *Ann Surg.* 2007;246:693–701.
17. Sebag-Montfiore D, Steele R, Quike P, et al. Short-course preoperative radiotherapy results improves outcome when compared with highly selective postoperative radiochemotherapy. Preliminary results of the MRC CR07 randomised trial. *Radiother Oncol.* 2006;81(suppl 1):s19 (abstract).
18. Bujko K, Richter P, Kolodziejczyk M, et al. Preoperative radiotherapy and local excision of rectal cancer with immediate radical re-operation for poor responders. *Radiother Oncol.* 2009;92(2):195–201.
19. Marijnen CA, Kapiteijn E, van de Velde CJ, et al. Acute side effects and complications after short-term preoperative radiotherapy combined with total mesorectal excision in primary rectal cancer: report of a multicenter randomized trial. *J Clin Oncol.* 2002;20:817–825.

20. Bujko K, Nowacki MP, Nasierowska-Guttmejer A, et al. Sphincter preservation following preoperative radiotherapy for rectal cancer: report of a randomised trial comparing short-term radiotherapy vs. conventionally fractionated radiochemotherapy. *Radiother Oncol.* 2004;72:15–24.
21. Pahlman L, Glimelius B, Graffman S. Pre-versus postoperative radiotherapy in rectal carcinoma: an interim report from a randomised multicentre trial. *Br J Surg.* 1985;72:961–966.
22. Swedish Rectal Cancer Trial. Initial report from a Swedish multicentre study examining the role of preoperative irradiation in the treatment of patients with resectable rectal carcinoma. *Br J Surg.* 1993;80:1333–1336.
23. Ngan S, Fisher R, Mackay J, et al. Acute adverse events in a randomised trial of short course versus long course preoperative radiotherapy for T3 adenocarcinoma of rectum: a Trans-Tasman Radiation Oncology Group trial (TROG 01.04). *Eur J Cancer.* 2007;5(suppl 4):237 (abstract).
24. Holm T, Rutqvist LE, Johansson H, Cedermark B. Postoperative mortality in rectal cancer treated with or without preoperative radiotherapy: causes and risk factors. *Br J Surg.* 1996;83:964–968.
25. Swedish Rectal Cancer Trial. Improved survival with preoperative radiotherapy in resectable rectal cancer. *N Engl J Med.* 1997;336:980–987.
26. Kapiteijn E, Marijnen CAM, Nagtegaal ID, et al. Preoperative radiotherapy combined with total mesorectal excision for resectable rectal cancer. *N Engl J Med.* 2001;345:638–646.
27. Birgisson H, Pahlman L, Gunnarsson U, Glimelius B. Adverse effects of preoperative radiation therapy for rectal cancer: long-term follow-up of the Swedish Rectal Cancer Trial. *J Clin Oncol.* 2005;23:8697–8705.
28. Birgisson H, Pahlman L, Gunnarsson U, Glimelius B. Late gastrointestinal disorders after rectal cancer surgery with and without preoperative radiation therapy. *Br J Surg.* 2008;95:206–213.
29. Peeters KCMJ, van de Velde CJ, Leer JWH, et al. Late side effects of short-course preoperative radiotherapy combined with total mesorectal excision for rectal cancer: increased bowel dysfunction in irradiated patients – a Dutch colorectal cancer group study. *J Clin Oncol.* 2005;23:6199–6206.
30. Marijnen CAM, van de Velde CJ, Putter H, et al. Impact of short-term preoperative radiotherapy on health-related quality of life and sexual functioning in primary rectal cancer: report of multicenter randomized trial. *J Clin Oncol.* 2005;23:1847–1858.
31. Frykholm JG, Sintorn K, Montelius A, Jung B, Pahlman S, Glimelius B. Acute lumbosacral plexopathy during and after preoperative radiotherapy of rectal adenocarcinoma. *Radiother Oncol.* 1996;38:121–130.
32. Holm T, Singnomklao T, Rutqvist LE, Cedermark B. Adjuvant preoperative radiotherapy in patients with rectal carcinoma. Adverse effects during long term follow-up in two randomised trials. *Cancer.* 1996;78:968–976.
33. Bujko K, Nowacki MP, Nasierowska-Guttmejer A, Michalski W, Bebenek M, Kryj M. Long-term results of a randomised trial comparing preoperative short-course radiotherapy vs. preoperative conventionally fractionated chemoradiation for rectal cancer. *Br J Surg.* 2006;93:1215–1223.
34. Bujko K, Kepka L, Michalski W, Nowacki MP. Does rectal cancer shrinkage induced by preoperative radio(chemo)therapy increase the likelihood of anterior resection? A systematic review of randomised trials. *Radiother Oncol.* 2006;80:4–12.
35. Wong RKS, Tandan V, De Silva S, Figueredo A. Pre-operative radiotherapy and curative surgery for the management of localized rectal carcinoma. *Cochrane Database Syst Rev.* 2007;(2):CD002102.
36. Bujko K, Nowacki MP, Kepka L, Oledzki J, B benek M, Kryj M. Postoperative complications in patients irradiated pre-operatively for rectal cancer: report of a randomised trial comparing short-term radiotherapy vs chemoradiation. *Colorectal Dis.* 2005;7:410–416.
37. Francois Y, Nemoz CJ, Bauliex J, et al. Influence of the interval between preoperative radiation therapy and surgery on downstaging and on the rate of sphincter-sparing surgery for rectal cancer: the Lyon R90-01 randomized trial. *J Clin Oncol.* 1999;17:2396–2402.
38. Suit HD, Gallager HS. Intact tumor cells in irradiated tissue. *Arch Pathol.* 1964;78:648–651.
39. Pietrzak L, Bujko K, Nowacki MP, et al. Quality of life, anorectal and sexual functions after preoperative radiotherapy for rectal cancer: report of a randomised trial. *Radiother Oncol.* 2007;84:217–225.
40. Marijnen CA, Nagtegaal ID, Klein Kranenbarg E, et al. No downstaging after short-term preoperative radiotherapy in rectal cancer patients. *J Clin Oncol.* 2001;19:1976–1984.

41. Mercury Study Group. Diagnostic accuracy of preoperative magnetic resonance imaging in predicting curative resection of rectal cancer: prospective observational study. *BMJ.* 2006;333:779.
42. Radu C, Berglund K, Pahlman L, Glimelius B. Short-course preoperative radiotherapy with delayed surgery in rectal cancer – a retrospective study. *Radiother Oncol.* 2008;87:343–349.
43. Sebag-Montfiore D, Hingorani M, Radhakrishna G, et al. Short-course pre-operative radiotherapy with elective delay prior to surgery, in frail and poor PS patients with unresectable rectal cancer. *Radiother Oncol.* 2008;88(2):S220 (abstr.).
44. Widder J, Herbst F, Scheithauer W. Preoperative sequential short-term radiotherapy plus chemotherapy can induce complete remission in T3N2 rectal cancer. *Acta Oncol.* 2005;44:921–923.
45. Rutten H, den Dulk M, Lemmens V, et al. Survival of elderly rectal cancer patients not improved: analysis of population based data on the impact of TME surgery. *Eur J Cancer.* 2007;43: 2295–2300.
46. Greenberg JA, Shibata D, Herndon JE II, Steele GD Jr, Mayer R, Bleday R. Local excision of distal rectal cancer: an update of cancer and leukemia group B 8984. *Dis Colon Rectum.* 2008;51: 1185–1191.
47. Bujko K, Sopylo R, Kepka L. Local excision after radio(chemo)therapy for rectal cancer: is it safe? *Clin Oncol (R Coll Radiol).* 2007;19:693–700.
48. Fowler JF. The linear-quadratic formula and progress in fractionated radiotherapy. *Br J Radiol.* 1989;62:679–694.
49. Colorectal Cancer Collaborative Group. Adjuvant radiotherapy for rectal cancer: a systematic overview of 8507 patients from 22 randomised trials. *Lancet.* 2001;358:1291–1304.
50. Birgisson H, Pahlman L, Gunnarsson U, Glimelius B. Occurrence of second cancers in patients treated with radiotherapy for rectal cancer. *J Clin Oncol.* 2005;23:6126–6131.

15 Chemoradiation Therapy: Nonoperative Approaches

Angelita Habr-Gama, Rodrigo Perez, Igor Proscurshim, and Joaquim Gama-Rodrigues

TUMOR RESPONSE TO RADIATION THERAPY AND SURGERY

Tumor-cell death appears to be significantly related to a process induced by ionizing radiation. Experimental studies have demonstrated that tumoral cellular proliferation is markedly reduced following delivery of dose of 44 Gy. It is believed that after such dose, the metastatic potential of irradiated cells is significantly compromised *(3)*. Indeed, tumor regression or cellular death may be observed not only in the primary tumor (within the rectal wall) but also in metastatic disease in perirectal lymph nodes. This has been supported by the observation of a shift toward earlier disease stage in patients receiving preoperative therapy, where the rates of pathologic stage II or III disease are markedly decreased when compared to patients managed by surgery alone *(1,2)*.

Ultimately, tumor regression following neoadjuvant therapy may be complete, leading to absence of residual neoplasia in the resected specimen, termed complete pathological regression or ypT0N0M0 (ypCR) *(4)*. In this setting, patients without microscopic residual disease would probably not benefit from radical surgery and instead, would be unnecessarily exposed to surgery-related morbidity, mortality, sexual/urinary dysfunction, and to the placement of permanent or temporary stomas.

Indeed, radical surgery for rectal cancer has been associated with high rates of acute morbidity and mortality. In terms of immediate morbidity, anastomotic leaks are probably the most feared complication and may occur in up to 12% of cases *(1,5)*. Even though it has been suggested that preoperative radiation therapy would lead to a significant increase in the risk of anastomotic leaks, prospective randomized trials have failed to demonstrate such differences previously observed in retrospective analyses *(1,6,7)*. Overall, perioperative

From: *Current Clinical Oncology: Rectal Cancer*,
Edited by: B.G. Czito and C.G. Willett, DOI: 10.1007/978-1-60761-567-5_15,

mortality rates may reach 2–3% in patients managed by radical surgery. These rates, however, are significantly higher in cases of anastomotic leak, reaching up to 13% *(6,7)*. In order to significantly decrease the incidence of anastomotic leaks, the adoption of routine, temporary diversion of patients undergoing low anterior resection, particularly when associated with total mesorectal excision (TME), has been recommended and was shown to be beneficial in a prospective randomized trial *(8)*. Finally, one must consider the cumulative morbidity and mortality of patients managed by temporary diversion since simple stoma closure may also be associated with significant morbidity rates, notably in patients with rectal cancer, who are often older and frequently have increased rates of medical comorbidities relative to patients with benign colorectal diseases *(9–11)*. Moreover, radical resection of the rectum may further lead to functional disabilities including fecal incontinence as well as variable rates of urinary and sexual dysfunction. Therefore, the finding of complete pathological response in up to 30% of neoadjuvantly irradiated cases raised the question regarding the benefits of a procedure in which not a single cancer cell was removed *(12)*. For these reasons, an alternative approach was suggested in highly selected patients with complete clinical response. With this approach, patients with no signs of residual disease at least 8 weeks following chemoradiation therapy completion would be managed by serial observation without immediate surgery *(12)*.

In order to fully understand this approach, several aspects should be discussed, including definitions of complete clinical response, the management algorithm itself, the timing and tools for assessment of tumor response, and the risks involved with an approach of serial observation following chemoradiotherapy.

Definition of Complete Clinical Response

Complete clinical response is defined by the absence of residual disease following neoadjuvant therapy. Even though this definition may seem straightforward, the term "absence of residual disease" may in fact be interpreted in different ways. Most authors argue that there is usually, if not always, some type of residual scar tissue at the site of the primary tumor, even following complete tumor regression. In our experience, a subtitle white discoloration of the mucosa may be detectable by proctoscopy in some of these patients, and requires no immediate surgical resection. If there is any suspicion of a residual scar that can be either seen by proctoscopy or palpated by digital rectal examination, a full-thickness local excision may be performed, primarily as a diagnostic approach. Any residual ulcer or mass should be interpreted as incomplete clinical response and surgery is the preferred approach *(13)* (Fig. 1a, b).

Timing of Response Assessment

One cannot define complete clinical response without defining the exact timing for assessment of such. Since the beginning of the author's experience with neoadjuvant chemoradiotherapy, the assessment of tumor response has been performed no less than 8 weeks following chemoradiation completion *(12,13)*. In contrast, most surgeons still recommend surgery 6 weeks following chemoradiotherapy completion *(1,5)*. Even though there is no good evidence indicating the optimal timing for response assessment for neoadjuvantly-treated rectal cancer, there is data indicating that waiting longer periods following chemoradiotherapy completion may be associated with higher rates of tumor downstaging. A retrospective study of patients managed by neoadjuvant chemoradiotherapy followed by radical surgery showed that patients who underwent resection beyond 45 days following chemoradiotherapy

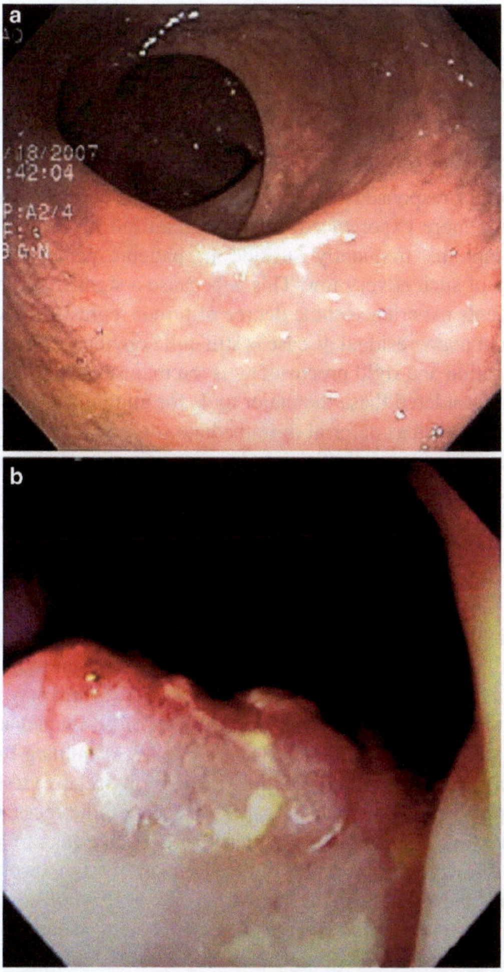

Fig. 1. (**a**) Endoscopic view of a patient with a complete clinical response at 8 weeks from CRT completion; (**b**) Endoscopic view of a patient with an incomplete clinical response at 8 weeks from CRT completion.

completion had slightly higher rates of complete pathological response *(14)*. Another retrospective study demonstrated that patients managed by radical surgery after a period greater than 7 weeks following chemoradiotherapy completion experienced increased rates of pCR. More interestingly, these patients also experienced improved disease-related outcomes *(15)*. Similarly, the interval between chemoradiotherapy completion and tumor response assessment has been a matter of interest in squamous cell cancer of the anus. Despite the obvious differences in histology, these tumors (anal and rectal cancer) share a close anatomical proximity and a somewhat similar treatment strategy (combined chemoradiotherapy). For anal cancer, tumor response assessment is generally performed at least 8–12 weeks following chemoradiotherapy completion. In one study in patients undergoing chemoradiotherapy for squamous cell carcinoma of the anus, tumor response assessment performed at 4 weeks following treatment completion resulted in a 12% complete clinical response rate as opposed to 80% when response assessment was performed at 8 weeks *(16)*.

Tools in Assessment of Tumor Response

Assessment of tumor response is not an easy task for the colorectal surgeon and may be challenging, even for more experienced, highly specialized rectal cancer surgeons. Even though clinical symptoms frequently subside in patients achieving complete clinical response, specificity of such is very low. This is because a significant proportion of neoadjuvantly treated patients experience some degree of tumor regression and associated symptom relief, although in many residual disease is still quite obvious. Clinical assessment using digital rectal examination and rigid proctoscopy is the mainstay of response assessment and up to now, we have considered these the major tools for guiding appropriateness of alternative treatment strategies such as deferral of immediate surgery. If there is any residual ulcer, mass, or even an excisable scar, full-thickness local excision should be attempted, primarily as a diagnostic procedure. In such cases, standard full-thickness local excision or transanal microscopic endoscopic surgery may be performed. Besides proper surgical technique, full pathological examination of the specimen is of paramount importance, since diagnosing microscopic residual disease may be also a challenge for the pathologist. These histologic analyses should be performed by an experienced pathologist, a critical member of the rectal cancer multidisciplinary management team. Since clinical assessment by rigid proctoscopy and digital rectal examination are probably still the most important tools in assessing tumor response to chemoradiotherapy, tumors located in the upper rectum may not be as amenable to assessment when considering an alternative approach of no immediate surgery. In addition, these tumors, which are inaccessible to the surgeon's examining finger, may be more amenable to anterior resection (with lower rates of morbidity relative to lower tumors) with improved rates of sphincter resection and local recurrence. Studies performed on the usefulness and accuracy of clinical assessment of patients with rectal cancer following neoadjuvant chemoradiotherapy showed disappointing rates of sensitivity and specificity. It should be noted, however, that these studies used a 6-week interval between chemoradiotherapy completion and response assessment, and therefore could have potentially detected clinically residual disease in patients with ongoing tumor regression. Additionally, the inclusion of varying examiners could have also biased these results, depending on individual's experience and perception of complete clinical response *(17)*.

Carcinoembryonic antigen (CEA) has been extensively used in colorectal cancer management for different purposes. One study of patients undergoing radical surgery alone for rectal cancer demonstrated that a decrease in CEA 7 days following rectal resection was associated with improved outcomes, suggesting that initial CEA levels were probably exclusively related to the primary tumor instead of undetected/microscopic metastatic disease *(18)*. In addition to clinical and surgical assessment of tumor response, determination of CEA levels before and after chemoradiotherapy may also be useful. In a study of over 500 patients with rectal cancer managed by neoadjuvant chemoradiotherapy, low CEA level prior to treatment was a predictor of complete pathological response at radical surgery on univariate analysis *(19)*. In our experience, the fall or difference between pre- and postchemoradiotherapy CEA levels was not a good predictor of complete tumor regression. Instead, patients with low postchemoradiotherapy CEA levels, irrespective of prechemoradiotherapy CEA levels, were significantly more likely to achieve complete clinical response and improved outcomes following neoadjuvant therapy *(20)*.

Radiological assessment of tumor response has been a significant challenge in rectal cancer management. Staging of primary (untreated) tumor depth of penetration and distance from the circumferential margin seems to be adequately assessed by endorectal ultrasound and magnetic resonance imaging. However, following neoadjuvant therapy, distinguishing between residual cancer and transmural fibrosis may be challenging as both ultrasonography and magnetic resonance imaging rely primarily on morphological features *(21–23)*.

The integration of PET imaging into standard radiologic evaluation has provided significant additional information through the incorporation metabolic activity data with standard morphologic assessment. In addition, PET imaging may also provide a useful and objective estimate of the metabolic activity of a specified area through the standard uptake value (SUV) measured at various phases of the study. One study of 25 rectal cancer patients compared the results of a baseline PET-CT (before chemoradiotherapy) with a second PET-CT performed at 6 weeks following chemoradiotherapy completion. All patients experienced a decrease in the maximum standard uptake value (SUVmax) between baseline and posttherapy PET-CT. Additionally, the posttherapy SUVmax was significantly associated with primary T-stage downstaging, as patients experiencing T-stage downstaging had significantly lower SUVmax values (1.9 vs. 3.3; $p=0.03$) *(24)*. However, even though SUVmax obtained posttherapy was associated with significant tumor downstaging, this did not correlate with ultimate disease-related outcomes. Other studies have also attempted to establish a correlation between PET response, including visual response scores with SUV values, with tumor downstaging and outcomes. In a study of 15 patients undergoing baseline PET (before chemoradiotherapy), followed by a second PET 6 weeks postchemoradiotherapy, the visual response score was shown to provide superior prediction of tumor downstaging as well as extent of pathological response to chemoradiotherapy *(25)*. This same group of patients was prospectively followed and outcome analyses showed that patients who ultimately developed recurrent disease had a significantly lower percent decrease between baseline and postchemoradiotherapy PET SUVmax values. A cutoff of a 62.5% decrease/difference between baseline and postchemoradiotherapy SUVmax values was a significant predictor of disease-free survival. Patients with a greater than 62.5% decrease in SUVmax were at lower risk for recurrence *(26)*. These same authors studied the prediction of tumor response by sequential PET imaging. In a study of 25 patients undergoing baseline PET, followed by an early (10 days after initiation of chemoradiotherapy) PET, the visual response score was able to predict patients who achieved complete pathological response following chemoradiotherapy. This knowledge could potentially be useful in tailoring the treatment of these patients by allowing change in treatment regimen during therapy *(27)*.

Besides small patient numbers, another limitation of these studies is that none addressed the influence of an increased time interval between chemoradiotherapy and tumor response assessment on results. A recent study evaluated 30 patients with rectal cancers less than 5 mm from the circumferential margin as determined by MRI. All patients underwent chemoradiotherapy (65.6 Gy of radiation). Baseline and 8-week posttherapy PET-CT results were compared. This study found a poor correlation between PET-CT results and final pathological findings. The sensitivity and specificity rates for complete pathological response were 75 and 40% respectively. Twelve patients out of 30 studied had a false negative PET-CT result *(28)*.

In an earlier study, we performed PET imaging in patients with complete clinical response who were managed nonoperatively. In all 22 patients, PET showed no signs of residual disease in the primary site, consistent with the findings of clinical, endoscopic, and radiological assessment. On the other hand, eight patients with known residual disease following chemoradiotherapy completion also underwent PET and served as a "control" group. All eight patients in the control group showed PET-avid disease within the rectal wall. This study suggests that PET may be useful in the late assessment of tumor response following nonoperative management of patients achieving complete clinical response following chemoradiotherapy and provides further evidence of durable long-term local control in these patients *(29)*. There is an ongoing study at our Institution evaluating the role of PET-CT in assessing tumor response after neoadjuvant chemoradiotherapy. In this study, all patients undergo a baseline, a 6-week, and a 12-week PET-CT following chemoradiotherapy completion. In addition, nonoperative patients with sustained complete clinical response will undergo further annual PET-imaging during follow-up. The results of this study may further define the role of PET-CT imaging in assessing tumor response and the significance of prolonged (6 weeks vs. 12 weeks) response of tumor metabolism and associated downstaging (Figs. 2 and 3).

The Effects of Radiation Therapy on Nodal Status

The inclusion of the mesorectum within the radiation field in patients undergoing neoadjuvant chemoradiotherapy for rectal cancer is standard practice. Therefore, one could anticipate that such an approach would have an effect on perirectal nodes similar to that observed in the primary tumor. In fact, it seems that downstaging of rectal cancer may not only be observed in the primary tumor, but also in involved perirectal nodes.

Available data suggests that radiation therapy may influence the overall number of pelvic and perirectal nodes of patients undergoing neoadjuvant therapy followed by radical surgery. Data obtained from the SEER (Surveillance, Epidemiology, and End-Results) database have indicated that patients undergoing neoadjuvant radiation therapy had significantly fewer nodes retrieved from the surgical specimen when compared to patients undergoing surgery without neoadjuvant therapy on multivariate analysis. Interestingly, the number of retrieved nodes was significantly higher in patients with N+ disease *(30)*. This observation of an overall reduction in the number of nodes of patients undergoing neoadjuvant therapy seems to be influenced by the time lapse between radiation completion and surgical resection.

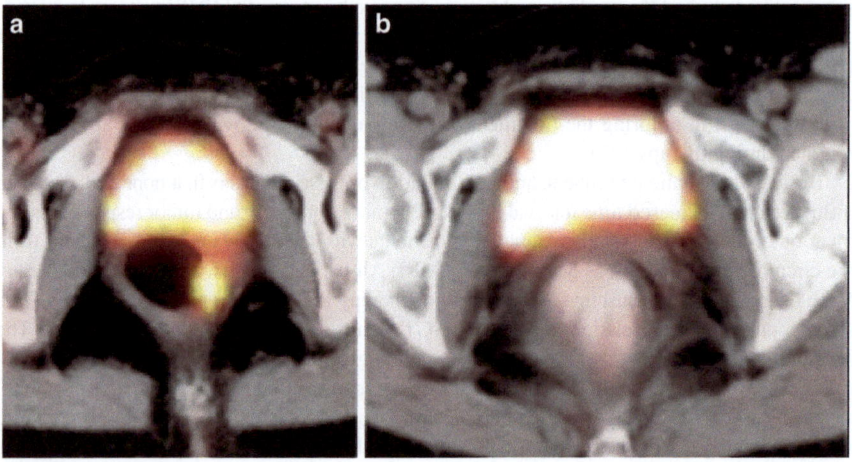

Fig. 2. (**a**) Shows an obvious abnormal uptake in the left lateral rectal wall. (**b**) Shows no uptake within the rectal wall. The rectum has been distended by the presence of intrarectal contrast to facilitate visualization of the rectal wall.

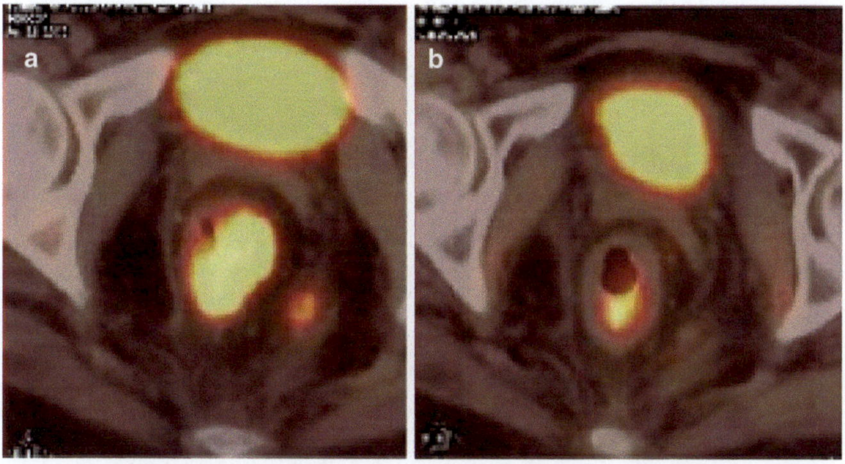

Fig. 3. (**a**) Shows abnormal rectal uptake within the rectal wall and (**b**) persistent uptake at 6 weeks from CRT completion (in the posterior aspect of the rectum).

Another study showed that the number of recovered nodes was significantly affected by the interval between chemoradiotherapy completion and surgery but not by total radiation dose. Patients with a longer interval between radiation and surgery had recovery of fewer nodes in their surgical specimens. This observation has at least two potential implications: first, the critical and required number of nodes for proper pathologic staging of rectal cancer may not be the same for patients undergoing neoadjuvant therapy; second, the effects of radiation on lymph nodes seem to be time-dependent, similar to what has been observed for primary tumor regression *(31)*.

Regarding this matter, we retrospectively reviewed the outcomes of patients without any recovered lymph nodes from the resected specimen following neoadjuvant chemoradiotherapy and radical surgery (only patients demonstrating incomplete clinical response). Surprisingly, outcomes of patients with no recovered nodes were slightly better than patients with node-negative disease and significantly better than patients with node-positive disease. This suggests that patients with no nodes retrieved from the resected specimen may represent a subset of patients with a particularly increased sensitivity to chemoradiotherapy *(32)*.

It seems, therefore, that neoadjuvant chemoradiotherapy leads to a fewer number of perirectal nodes, that this effect is time-dependent (interval between chemoradiotherapy and surgery) and that the reduction of lymph node number may reflect increased sensitivity to chemoradiotherapy.

Besides the effects of neoadjuvant chemoradiotherapy on the number of perirectal nodes, studies have consistently demonstrated decreased rates of lymph node metastases among patients undergoing preoperative radiotherapy/chemoradiotherapy. In addition to this observation, the risk of lymph node micrometastases also seems to be decreased in neoadjuvantly treated patients. However, nodal sterilization secondary to neoadjuvant chemoradiotherapy remains highly controversial. The interesting finding of mucin deposits within lymph nodes of patients with rectal cancer following neoadjuvant therapy without any residual cancer cells, facilitated by the use of anticytokeratin stains, may provide indirect evidence of such sterilization *(33)* (Fig. 4).

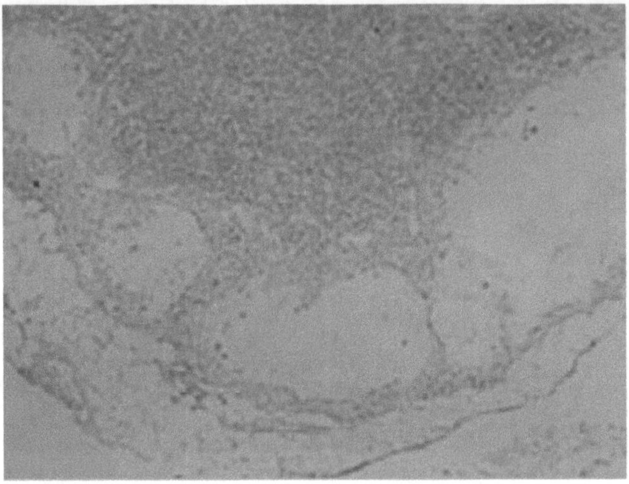

Fig. 4. Microscopic view of a lymph node with significant mucin deposits but no cancer cells detected.

Finally, one of the major concerns following neoadjuvant chemoradiotherapy is that even though the primary tumor may have completely regressed, there is still a risk of residual nodal positivity. The rates of nodal disease (N+) in patients with complete primary tumor regression (ypT0) vary between 0 and 7% *(34–37)*. Again, these rates might reflect differences in timing of surgery and doses of radiation therapy. In support of this, the higher rates of ypT0N+ disease are consistently associated with patients undergoing surgery at 6 weeks following chemoradiotherapy completion and could be detecting lymph node metastases that are in the process of cancer cell death. Additionally, the clinical relevance of microscopic residual lymph node metastases is still poorly understood. The presence of lymph node micrometastases has not been completely accepted as a clinically relevant finding as conflicting results have been observed in these patients *(38,39)*. To keep things in perspective, however, is the fact that the risk of residual microscopic nodes with ypT0 disease remains less than the risk of lymph node metastases of patients with pT1 rectal cancer (around 12–13%), who are frequently managed by transanal local excision alone *(40)*.

Follow-Up Algorithm

Patients with complete clinical response, either after clinical assessment or after transanal local excision (ypT0), are enrolled in a strict follow-up program (Fig. 5). This algorithm includes monthly follow-up visits with digital rectal examination and rigid proctoscopy at every visit. Repeat local excision is sometimes required. CEA levels are also determined every 2 months. As discussed previously, the relationship of PET-CT to tumor response assessment is currently being investigated in a prospective study. Other radiological studies such as pelvic CT scans or magnetic resonance imaging are performed at initial tumor response assessment and every 6 months if there are no signs of tumor recurrence. The main objective of these radiological studies is to rule out any sign of residual extrarectal disease (such as residual nodal disease) that would require further investigation or even radical resection.

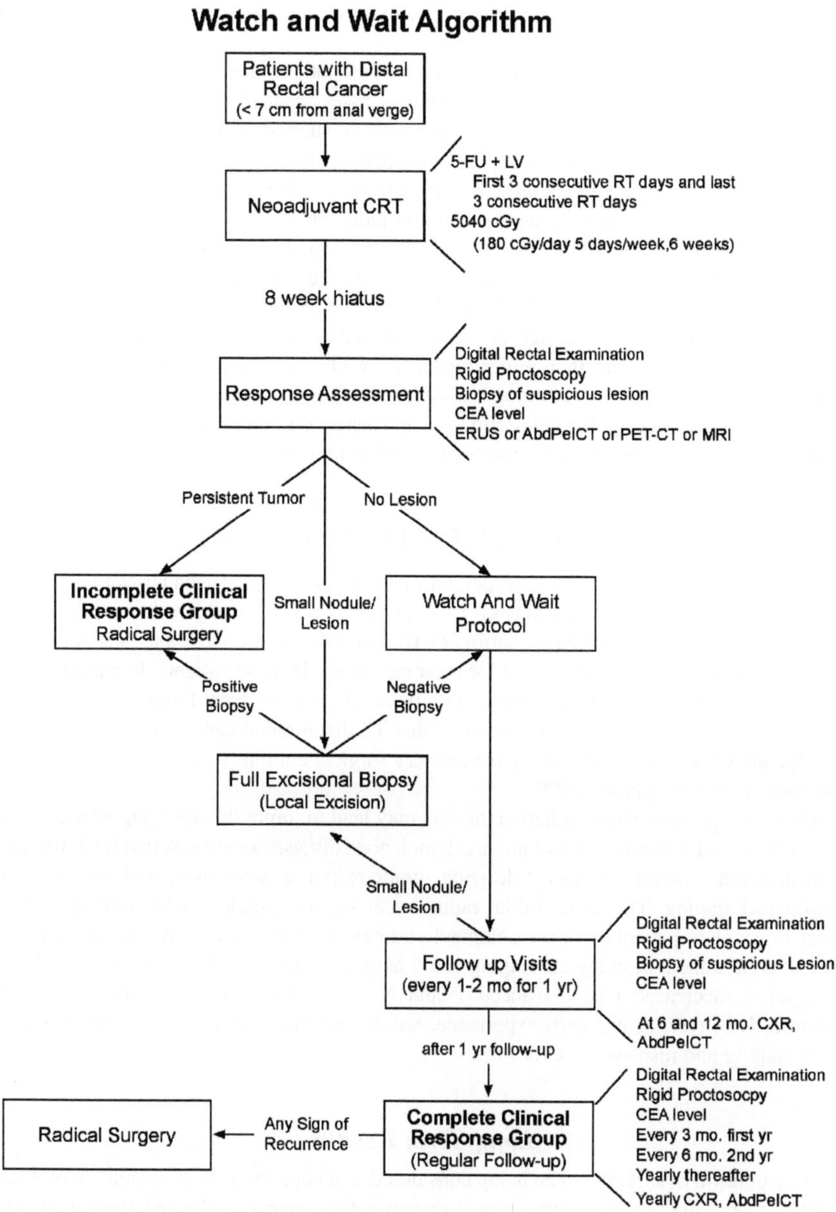

Fig. 5. Algorithm for a "watch and wait" strategy following complete clinical response in patients with rectal cancer receiving neoadjuvant chemoradiotherapy.

Patients are fully informed that complete clinical regression of their primary tumor may be temporary and disease recurrence or tumor regrowth may occur at any time during follow-up. In the case of overt recurrence or tumor regrowth, radical surgery is strongly recommended. Small nodules or scar may develop over time and can be managed by full-thickness transanal excision (either standard or microscopic endoscopic surgery), primarily as a diagnostic approach.

After 1 year of sustained complete clinical response, patients are recommended for follow-up visits every 3 months using the same clinical assessment tools described above. This arbitrary 12-month initial observation period has been suggested by us as an interval long enough for one to decide between complete, incomplete, and near-complete response in these patients. One must remember that this treatment strategy evolved during over the last 15 years and that our accuracy in clinical assessment and judgment has significantly improved over this period. During the early period using this approach, patients were followed without immediate surgery more often, even after a near-complete clinical response, with the hope that a longer time interval would ultimately lead to a complete clinical response. More recently, these patients are more aggressively evaluated using full-thickness local excision as a diagnostic procedure and then either managed by observation or referred to immediate radical surgery depending on histologic findings. As above, we are currently investigating the role of PET-CT in assessing long-term local and distant disease control following complete clinical response and nonoperative management of rectal cancer.

PATIENT SELECTION

Initial radiological assessment is crucial for patient selection for neoadjuvant CRT. It has been shown that radiologically staged T3–4 and/or N± rectal cancers benefit from this approach in terms of local disease control *(1)*. However, in addition to T and N status, tumor location is also a significant predictor for local recurrence in these patients. In particular, the most distal rectal cancers are associated with increased risk for local failure, even in T2N0 disease *(39)*. In this setting, we recommend that T2 distal rectal cancers be considered for neoadjuvant CRT, particularly where the primary surgical alternative would otherwise be an abdominoperineal resection (APR).

Since neoadjuvant chemoradiation therapy may lead to tumor downstaging or regression in both the primary (within the rectum) and lymph node disease, we suggest that final management decisions should be made following tumor response assessment and not at initial radiological staging. Therefore, initial radiological staging should not be used upfront to select or exclude patients from a treatment strategy of CRT with no immediate surgery. Indeed, pretreatment radiological staging could help select patients at increased (early T and N stage) or decreased risk (advanced T and N stage) for achieving complete clinical response. However, in our own experience, we did not observe any correlation between initial staging and response to CRT *(40)*.

Long-Term Results

Once deferral of surgery began being considered as an option in the management of distal rectal cancer achieving complete clinical response following neoadjuvant therapy, it was truly difficult to argue to proceed with resection given both patients and physicians were unwilling to pursue radical surgery unless residual tumor was strongly suspected. Ideally, a prospective randomized trial comparing radical surgery vs. observation alone could potentially provide definitive answers in terms of long-term local control, survival, associated morbidity, and functional outcomes using this approach.

Even though deferred surgery was considered an alternative approach by our group, some patients were still managed with radical surgery even though residual cancer could

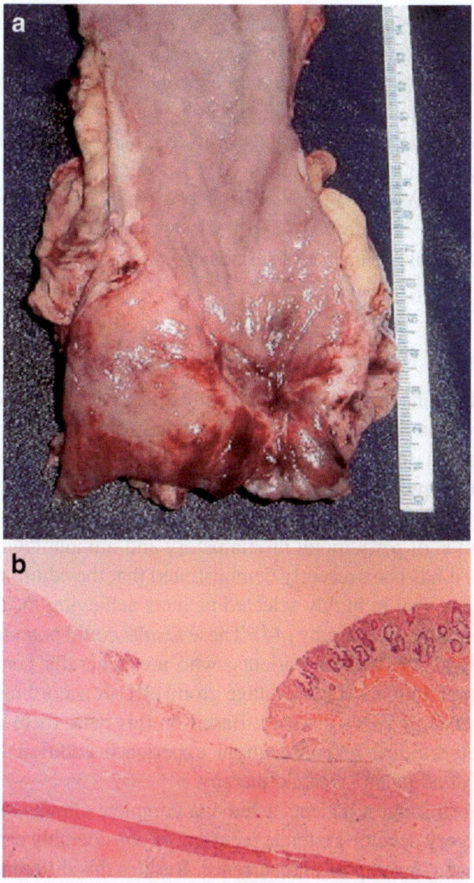

Fig. 6. (**a**) Specimen after radical rectal resection showing residual rectal ulcer. (**b**) Despite macroscopic ulcer, no cancer cells were identified at microscopy.

neither be confirmed nor ruled out. This includes patients with residual scars that were not amenable to local excision as well with partial narrowing of the rectum impeding complete and adequate rectal visualization. In this setting, several patients ultimately underwent radical surgery and were found to have complete pathological response (Fig. 6).

Patients achieving complete clinical response and managed nonoperatively were compared to similar patients with complete pathological response following radical surgery (ypT0N0M0) in order to understand the benefits of radical surgery in both survival and local disease control *(41)*. Surprisingly, patients managed by observation alone fared (oncologically) no worse than patients managed by radical surgery. Systemic recurrences and long-term survival were both similar. However, local relapse was (expectedly) higher in the group of patients managed nonoperatively. Interestingly, these local failures were confined to the rectal wall exclusively, all were amenable to salvage therapy and no pelvic relapse was observed. These results suggested that, in the absence of any benefit in terms of overall and disease-free survival, serial observation following a complete clinical response might be preferred to immediate radical surgery by avoiding potential unnecessary morbidity, mortality, sexual and urinary dysfunction, and the requirement for temporary or definitive stomas.

Long-term results of patients achieving complete clinical response managed nonoperatively were also compared to patients with incomplete clinical response and managed by radical surgery. Patient survival was closely associated with final (clinical or pathological) staging. In this setting, patients with clinical complete response (stage c0) had similar long-term results to patients with complete pathological response (stage p0). Accordingly, these survival rates were significantly better than those observed for patients with stage group ypII and ypIII disease. Patients with stage group ypI experienced intermediate long-term survival rates.

Survival and Recurrences

Recurrence in rectal cancer following any form of therapy should be stratified into local and systemic recurrence. In fact, prospective randomized studies have failed to demonstrate a survival benefit in patients undergoing neoadjuvant chemoradiotherapy when compared to adjuvant chemoradiotherapy. One of the possible explanations for this could be the detrimental effect of neoadjuvant therapy on host immunological response against rectal cancer, such as the potential inhibition of peritumoral inflammatory and immunological response *(42,43)*.

On the other hand, it has been recently demonstrated that the addition of adjuvant chemotherapy can improve survival in highly selected patients achieving local tumor downstaging (ypT0-2) following neoadjuvant therapy *(44)*. These results could potentially lead to a significant change in management of these patients, who are generally considered for adjuvant therapy according to pretreatment staging (stage group cIII) or according to final pathological staging (i.e., the presence of ypN+ disease). Based on this data, there is the possibility that patients with complete clinical response might experience additional benefit in terms of survival with the use of adjuvant systemic therapy.

Interestingly, our data suggest patients achieving complete clinical response and managed with no immediate surgery develop systemic recurrences considerably earlier during follow-up compared to patients who develop local recurrence. Besides this difference being attributed to intrinsic tumor behavior, this discrepancy may be partly explained by the recognized limitations with contemporary imaging modalities, which are incapable of detecting microscopic foci of metastatic disease at initial presentation. Again, in this particular series of patients, adjuvant systemic therapy was considered only in patients with stage group ypIII disease *(45)*.

Local recurrences may occur in nearly 10% of patients managed nonoperatively following complete clinical response. Interestingly, in all of these patients, local recurrences were exclusively confined to the rectal wall. There were no extra-rectal pelvic recurrences. In addition, even though some recurrences within the rectal wall may develop deep in the outer layers of the bowel, in all cases, there was some expression of recurrence in the lumen that could be detected by clinical assessment. Therefore, it seems likely that these recurrences or regrowths may develop from microscopic residual foci in the outer layers rectum and should be detectable by clinical assessment, given the fact that close follow-up and thorough examination is rigorously performed (Fig. 7).

Second, local recurrences may develop many years later during follow-up period. In addition to our series, this has been observed in other series as well, where more than one-third of patients who developed local recurrences following neoadjuvant chemoradiotherapy and radical surgery did so beyond 5 years of follow-up. In contrast, over 75% of patients who develop local recurrences after radical surgery alone do so within 2 years of follow-up. Besides providing improved understanding of tumor behavior following chemoradiotherapy,

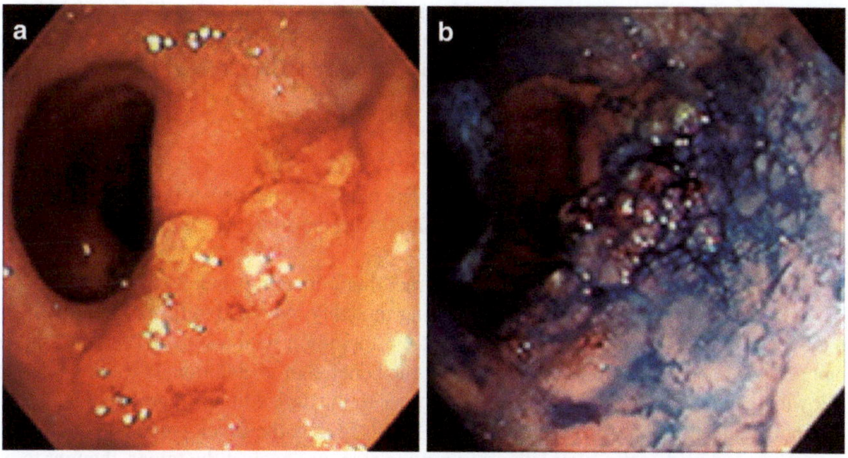

Fig. 7. Endoscopic view of a local recurrence in a patient with an initial complete clinical response detected after 12 months of follow-up during regular flexible proctoscopy (**a**) and after indigo-carmine instillation (**b**).

this information may have additional implications in terms of follow-up and surveillance strategies in these patients, where considerably later recurrences are expected.

Salvage Therapy

The fact that all local recurrences following nonoperative treatment of patients achieving complete clinical response following neoadjuvant therapy were amenable to salvage therapy is quite important. These recurrences and their salvage procedures were identified/performed after a considerably long interval following chemoradiotherapy completion (mean interval >50 months) and included APR in almost half of these patients. Interestingly, nearly one-third of these patients presented with anatomically low, superficial recurrences, amenable to full-thickness transanal excision. In these particular patients, APR was refused as a definitive surgical alternative and local excision was performed *(45)*.

Finally, there was a subset of patients that developed early tumor regrowth, within the initial 12-month "probation" period after complete clinical response was suspected and surgery deferred. These patients were frequently misdiagnosed as achieving complete clinical response with resultant delay of definitive surgical resection for variable periods of time. One issue raised was whether these patients could have a negative outcome from an oncological point of view, including inferior recurrence-free and long-term survivals. However, these patients fared no worse than patients with incomplete clinical response detected immediately following chemoradiotherapy and managed by radical surgery 8 weeks following chemoradiotherapy completion. Interestingly, patients initially suspected to have a cCR and who later underwent delayed surgery had significantly earlier pathological staging (including lower rates of lymph-node positivity), further supporting the idea that downstaging is a time-dependent phenomena. In addition, these patients were more frequently managed by abdominal perineal excision. This could reflect, in part, a motivation both by the surgeon and the patient to delay a final decision based upon response assessment, with the knowledge that tumor regression may occur over a long-duration. Indeed, the exact point in time for the surgeon to decide whether surgery should be performed is still unknown. The available data suggests that in patients with high suspicion of achieving a cCR, waiting more than the standard 8 weeks seems to have no adverse disease-related consequences *(46)*.

Perspectives

Several aspects in the management of complete clinical responders following neoadjuvant chemoradiotherapy remain unresolved and should be the topic of clinical and molecular genetics investigation in the future.

The development of new technologies in radiologic imaging such as the association of PET and MRI into a single radiological imaging modality may lead to further improvement in the identification of patients achieving cCR. Furthermore, final results of ongoing studies may provide additional information regarding the benefits of an additional "waiting" period following chemoradiotherapy completion in order to maximize tumor regression and minimize potential detrimental effects of radiation. In this setting, the development of novel drugs or vaccines may aid in the stimulation of immune response against the tumor, thought to be blocked by the effects of neoadjuvant chemoradiotherapy.

Another area of significant interest is the development of novel radiotherapeutic regimens including alternative radiation doses, delivery methods and technical variants in efforts to further increase the potential effects of radiation-related tumor cell death and minimize side effects. Additionally, the search for alternative chemotherapy regimens may potentially lead to an increase in the rates of cCR and possibly survival. For these reasons, some authors have suggested the use of induction aggressive chemotherapy prior to the delivery of radiation therapy in order to provide optimal, immediate treatment for undetected microscopic metastatic foci in addition to the primary tumor *(47)*. These regimens are currently under investigation in controlled trials in order to provide clear data on safety and long-term benefits. Another strategy involving the use of alternative chemotherapy regimens in neoadjuvant chemoradiotherapy is the delivery of chemotherapy during the "waiting" or "resting" period between radiation completion and tumor response assessment. Our group is currently studying this alternative treatment strategy, and these results will be available in the near future.

Finally, the greatest challenge in rectal cancer management will be the incorporation of molecular biology data into clinical practice, potentially allowing oncologists and surgeons to identify patients whose tumors are more likely to achieve downsizing, downstaging, or even for complete pathological regression. In an interesting study using DNA microarray technology, a set of 95 genes was able to identify patients who would develop complete pathological response following neoadjuvant chemoradiotherapy with 85% accuracy. Future studies will likely attempt to identify a subset of genes capable of identifying patients achieving complete pathologic response, with the endpoint of avoiding radical surgery in a significant number of patients (*48*).

REFERENCES

1. Sauer R, Becker H, Hohenberger W, et al. Preoperative versus postoperative chemoradiotherapy for rectal cancer. *N Engl J Med*. 2004;351:1731–1740.
2. Habr-Gama A, Perez RO, Kiss DR, et al. Preoperative chemoradiation therapy for low rectal cancer. Impact on downstaging and sphincter-saving operations. *Hepatogastroenterology*. 2004;51:1703–1707.
3. Withers HR, Haustermans K. Where next with preoperative radiation therapy for rectal cancer? *Int J Radiat Oncol Biol Phys*. 2004;58:597–602.

4. Greene FL, American Joint Committee on Cancer, American Cancer Society. *AJCC Cancer Staging Manual*. 6th ed. New York: Springer; 2002.
5. Chessin DB, Enker W, Cohen AM, et al. Complications after preoperative combined modality therapy and radical resection of locally advanced rectal cancer: a 14-year experience from a specialty service. *J Am Coll Surg*. 2005;200:876–882. discussion 82–84.
6. Eriksen MT, Wibe A, Norstein J, et al. Anastomotic leakage following routine mesorectal excision for rectal cancer in a national cohort of patients. *Colorectal Dis*. 2005;7:51–57.
7. Matthiessen P, Hallbook O, Andersson M, et al. Risk factors for anastomotic leakage after anterior resection of the rectum. *Colorectal Dis*. 2004;6:462–469.
8. Matthiessen P, Hallbook O, Rutegard J, et al. Defunctioning stoma reduces symptomatic anastomotic leakage after low anterior resection of the rectum for cancer: a randomized multicenter trial. *Ann Surg*. 2007;246:207–214.
9. Edwards DP, Leppington-Clarke A, Sexton R, et al. Stoma-related complications are more frequent after transverse colostomy than loop ileostomy: a prospective randomized clinical trial. *Br J Surg*. 2001;88:360–363.
10. Law WL, Chu KW, Choi HK. Randomized clinical trial comparing loop ileostomy and loop transverse colostomy for faecal diversion following total mesorectal excision. *Br J Surg*. 2002;89:704–708.
11. Perez RO, Habr-Gama A, Seid VE, et al. Loop ileostomy morbidity: timing of closure matters. *Dis Colon Rectum*. 2006;49:1539–1545.
12. Habr-Gama A, de Souza PM, Ribeiro U Jr, et al. Low rectal cancer: impact of radiation and chemotherapy on surgical treatment. *Dis Colon Rectum*. 1998;41:1087–1096.
13. Habr-Gama A. Assessment and management of the complete clinical response of rectal cancer to chemoradiotherapy. *Colorectal Dis*. 2006;8(suppl 3):21–24.
14. Moore HG, Gittleman AE, Minsky BD, et al. Rate of pathologic complete response with increased interval between preoperative combined modality therapy and rectal cancer resection. *Dis Colon Rectum*. 2004;47:279–286.
15. Tulchinsky H, Shmueli E, Figer A, et al. An interval >7 weeks between neoadjuvant therapy and surgery improves pathologic complete response and disease-free survival in patients with locally advanced rectal cancer. *Ann Surg Oncol*. 2008;15:2661–2667.
16. Deniaud-Alexandre E, Touboul E, Tiret E, et al. Results of definitive irradiation in a series of 305 epidermoid carcinomas of the anal canal. *Int J Radiat Oncol Biol Phys*. 2003;56:1259–1273.
17. Hiotis SP, Weber SM, Cohen AM, et al. Assessing the predictive value of clinical complete response to neoadjuvant therapy for rectal cancer: an analysis of 488 patients. *J Am Coll Surg*. 2002;194:131–135. discussion 5–6.
18. Park YA, Lee KY, Kim NK, et al. Prognostic effect of perioperative change of serum carcinoembryonic antigen level: a useful tool for detection of systemic recurrence in rectal cancer. *Ann Surg Oncol*. 2006;13:645–650.
19. Das P, Skibber JM, Rodriguez-Bigas MA, et al. Predictors of tumor response and downstaging in patients who receive preoperative chemoradiation for rectal cancer. *Cancer*. 2007;109:1750–1755.
20. Perez RO, Sao Juliao GP, Habr-Gama A, et al. The role of carcinoembriogenic antigen in predicting response and survival to neoadjuvant chemoradiotherapy for distal rectal cancer. *Dis Colon Rectum*. 2009;52(6):1137–1143.
21. Brown G. Staging rectal cancer: endoscopic ultrasound and pelvic MR. *Cancer Imaging*. 2008;8 (suppl A):S43-S45.
22. Koh DM, Chau I, Tait D, et al. Evaluating mesorectal lymph nodes in rectal cancer before and after neoadjuvant chemoradiation using thin-section T2-weighted magnetic resonance imaging. *Int J Radiat Oncol Biol Phys*. 2008;71:456–461.
23. Shihab OC, Moran BJ, Heald RJ, et al. MRI staging of low rectal cancer. *Eur Radiol*. 2009;19(3):643–650.
24. Calvo FA, Domper M, Matute R, et al. 18F-FDG positron emission tomography staging and restaging in rectal cancer treated with preoperative chemoradiation. *Int J Radiat Oncol Biol Phys*. 2004;58:528–535.
25. Guillem JG, Puig-La Calle J Jr, Akhurst T, et al. Prospective assessment of primary rectal cancer response to preoperative radiation and chemotherapy using 18-fluorodeoxyglucose positron emission tomography. *Dis Colon Rectum*. 2000;43:18–24.

26. Guillem JG, Moore HG, Akhurst T, et al. Sequential preoperative fluorodeoxyglucose-positron emission tomography assessment of response to preoperative chemoradiation: a means for determining longterm outcomes of rectal cancer. *J Am Coll Surg*. 2004;199:1–7.
27. Chessin DB, Kiran RP, Akhurst T, et al. The emerging role of 18F-fluorodeoxyglucose positron emission tomography in the management of primary and recurrent rectal cancer. *J Am Coll Surg*. 2005;201:948–956.
28. Kristiansen C, Loft A, Berthelsen AK, et al. PET/CT and histopathologic response to preoperative chemoradiation therapy in locally advanced rectal cancer. *Dis Colon Rectum*. 2008;51:21–25.
29. Perez RO, Bresciani BH, Bresciani C, et al. Mucinous colorectal adenocarcinoma: influence of mucin expression (Muc1, 2 and 5) on clinico-pathological features and prognosis. *Int J Colorectal Dis*. 2008;23:757–765.
30. Baxter NN, Morris AM, Rothenberger DA, et al. Impact of preoperative radiation for rectal cancer on subsequent lymph node evaluation: a population-based analysis. *Int J Radiat Oncol Biol Phys*. 2005;61:426–431.
31. Sermier A, Gervaz P, Egger JF, et al. Lymph node retrieval in abdominoperineal surgical specimen is radiation time-dependent. *World J Surg Oncol*. 2006;4:29.
32. Habr-Gama A, Perez RO, Proscurshim I, et al. Absence of lymph nodes in the resected specimen after radical surgery for distal rectal cancer and neoadjuvant chemoradiation therapy: what does it mean? *Dis Colon Rectum*. 2008;51:277–283.
33. Perez RO, Habr-Gama A. Nishida Arazawa ST, et al. Lymph node micrometastasis in stage II distal rectal cancer following neoadjuvant chemoradiation therapy. *Int J Colorectal Dis*. 2005;20:434–439.
34. Stipa F, Zernecke A, Moore HG, et al. Residual mesorectal lymph node involvement following neoadjuvant combined-modality therapy: rationale for radical resection? *Ann Surg Oncol*. 2004;11:187.
35. Pucciarelli S, Capirci C, Emanuele U, et al. Relationship between pathologic T-stage and nodal metastasis after preoperative chemoradiotherapy for locally advanced rectal cancer. *Ann Surg Oncol*. 2005;12:111–116.
36. Zmora O, Dasilva GM, Gurland B, et al. Does rectal wall tumor eradication with preoperative chemoradiation permit a change in the operative strategy? *Dis Colon Rectum*. 2004; 47:1607–1612.
37. Fleming FJ, Hayanga AJ, Glynn F, et al. Incidence and prognostic influence of lymph node micrometastases in rectal cancer. *Eur J Surg Oncol*. 2007;33:998–1002.
38. Nascimbeni R, Burgart LJ, Nivatvongs S, et al. Risk of lymph node metastasis in T1 carcinoma of the colon and rectum. *Dis Colon Rectum*. 2002;45:200–206.
39. Petersen S, Hellmich G, von Mildenstein K, et al. Is surgery-only the adequate treatment approach for T2N0 rectal cancer? *J Surg Oncol*. 2006;93:350–354.
40. Habr-Gama A, Perez RO, Nadalin W, et al. Long-term results of preoperative chemoradiation for distal rectal cancer correlation between final stage and survival. *J Gastrointest Surg*. 2005;9:90–99. discussion 9–101.
41. Habr-Gama A, Perez RO, Nadalin W, et al. Operative versus nonoperative treatment for stage 0 distal rectal cancer following chemoradiation therapy: long-term results. *Ann Surg*. 2004;240:711–717. discussion 7–8.
42. Wichmann MW, Meyer G, Adam M, et al. Detrimental immunologic effects of preoperative chemoradiotherapy in advanced rectal cancer. *Dis Colon Rectum*. 2003;46:875–887.
43. Perez RO, Habr-Gama A, dos Santos RM, et al. Peritumoral inflammatory infiltrate is not a prognostic factor in distal rectal cancer following neoadjuvant chemoradiation therapy. *J Gastrointest Surg*. 2007;11:1534–1540.
44. Collette L, Bosset JF, den Dulk M, et al. Patients with curative resection of cT3–4 rectal cancer after preoperative radiotherapy or radiochemotherapy: does anybody benefit from adjuvant fluorouracil-based chemotherapy? A trial of the European Organisation for Research and Treatment of Cancer Radiation Oncology Group. *J Clin Oncol*. 2007;25:4379–4386.

45. Habr-Gama A, Perez RO, Proscurshim I, et al. Patterns of failure and survival for nonoperative treatment of stage c0 distal rectal cancer following neoadjuvant chemoradiation therapy. *J Gastrointest Surg*. 2006;10:1319–1328. discussion 28–9.
46. Habr-Gama A, Perez RO, Proscurshim I, et al. Interval between surgery and neoadjuvant chemoradiation therapy for distal rectal cancer: does delayed surgery have an impact on outcome? *Int J Radiat Oncol Biol Phys*. 2008;71:1181–1188.
47. Chau I, Brown G, Cunningham D, et al. Neoadjuvant capecitabine and oxaliplatin followed by synchronous chemoradiation and total mesorectal excision in magnetic resonance imaging-defined poor-risk rectal cancer. *J Clin Oncol*. 2006;24:668–674.
48. Kim IJ, Lim SB, Kang HC, et al. Microarray gene expression profiling for predicting complete response to preoperative chemoradiotherapy in patients with advanced rectal cancer. *Dis Colon Rectum*. 2007;50:1342–1353.

16 Contact X-Ray Therapy

Jean-Pierre Gérard, Robert Myerson, and A. Sun Myint

DEFINITION

In this chapter, the term "contact X-ray therapy" (CXRT) will be restricted to irradiation given by means of an X-ray tube using a short skin–source distance (close to 4 cm). The maximum beam energy is, in most instances, 50 kV with some degree of aluminum filtration. The treatment is delivered by an endoluminal approach with the help of a metallic applicator (rectoscope). For the past fifty years, the Philips RT 50® unit has been the most widely used machine for this purpose.

BRIEF HISTORICAL BACKGROUND

The first CXRT machine was designed by Chaoul in Germany with the Siemens Company in 1939. It was used primarily to treat uterine cervix carcinoma. Larmarque from Montpellier, France *(1)* was the first to use the Philips RT 50® unit to treat rectal adenocarcinoma. It was Papillon in Lyon, France who popularized CXRT in the treatment of rectal tumors and also demonstrated for the first time that rectal adenocarcinoma could be locally controlled and cured with radiotherapy alone *(2,3)*. Following his pioneering work, CXRT has been used in many centers in France, Europe, and North America *(4–11)*.

TECHNICAL DESCRIPTION

The RT 50 Machine® contains an X-ray tube that produces a 50 kV beam, which is connected to a generator and a dosimetric electric supply. The anode is located 2 cm from the thin mica beryllium exit window. Extra filtration consisting of 0.5 mm Al is routinely used. For rectal tumor treatment, the tube is used in conjunction with an applicator with a diameter of 3 cm. An applicator with a reduced diameter of 2 cm can be used for small lesions. The overall source–skin distance with the applicator is 4 cm. In approximately one-third of cases, an applicator with a visor (1.5 cm long) is used to prevent the contralateral rectal wall

From: *Current Clinical Oncology: Rectal Cancer*,
Edited by: B.G. Czito and C.G. Willett, DOI: 10.1007/978-1-60761-567-5_16,

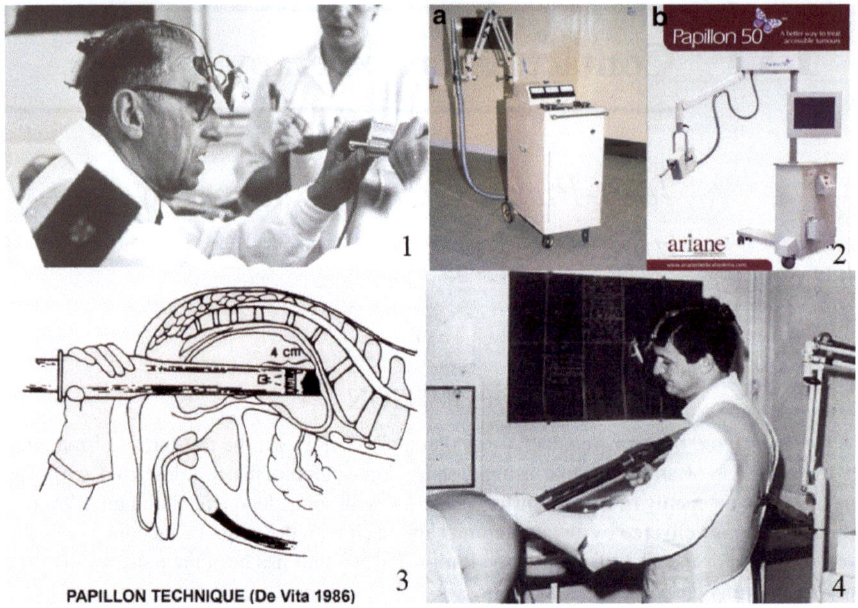

Fig. 1. Technique of contact X-ray therapy. (1) Papillon performing a rectoscopy with a rigid rectoscope before CXRT. (2) Contact X-ray machine: (**a**) The Philips RT50® and (**b**) The Papillon 50®. (3) Scheme of the accurate irradiation with the applicator on the tumor and control under direct visualization. (4) A CXRT session with patient in the knee chest position (duration 1–3 min). (Reproduced from Clinical Oncology 2007 with permission from Saunders Company Ltd).

from collapsing in front of the beam. The radiation output is very high at approximately 20 Gy/min, and the session duration does not generally exceed 2 or 3 min. The treatment is performed in the knee chest position with an empty rectal ampulla. It is performed in the ambulatory setting and is feasible at any age. If dilatation with the 3 cm diameter applicator is painful, local anesthesia of the anal sphincter may be performed and usually makes the applicator insertion feasible (required in about 10% of cases). The percentage depth dose is 100% at 0 mm, 45% at 5 mm, and 10% at 20 mm. One of the most important aspects of CXRT is the fact that the radiation treatment is carried out under direct visual inspection. This view-guided approach of radiotherapy delivery allows a highly accurate (1 mm precision) beam delivery. In cases of large tumors exceeding 3 cm, it is possible to initially treat with two overlapping fields, facilitating proper coverage of tumors up to 5 cm in diameter (Fig. 1). From an exposure point of view, CXRT is very safe. The dose delivered at the handgrip of the tube is less than 0.001 mSv for 10 Gy delivered at the tumor.

TREATMENT PROTOCOLS

T1 N0 Disease: CXRT Alone for Cure

These tumors are usually polypoid, measuring less than 3 cm in diameter. The standard treatment regimen is as follows: Day 1: 35 Gy, Day 7: 25–30 Gy, Day 21: 15 Gy in cases of complete clinical response, 20–25 Gy (using a shrinking field) if partial response is seen, and

Day 35: 15 Gy (generally delivered on a normal-appearing mucosa). The total dose ranges between 90 and 110 Gy in four fractions over a 1 month period.

As Papillon very elegantly described, "The tumor is destroyed layer by layer. The reduction in volume affects both the width and the thickness of the lesion. The tumor always shrinks centripetally and is brought back to its point of origin. The rapidity of the shrinkage serves as a guideline at each treatment to define the dose to be given and the interval before the next application." The response following three sessions is highly predictive of the final outcome. In the case of a complete clinical response (no visible tumor, rectal wall supple), the likelihood of cure is very high (and the risk of metastatic lymph node involvement very low). These statements are also valid when combining CXRT with external beam radiotherapy (EBRT) in the treatment of T2 or small T3 lesions (with or without local excision) with curative intent *(2,11)*.

Adjuvant CXRT After Local Excision for T1 N0 Disease

In such a situation, CXRT is performed in an effort to sterilize potential residual microscopic disease in the tumor bed of the rectal wall. The rectal wall thickness is usually 5 mm (mucosa + muscularis propria). Irradiation is performed on a clinically normal mucosa. The standard treatment is as follows: Day 1: 20 Gy, Day 7 (or 14): 15 Gy, and Day 21 (or 28): 15 Gy. The total dose is 50 Gy delivered in three fractions over 3 or 4 weeks. Usually, an asymptomatic, acute proctitis can be seen with the rectoscope at the end of the treatment, which usually subsides within 3 weeks. At Washington University, following en bloc local resection (R0) of a pT1 lesion, adjuvant CXRT is delivered to a total dose of 60 Gy (surface dose of 30 Gy for each of two treatments, 2 weeks apart) *(7,13)*.

T2–3 N0 Disease: CXRT Combined with EBRT

In such cases, the tumor is often ulcerated, close to 3 cm in diameter (sometimes more but usually not exceeding 5 cm) and involves less than half of the rectal circumference. Although, CXRT following EBRT seems attractive, initiating the treatment with CXRT has some advantages, namely that there is no treatment delay as CXRT can be started immediately. A very high dose can be delivered to the tumor as minimal to no normal rectal tissue is included in the X-ray beam. As in the previous setting, response at day 21 can be used as a good indicator of tumor radiosensitivity and also used to adapt the total radiation dose. There is generally no discomfort due to the radiation-induced proctitis. It is always possible to add an additional session of CXRT, 4–5 weeks following EBRT, if the gross residual disease persists (Fig. 2).

The usual treatment protocol in this setting is as follows: day 1: 35–45 Gy (delivered over 2 or 3 min); if necessary, two overlapping fields each receiving 35 Gy are used; day 7 (or 14 – the longer time interval allows for additional tumor shrinkage): 30–35 Gy; and day 21 (or 28): 20–30 Gy. Note that this dose is adapted according to tumor regression. If the tumor is 2 cm in diameter, a dose of 30 Gy can be given with 15 Gy delivered with the 3 cm applicator encompassing some normal rectal mucosa and 15 Gy with the 2 cm applicator encompassing gross disease only; day 36 (or 43): Usually EBRT is initiated on day 21 or 28, and CXRT (15–20 Gy) can be applied concurrently without any difficulty. A complete or nearly complete clinical response is often observed at that time. If the tumor does not demonstrate a complete clinical response, it is possible to escalate the CXRT dose. The normal mucosa dose should not exceed 10–15 Gy per session. The 2 cm applicator is well adapted for delivery of 20–25 Gy to gross residual disease. The total CXRT dose is between 100 and

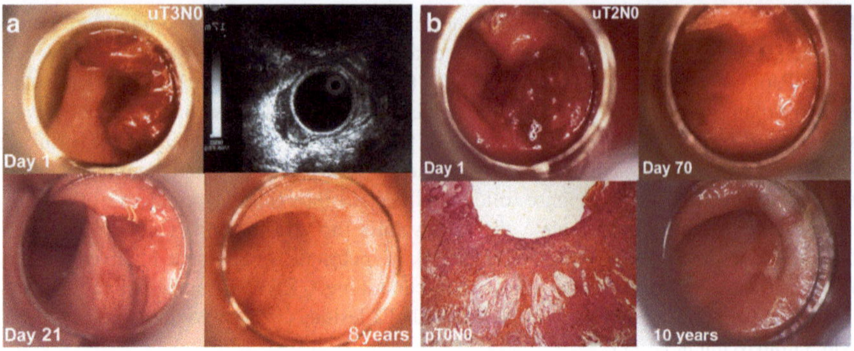

Fig. 2. Clinical results obtained with contact X-ray therapy. (**a**) T3 N0 adenocarcinoma in an elderly, inoperable patient treated with combined CXRT and EBRT (EUS *upper right panel*). (**b**) Low lying T2 N0 adenocarcinoma juxtaposing the anal canal. This patient was randomized in the Lyon R96.02 trial, receiving CXRT+EBRT. Complete clinical response was noted, followed by transanal local excision. The operative specimen revealed ypT0 disease. This patient had good clinical and functional results after 10 years follow-up. (Reproduced from Clinical Oncology 2007 with permission from Saunders Company Ltd).

120 Gy, delivered in four to six fractions when combined with EBRT, with or without chemotherapy. The total treatment time is usually 6 weeks but can be longer than this. Further treatment usually includes surgery (anterior resection or TLE), or if inoperable, brachytherapy may be used (usually interstitial implant with high-, low- or pulse-dose-rate). At Washington University and at Clatterbridge Centre for Oncology, The United Kingdom, CXRT has been used as a "delayed" boost following EBRT. Pelvic radiotherapy dose is 45 Gy delivered in 25 fractions concurrently with chemotherapy. Patients receive CXRT 6–8 weeks following EBRT completion. By that point, most patients have only a small scar at the tumor site, small enough to be encompassed within the treatment applicator. CXRT consists of two treatments, 2 weeks apart. The mucosal surface dose is 30 Gy for each treatment. This radiotherapy regimen can also be used after full-thickness local excision *(7,10,13)*.

Other Protocols

CXRT can be used palliatively to induce tumor shrinkage, to reduce discharge, or to stop bleeding. Usually, one or two sessions (50–60 Gy total dose) are prescribed. It can also be used to irradiate a rectal tumor that has been previously subjected to pelvic irradiation (carcinoma of prostate or uterine cervix). It is also possible to reirradiate a rectal tumor following local recurrence and to deliver two or three CXRT treatments to "stabilize" the recurrent tumor.

TOXICITY

Early Toxicity

The introduction of the CXRT applicator may be painful in approximately 10% of patients. In such cases, local anesthesia of the anal region with 20 ml of 2% lidocaine makes the insertion of applicator possible in most of the cases. When irradiating a normal rectal mucosa after local excision, an acute proctitis delineating the field of CXRT is seen after 45 Gy/4 weeks. It is not painful and heals without treatment in a month. When irradiating a T2 or T3 tumor penetrating the rectal wall, ulceration can occur after complete disappearance of the tumor, usually 3–4 months after the first session. It is usually not painful and will usually heal within 2–3 months without any treatment.

Late Toxicity

Two to three years after CXRT (with or without EBRT), telangiectasias will manifest in the irradiated area in approximately 50% of cases. Bleeding can occur, especially if exacerbated by constipation and hard stools. If the bleeding becomes distressing to the patient, local treatment can reduce or stop the bleeding (formalin acid, Argon plasma therapy). Usually, there is no or moderate fibrosis of the rectum and no stenosis. Anorectal function is well preserved, allowing normal bowel habits with the exception of some frequency and urgency in some patients, usually in the morning. No rectal perforation, fistula, or rectal injuries requiring major surgery have been reported.

PRIMARY ADVANTAGES OF CXRT

CXRT is a unique approach to treat rectal cancer with irradiation. The main advantages are as follows: (1) High accuracy of beam delivery: Taking advantage of the direct visual guidance allows delivery of dose to the gross tumor alone and completely spares the normal rectal mucosa, allowing delivery of very high doses without associated toxicity. (2) Small irradiation volume: As the dose falls off very rapidly beyond 5 mm depth, the volume of rectal wall irradiated is less than 5 cm^3. The small irradiation volume, along with the accuracy of this technique, explains why the doses can be very high with minimal or no toxicity.

Additional advantages of CXRT include the following: (1) It is a highly adaptive technique. It is possible to compensate for patient movement and rectal contraction during the radiotherapy session. It is also possible to very precisely assess tumor response and to adapt the irradiated volume to the shrinkage of the tumor after each fraction. (2) It is simple and well tolerated at any age. It is a fully ambulatory treatment of very short duration. It can be performed at any age. If the knee position is not adaptable, CXRT can also be delivered in the gynaecologic position. The tolerance is generally very good. (3) It is a cost-effective treatment: Depending on the country and the economic system, a full treatment of four to six sessions is estimated to cost between 1,000 and 2,000 € (1,250–2,500 US$). The CXRT machine can be used to treat many other lesions (cancers of the skin, eyelid, cornea, oral cavity, and vagina) that are accessible to the X-ray tube. With a total of 30–50 patients per year, the machine should generate revenue sufficient to cover its cost in less than 10 years. Maintenance of the machine is simple, inexpensive, and machine malfunctions are rare.

CLINICAL RESULTS

More than 1,300 patients with T1 N0 (or early T2) rectal tumors have been treated with CXRT alone. The results are shown in Table 1. Local control (85–90%) and survival are comparable with surgical data using local excision alone. Adjuvant CXRT after local excision for pT1 tumors also results in excellent long-term control (90–95%) and survival *(12)*.

A smaller group of patients (usually elderly patients with comorbidities) has been treated with curative intent for T2–3 M0 tumors, using a combination of CXRT and EBRT.

Table 1
Results of patients treated with CXRT alone for T1 (some T2) N0 M0 rectal adenocarcinomas

City	*Country*	*Reference*	*Years*	*No. of patients*	*Local failure (%)*	*Survival % (5 years)*
Lyon–Papillon	F	*(2,3)*	1951–1987	312	9	75
Rochester	USA	*(8)*	1973–1990	244	9	76
Dijon	F	*(5)*	1970–1995	100	15	63
Lyon–Sud	F	*(4)*	1980–1999	116	10	83
St. Louis	USA	*(7)*	1980–1997	22	16	94 (DFS 3)
Liverpool	UK	*(10)*	1992–2007	20	7	70
Nancy	F	*(6)*	1981–1996	97	10	64
Lyon–Sud[a]	F	*(12)*	1980–1997	37	3	82

DFS 3 disease-free survival at 3 years, *F* France, *USA* The United States of America, *UK* The United Kingdom

[a]Lyon Sud: CXRT alone after local excision for T1 N0

Table 2
Results of patients treated with combination of CXRT + EBRT for T2 and early T3 rectal adenocarcinoma (radiotherapy alone with curative intent)

City	*Country*	*Reference*	*Year*	*No. of Patients*	*Stage*	*Local failure (%)*	*Survival % (5 years)*
Lyon–Papillon	F	*(3)*	1975–1987	43	T2–3	30	52
St. Louis	USA	*(7,13)*	1980–2004	152	T2–3	35[a]	56
Dijon	F	*(5)*	1980–1995	34	T2–3	28	48
Lyon–Sud	F	*(11)*	1985–1999	63	T2	20	80
					T3	39	50
Liverpool	UK	*(10)*	1993–2007	104	T2–3	11[b]	62
St. Louis	USA	*(13)*	1980–2004	89	T1–2–3	9[c]	58

F France, *USA* The United States of America, *UK* The United Kingdom

[a]Local failure 3% for T1 lesions (18 patients)

[b]Some patients with large T1 (>3cm) tumors are included

[c]Patients treated with local excision first (all macroscopic disease removed) followed by EBRT + CX

Long-term control has been shown to be feasible in this group of nearly 300 patients. The results are shown in Table 2. In T2 lesions, local control can be achieved in up to 80% of patients. In T3 lesions, the local control rate is close to 50%. It must be stressed that in these series, the rate of perirectal lymph node failure has been very low (<10%). This tends to suggest that EBRT (± concurrent chemotherapy) using doses of 45–50 Gy delivered over 5–6 weeks should be able to sterilize a high percentage of subclinical, metastatic perirectal lymph nodes *(3,5,7,10,11,13)*.

The Lyon R96.02 randomized trial has provided good evidence of the benefits of dose escalation with CXRT. Between 1996 and 2001, 88 patients with T2/early T3 tumors of the distal rectum were randomized between preoperative EBRT alone and preoperative EBRT with CXRT (90 Gy/three fractions). In the CXRT group, a complete clinical response and a complete pathological response was seen in 29% vs. 2% and 35% vs. 10% of patients, respectively. Sphincter preservation was performed in 76% vs. 44% of patients ($p<0.05$).

In three cases of complete clinical response, the surgeon was able to perform a TLE instead of abdominoperineal resection or low anterior resection *(14)*.

PRESENT PERSPECTIVES

Surgery remains the cornerstone of rectal cancer treatment. In cases of malignant polyps or early, polypoid T1 adenocarcinomas, TLE is considered standard therapy. The standard treatment for T2 lesions is usually radical surgery, with low anterior resection performed in most cases. Following results from randomized trials, *(15–17)* T3 lesions are usually treated with preoperative chemoradiation therapy followed by radical surgery. Within this general frame, CXRT may be indicated in three situations.

CXRT After Local Excision for T1 N0 Lesions

The indications for adjuvant treatment following local excision depend on a careful pathological examination of the operative specimen. In cases of pT1 R0 disease with no adverse pathologic features (no piecemeal removal, good differentiation, no vascular or perineural invasion), a close follow-up alone is indicated. In cases of pT3 or pT2 R1 resected disease, radical surgery is mandatory, usually with low anterior resection. In between, where a small risk of microscopic residual disease in the tumor bed exists, it is appropriate to use CXRT, delivering to a total dose of 45–50 Gy in three fractions over 3 or 4 weeks. In elderly patients with a high surgical risk, if there is an increased risk of residual disease in the mesorectum, a combination of CXRT (40 Gy/two fractions) and EBRT (45–50 Gy ± chemotherapy) can be discussed.

Elderly Patients

With aging of the population, it is quite frequent to encounter patients of 80 years and above with rectal cancer. Quite often, these patients are found with comorbidities and are at a high surgical risk. Data from the Dutch cancer registry *(18)* show that after 80 years of age the risk of dying within 6 months following surgery is greater than 10% and can reach 29% between 85 and 95 years of age. Similarly, the rates of anastomotic leakage increase after 75 years of age as do the rates of incontinence. These are reasons why less invasive treatment options are gaining increased attention in this age group, where it may be reasonable to avoid surgical trauma as much as possible. As stated by the Dutch authors, "Radical radiotherapy appears as a good alternative, especially using CXRT which enables the delivery of high doses of radiation in the tumor with low dose to normal tissue and good tolerance" *(18)*.

In this group of elderly patients with comorbidities, radical radiotherapy combining CXRT with EBRT and concurrent chemotherapy should be considered for patients with T2 N0 tumors, early T3 N0 tumors (not exceeding 5 cm), and large T1 tumors (2 cm or more in diameter). In a recent small series of 12 patients treated in Nice, France, no deaths occurred during the first 6 months posttherapy period, and 11 patients were locally controlled *(19)*.

T2 N0 Disease: Neoadjuvant CXRT ± EBRT Followed by TLE

This approach is a new field of clinical research and requires strict patient selection. An Italian randomized trial *(20)* that included T2 (less than 4 cm) N0 tumors compared laparoscopic surgery with local excision following neoadjuvant CT-RT (50.4 Gy/6 weeks + fluorouracil). Out of 70 patients, nine required permanent stomas in the laparoscopic group versus none in the local excision group. Other small series using a similar regimen have shown this approach to be a feasible one *(21–23)*. To perform a local excision, it is sometimes necessary to achieve a good tumor response, with the tumor optimally measuring less than 2 cm at the time of the local excision. As CXRT achieves a very high rate of complete clinical response in T2 N0 tumors, its use in such situations is very appealing so as to increase the likelihood of a sterilized specimen after neoadjuvant treatment.

THE PAPILLON 50® MACHINE AND THE CONTEM TRIAL

One of the main reasons for the decreasing use of CXRT is the obsolescence of the Philips RT 50® unit, which is no longer manufactured. Fortunately, a new contact X-ray machine named the Papillon 50® will be available for clinical use in Denmark, England, France and probably in Sweden. This machine will reproduce the characteristics of the previous Philips unit with some new advantages. A miniaturized fiberscope with a camera positioned in the applicator will allow real time visualization of the tumor during irradiation and will further improve the accuracy of the dose delivery. The machine will be fully computerized and will increase the reliability and reproducibility of the treatment. Radiotherapy departments using the Papillon 50® machine will be participating in a prospective rectal trial in collaboration with colorectal surgeons and other specialists of the multidisciplinary team. The CONTEM (Contact and Transanal Endoscope Microsurgery) trial encompasses the three previously described indications for CXRT as follows: *(24)* The CONTEM 1 trial will evaluate CXRT after local excision of malignant polyps/early T1 disease with a moderate risk of sub clinical residual disease in the tumor bed. The CONTEM 2 trial inclusion criteria include T2 N0 ≤4 cm in maximum diameter. The patients will be treated with CXRT (90 Gy/three fractions) followed by concurrent chemoradiation using EBRT (50 Gy/25 fractions/5 weeks) and chemotherapy (capecitabine) followed by local excision 6 weeks later if the tumor is (clinically assessed by digital rectal examination and rigid rectoscopy) less than 2 cm in diameter. In the CONTEM 1 and 2 trials, 150 patients will be enrolled to demonstrate an estimated risk of local recurrence of less than 8%. The CONTEM 3 trial will enroll elderly patients with comorbidities. The inclusion criteria include T2, N0, early T3 N0, and T1 N0 tumors > 2 cm in diameter. A combination of CXRT and EBRT (±CT) will be used.

CONCLUSION

Rectal cancer is a disease with many different clinical presentations. Careful staging is critical to optimize and individualize treatments. One important field of research centers on the improvement of the quality of life of rectal cancer patients and increase in rates of sphincter preservation and, if possible, rates of rectal preservation. Contemporary treatment approaches involve tailoring treatment to each clinical situation. Contact X-ray treatment can play an important role in conservative approaches, especially in elderly patients. Careful and prospective clinical trials should provide ample evidence for the feasibility of this approach.

REFERENCES

1. Lamarque PL, Gros CG. La radiothérapie de contact des cancers du rectum. *J Radiol Electrol.* 1946;27:333–348.
2. Papillon J. *Rectal and anal cancer. Conservative treatment by irradiation: an alternative to radical surgery.* Berlin: Springer; 1982.

3. Papillon J. Present status of radiation therapy in the conservative management of rectal cancer. *Radiother Oncol.* 1990;17(4):275–283.
4. Gérard JP, Ayzac L, Coquard R, et al. Endocavitary irradiation for early rectal carcinomas T1 (T2). A series of 101 patients treated with the Papillon technique. *Int J Radiat Oncol Biol Phys.* 1996;36:775–783.
5. Maingon P, Guerif S, Darsouni R, et al. Conservative management of rectal adenocarcinoma by radiotherapy. *Int J Radiat Oncol Biol Phys.* 1998;40(5):1077–1085.
6. Rauch P, Bey P, Peiffet D, Conroy T, Bresler L. Factors affecting local control and survival after treatment of carcinoma of the rectum by endocavitary radiation. *Int J Radiat Oncol Biol Phys.* 2001;49:117–124.
7. Aumock A, Birnbaum EH, Fleshman JW, et al. Treatment of rectal adenocarcinoma with endocavitary and external beam radiotherapy: results for 199 patients with localized tumors. *Int J Radiat Oncol Biol Phys.* 2001;51(2):363–370.
8. Sischy B, Graney MJ, Hinson EJ. Endocavitary irradiation for adenocarcinoma of the rectum. *CA Cancer J Clin.* 1984;34(6):333–339.
9. Mendenhall WM, Rout WR, Vauthey JN, Haigh LS, Zlotecki RA, Copeland EM. Conservative treatment of rectal adenocarcinoma with endocavitary irradiation or wide local excision and postoperative irradiation. *J Clin Oncol.* 1997;15(10):3241–3248.
10. Sun Myint A, Grieve RJ, McDonald AC, et al. Combined modality treatment of early rectal cancer: the UK experience. *Clin Oncol (R Coll Radiol).* 2007;19(9):674–681.
11. Gerard JP, Chapet O, Ramaioli A, Romestaing P. Long-term control of T2–T3 rectal adenocarcinoma with radiotherapy alone. *Int J Radiat Oncol Biol Phys.* 2002;54(1):142–149.
12. Gerard JP, Chapet O, Romestaing P, Favrel V, Barbet N, Mornex F. Local excision and adjuvant radiotherapy for rectal adenocarcinoma T1-2 N0. *Gastroenterol Clin Biol.* 2000;24(4):430–435.
13. Myerson RJ, Hunt SR. Conservative alternative to extirpative surgery for rectal cancer. *Clin Oncol.* 2007;19:682–686.
14. Gerard JP, Chapet O, Nemoz C, et al. Improved sphincter preservation in low rectal cancer with high-dose preoperative radiotherapy: the Lyon R96-02 randomized trial. *J Clin Oncol.* 2004;22(12):2404–2409.
15. Sauer R, Becker H, Hohenberger W, et al. Preoperative versus postoperative radiochemotherapy for rectal cancer. *N Engl J Med.* 2004;351(17):7131–7140.
16. Bosset JF, Collette L, Calais G, et al. Chemotherapy with preoperative radiotherapy in rectal cancer. *N Engl J Med.* 2006;355(11):1114–1123.
17. Gerard JP, Azria D, Gourgou-Bourgade S, et al. Comparison of two neoadjuvant chemoradiotherapy regimens for locally advanced rectal cancer: results of the phase III trial ACCORD 12/0405-Prodige 2. *J Clin Oncol.* 2010;28:1638–1644.
18. Rutten HJ, den Dulk M, Lemmens VE, van de Velde CJ, Marijnen CA. Controversies of total mesorectal excision for rectal cancer in elderly patients. *Lancet Oncol.* 2008;9(5):494–501.
19. Gérard JP, Ortholan C, Benezery K, et al. Contact X-ray therapy for rectal cancer: experience in Centre Antoine-Lacassagne, Nice, 2002–2006. *Int J Radiat Oncol Biol Phys.* 2008;72(3):665–670.
20. Lezoche G, Baldarelli M, Guerrieri M, et al. A prospective randomized study with a 5-year minimum follow-up evaluation of transanal endoscopic microsurgery versus laparoscopic total mesorectal excision after neoadjuvant therapy. *Surg Endosc.* 2008;22(2):352–358.
21. Kim CJ, Yeatman TJ, Coppola D, et al. Local excision of T_2 and T_3 rectal cancers after down staging chemoradiation. *Ann Surg.* 2001;34:352–358.
22. Ruo L, Guillem JG, Minsky BD, et al. Preoperative radiation with or without chemotherapy and full-thickness transanal excision for selected T_2 and T_3 distal rectal cancers. *Int J Colorectal Dis.* 2002;17:54–58.
23. Bonnen M, Crane C, Vouthey JN, et al. Long-term results using Local excision after preoperating chemoradiation among selected T3 rectal cancer patients. *Int J Radiat Oncol Biol Phys.* 2004;60:1098–1105.
24. Lindegaard J, Gerard JP, Sun Myint A, Myerson R, Thomsen H, Laurberg S. Whither papillon? Future directions for contact radiotherapy in rectal cancer. *Clin Oncol (R Coll Radiol).* 2007;19(9):738–741.

17 High-Dose-Rate Preoperative Endorectal Brachytherapy for Patients with Rectal Cancer

Té Vuong, Slobodan Devic, and Ervin Podgorsak

INTRODUCTION

Contact X-ray therapy for treatment of rectal cancer, introduced by Papillon (*1*) in the early 1970s, is highly effective and well tolerated for radical treatment of early stage rectal cancer (T1 and favorable T2 lesions) *(2,3)*. On the other hand, high-dose-rate endorectal brachytherapy (HDREBT) was mainly used in the past as a palliative treatment modality *(4,5)*.

In our center, we have developed a treatment protocol which we use to select eligible patients and also to improve tumor visualization for target outlining, based on magnetic resonance tumor imaging. Treatment planning is performed using 3D CT simulation in conjunction with conformal 3D treatment planning. In this chapter, we describe the technical aspects of HDREBT and discuss the ongoing institutional review board (IRB) approved studies exploring the clinical applications of this treatment modality for patients with rectal cancer *(6)*.

CLINICAL STUDY OF HDREBT

Beginning in 1998, we conducted a phase I/II study to evaluate the use of HDREBT as an alternative preoperative, downstaging modality to conventional external beam radiation therapy. Patients with T2–3 Nx tumors and no evidence of necrotic or extramesorectal nodes larger than 1 cm were selected for study participation. Over this period, techniques for imaging, treatment planning, and dose delivery have evolved into the currently used HDREBT technique and are discussed below.

From: *Current Clinical Oncology: Rectal Cancer*,
Edited by: B.G. Czito and C.G. Willett, DOI: 10.1007/978-1-60761-567-5_17,

Pretreatment Imaging

Patients eligible for preoperative endorectal HDRBT undergo endoscopic endorectal ultrasound (EUS) for tumor staging (to assess transmural extension) and magnetic resonance imaging (MRI) of the pelvis for gross tumor measurements (length and bulk evaluation). After the completion of clinical and radiological evaluations, radio-opaque clips are placed using direct rectoscopy to mark the proximal and distal margins of the tumor for subsequent positioning, simulation quality control, and treatment applications.

HDREBT Equipment

Several days following completion of clinical and radiological evaluations (Fig. 1), at least four radio-opaque clips (QuickClip2, model: HX-201LR-135; Olympus, Southend-on-Sea, Essex, UK) are placed during endoscopy on day 1 to mark the proximal and distal margins of the tumor (Fig. 2). The clips are of cylindrical shape with a length of 5 mm and a diameter of 1.5 mm. They are subsequently used for image guidance prior to daily treatments. We commonly use two clips to mark the proximal limit and two clips to mark the distal limit of the tumor volume. On occasion, more than four clips are inserted if there is a concern that some of the inserted clips may migrate during the 4-day course of treatment; however, usually at least one of the four clips remains inside the rectal lumen until the last treatment fraction is complete. In our experience to date, on only two occasions have all the clips migrated prior to treatment completion. Although performing longitudinal shifts based on bony anatomy was an alternate approach, we opted to insert new clips and repeated the treatment planning for the remaining treatment fractions.

An intracavitary mold applicator (Nucletron; Veenendaal, the Netherlands) of cylindrical shape (27 cm long and 2 cm in diameter) is used for treatment application. As shown in Fig. 3, eight catheter channels are distributed equally over the circumference of the applicator in

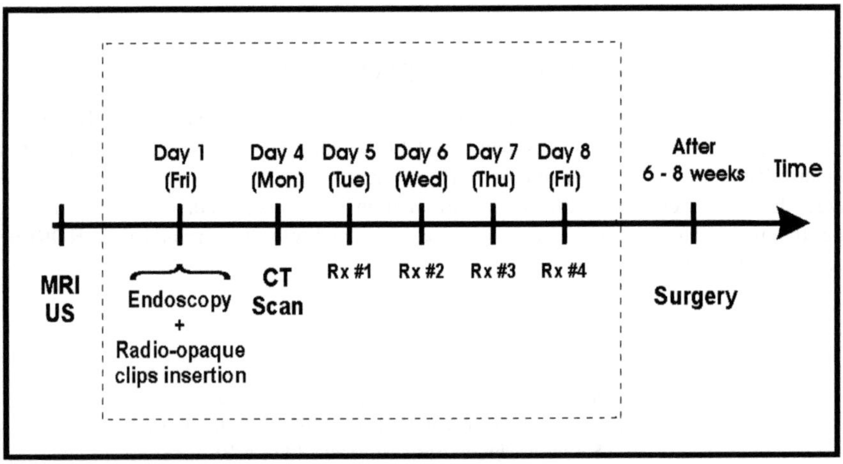

Fig. 1. Time scheme for preoperative endorectal HDR brachytherapy; the days of the week in parentheses represent the most suitable days not only from a logistical point of view but also for a reliable reproduction of the daily dose distribution.

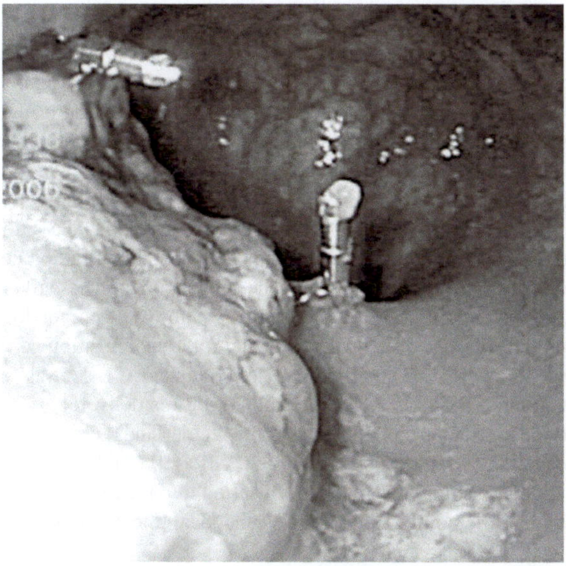

Fig. 2. Marking proximal and distal limit of a tumor using radio-opaque clips under direct rectoscopy.

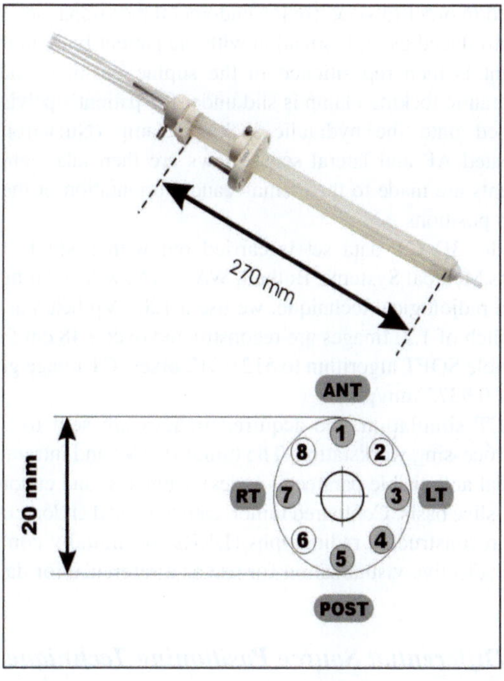

Fig. 3. Intracavitary mold applicator; the *bottom* schematics represents the catheter convention (*1–8*) as well as the catheters coded with X-ray markers (*1, 3, 4, 5, and 7*; *gray shaded circles*).

equal angular increments, and a central lumen is also available for insertion of an additional central catheter. The applicator is made of a pliable silicone rubber material, which allows easy insertion and navigation through the rectum and sigmoid colon. Figure 3 also indicates schematically the convention we are using with respect to the loading of the channels (from 1 to 8) as well as the catheters loaded with uniquely coded X-ray markers (gray circles: 1, 3, 4, 5, and 7) that are used for ensuring the daily rotational reproducibility.

Prior to applicator insertion into the rectal lumen, an endocavity balloon (CIVCO, Latex-Free Endocavity Balloon, 610-898 (BS3000)) is placed over the rectal applicator. This facilitates a snug fit to the mold applicator and contains an adjustable inflation control to provide proper fixation of the mold applicator within the rectal lumen. The balloon is oriented in such a way that its expanding section is placed opposite to the tumor location. Once the necessary longitudinal shift has been determined and rotational position verified, the balloon is inflated by water injection. A small amount of iodinated CT contrast can be added to facilitate visualization on a CT scan. The prescribed dose is delivered using a micro-Selectron remote afterloader (Nucletron, Veenendaal, the Netherlands) employing an iridium-192 source with a nominal activity at installation of 370 GBq (10 Ci). Daily radiographs with the patient in the treatment position and applicator inserted into the rectal lumen are acquired on a radiotherapy simulator (Simulix, Nucletron, Veenendaal, the Netherlands).

3D Treatment Planning

The details of treatment planning procedure have been described previously *(6,7)*. Prior to CT simulation, an initial anteroposterior (AP) scout view of the patient lying in the supine position is performed in order to visualize the endorectal radio-opaque clips. The endorectal applicator is then introduced using lubrication with the patient lying in the lateral decubitus position. The patient is then repositioned in the supine position, and a Plexiglas plate mounted with a hydraulic locking clamp is slid under the patient's pelvis, and the intracavitary mold is latched onto the hydraulic locking clamp (Nucletron, Veenendaal, the Netherlands). Repeated AP and lateral scout views are then taken and examined. When necessary, adjustments are made to the cranial–caudal orientation of the applicator relative to radio-opaque clip positions.

Acquisition of the 3D CT data set is carried out with a single slice CT simulator (AcQsim CT, Philips Medical Systems, Bothell, WA, USA) with a 3 mm slice thickness and 3 mm spacing. As a radiological technique, we use a 120 kVp beam at 250 mA and spiral acquisition with a pitch of 1.3. Images are reconstructed over a 48 cm field of view using a commercially available SOFT algorithm to 512 × 512 pixels CT image giving an axial plane spatial resolution of 0.9375 mm/pixel.

Following the CT simulation, the acquired images are sent to a dedicated virtual simulation image processing workstation. The tumor (GTV) and intramesorectal extension (including extra nodal and visible pararectal nodes), catheters, and endorectal clips are contoured on a slice-by-slice basis. Contoured tumor, catheters, and endorectal clips are incorporated into digitally reconstructed radiographs (DRRs) or digitally composite radiographs (DCRs) to enhance selective visualization for use as a reference for daily treatments.

Differential Source Positioning Technique

Source positions and engaged channels for brachytherapy (BT) are determined with respect to contoured tumor. Catheters are loaded in a differential manner so that only those

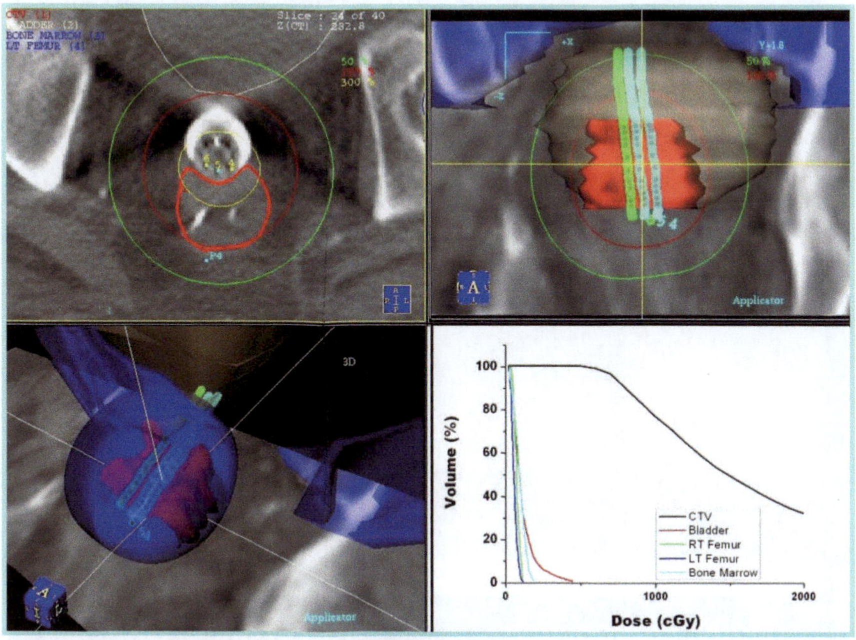

Fig. 4. Dose distribution obtained by treatment planning system.

in direct contact with the tumor contain active source dwell positions. Following the source position determination, CT-aided BT treatment planning is carried out so as to fully optimize the dose to the tumor, while limiting the dose to immediate adjacent tissues beyond the rectal wall. Isodose distributions are generated by commercially available Plato treatment planning software (Nucletron, Mayland, USA).

A total dose of 26 Gy, delivered in four daily fractions of 6.5 Gy, is prescribed at the CTV, defined as the GTV and intramesorectal deposits seen on the prestaging MRI. Figure 4 represents an example of the dose distribution obtained during treatment planning optimization. The 100% isodose cloud (Fig. 4, bottom-left) completely covers the CTV. The plan is checked prior to treatment by inspecting prescription dose to the CTV coverage on a slice-by-slice basis (Fig. 4, upper-left). Dose coverage can also be inspected within different planes (Fig. 4, upper-right). The bottom-right section of Fig. 4 shows a dose-volume histogram illustrating the difference between dose coverage to the CTV and sparing of the surrounding critical structures.

Daily Image Guidance

Reproduction of the treatment planned dose distribution on a daily basis is crucial for the success of fractionated 3D based BT treatments *(8,9)*. Due to the cylindrical symmetry of the applicator used for preoperative HDREBT, two types of adjustments are necessary: applicator rotation and dwell positions shift along the applicator's longitudinal axis.

During each treatment session, the applicator might not be positioned inside the rectal lumen in the same manner as it was placed during the 3D CT volume acquisition used for

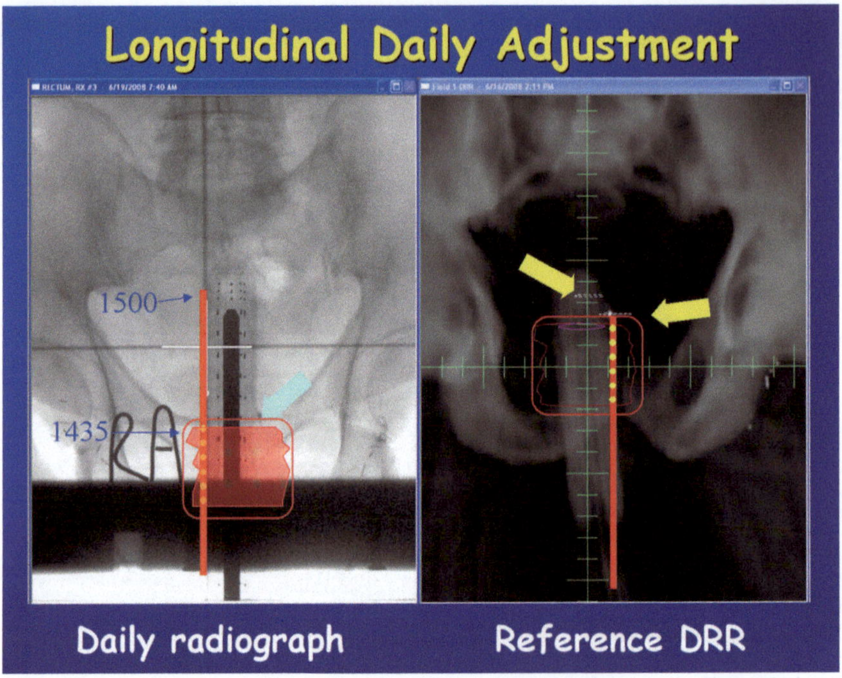

Fig. 5. Daily longitudinal treatment adjustment.

treatment planning; therefore, a shift along the catheter axis may have to be performed. The required shift is determined by comparison of a daily radiograph with the treatment planning DRR (see Fig. 5).

Accurate catheter identification is a crucial step in the treatment planning process to assure proper rotational reproducibility of the planned dose distribution on a daily basis. During the outlining procedure, catheters are assumed to follow their "ideal" positions, equally spaced by 45° and starting with the catheter number one at the "12 o'clock" position. We do not follow the actual catheter positions seen on the planning CT study, since, for daily treatments, we will only be able to reproduce the ideal angular positions of the catheters. Once the longitudinal shift has been determined, the applicator is rotated and subsequently reimaged using the fluoroscopic mode (low milliampere second) on the radiotherapy simulator, until an acceptable alignment is achieved. The final acceptable radiograph that confirms the proper rotational position is shown in Fig. 6b. In this figure, to achieve the "ideal" rotational position, the applicator was rotated counterclockwise.

CLINICAL APPLICATIONS OF HDREBT

Neoadjuvant Treatment for Patients with Operable Rectal Cancer

One hundred patients were treated for the study from 1998 to 2002. Patient and tumor characteristics are described in Table 1. All patients completed their planned treatment.

Acute proctitis was observed in all 100 patients for 7–10 days following treatment completion. In 99 patients, the proctitis was of grade 2, while one patient with grade 3 proctitis

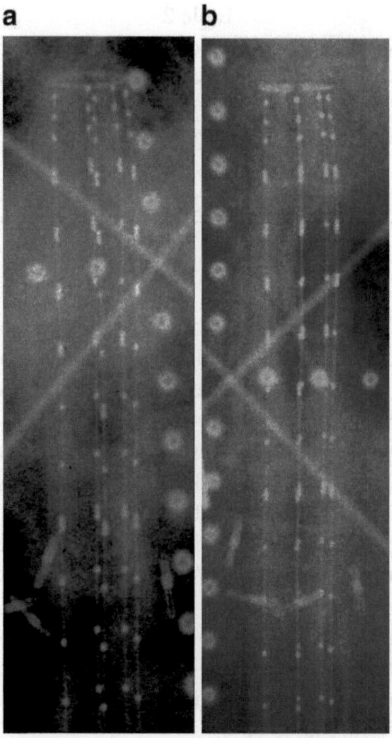

Fig. 6. Rotational alignment of the applicator: (**a**) initial position; (**b**) final position after appropriate applicator rotation.

Table 1
Tumor and patient characteristics (n = 100)

Tumor characteristics	*No. of patients*
T2	3
T3	93
T4	4
N0	58
N1	42
Tumor location	*(%)*
Upper third	6
Middle third	45
Lower third	49
Patient gender	
Male	62
Female	38

required a blood transfusion. There was no hospitalization for treatment related toxicity. Two patients refused planned abdominal resection based on a normal restaging EUS. Two patients died before surgery: one of a stroke and the other of a myocardial infarction. During the

Table 2
Comparative tumor sterilization rate by treatment modality

Treatment modality	*pT0 TRG1 (%)*	*Micro foci TRG2*
XRT alone	3.7	19
CT-XRT	8–12	15
HDR brachytherapy (MUHC)	29	37

period of the study, TME surgery was performed on 30 patients, and the remaining 66 patients were operated in community hospitals by general surgeons with no TME training. A postoperative leak rate of 9% was observed. The abdominoperineal resection rate was 53%, and the sphincter preservation rate was 47%.

Following the tumor response grade (TRG) scale *(10)*, we observed that among the surgical specimens, 29% were ypT0N0–2 (TRG1), 37% showed microscopic foci only (TRG2), and 34% showed residual tumor (TRG3–5) (Table 2). Postoperative external beam therapy and chemotherapy were delivered in 27 of the 31 patients with positive nodes in the pathological specimen as per the NIH recommendation *(11)*. Whether or not this is necessary is unclear, as we observed a 68% systemic relapse rate in this subgroup of patients. Since 2006, the treatment protocol was altered to deliver FOLFOX (5-fluorouracil, leucovorin and oxaliplatin) chemotherapy alone in patients treated with adjuvant therapy. At a median follow up time of 60 months, the actual 5-year local recurrence rate is 5%, the disease-free survival rate is 65%, and the overall survival rate is 70%.

In the quest for treatment with reduced morbidity relative to the current standard of care in North America (external beam radiation therapy and chemotherapy), BT is an exciting alternative. It offers the advantage of delivering a high radiation dose with a sharp dose falloff in comparison to external beam radiation therapy around the site of interest (tumor target). This advantage results in the sparing of normal tissues, in particular, the small bowel, as well as the bladder, the prostate, and the skin.

The physical conditions inherent to the BT technique offer several advantages over the external beam radiation therapy techniques. Within the tumor bed, a much larger radiation dose can be delivered (see Fig. 7), reducing the need for the sensitizing effect of chemotherapy. In addition, tissues peripheral to the target volume are better spared. Lastly, since the treatment volume is smaller than that in external beam radiation, the total treatment time can be shortened to 1 week. Irradiation of the tumor bed, identified intramesorectal deposits and immediate perirectal nodes to a high dose (in order to achieve downstaging/downsizing) may, in turn, lead to negative circumferential mesorectal margins and facilitate sphincter preservation surgery (SPS). Residual tumor cells and heavily irradiated tissues are removed during surgery. Consequently, it is reasonable to predict that the long-term toxicity on normal tissues is low.

As expected, proctitis was the main toxicity incurred by this approach, although no treatment related death occurred. As reported previously *(6)*, subsequent surgical complications were not increased with this approach and a 9% incidence of anastomotic leak was seen. The most common surgical difficulty was localizing the initial tumor bed since, in two-thirds of patients, there was no palpable residual tumor. Presently, surgeons measure the distal tumor margins during the initial evaluation. When the tumor is located in the lower third of the rectum, margin adequacy is decided after careful endoscopic examination, prior to coloanal anastomosis and ileostomy placement.

The mean dose delivered to the tumor bed volume in our series was 40 Gy in four fractions over 1 week and thus contributed to our low recurrence rate. This is in keeping with data

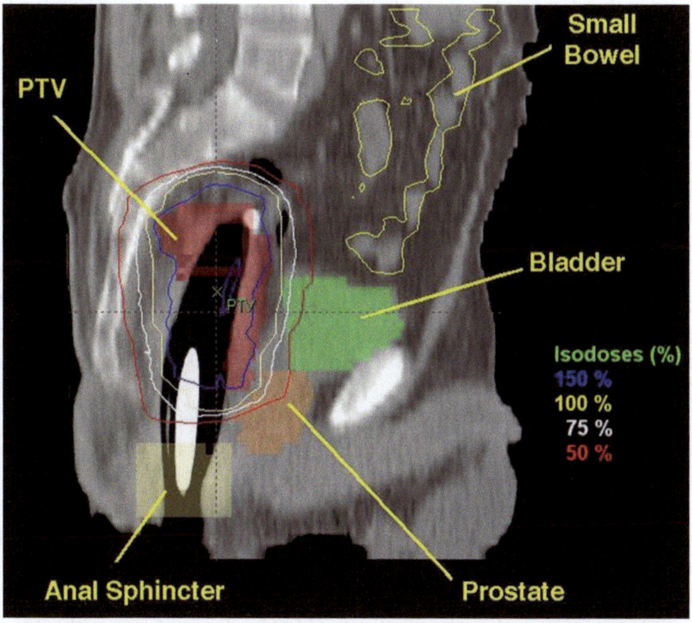

Fig. 7. Sagittal plane dose distribution using the endorectal brachytherapy treatment technique.

from a report by Glimelius et al *(12)* showing a dose–response relationship between radiation dose and reduction in local recurrence.

Our low recurrence rate of 5% during a median follow-up time of 60 months is significant, considering that in our study, TME surgery was performed in only 30% of resections. Local recurrence was found at the tumor bed in four patients. Two of these patients received postoperative external beam radiation therapy and adjuvant chemotherapy. Systemic relapse antedated local relapse in one patient and occurred subsequently in the second. Two other patients recurred after HDREBT alone. One had persistent tumor that was documented 1 month after surgery at the anastomosis, and the second patient recurred in the inguinal and external iliac nodes. In contrast to other studies, our patient selection excluded patients with (1) stenotic tumors not evaluable by EUS (three patients) due to the technical limitations of the treatment catheter, (2) bulky T4 tumors (six patients), (3) T1-small T2 lesions (nine patients), and (4) either suspicious paraaortic nodes or highly suspicious pelvic nodes (necrotic or ≥1.5 cm). Nevertheless, our group of patients exhibited bulky tumors (49% had tumors ≥5 cm), and 94% of tumors were within 10 cm of the anal verge.

An international, multicenter, randomized phase III trial that compares the HDREBT to standard chemotherapy/external beam radiation therapy is underway.

HDREBT as a Boost Treatment After External Beam Radiation for Patients with Medically Inoperable, Localized T2–3 Tumors

From February 2004 to October 2007, we treated 18 elderly patients whose tumors were inoperable or who refused surgery. All were diagnosed with adenocarcinoma of the rectum with no evidence of distant metastases.

The treatment of these patients combined an initial course of external beam radiotherapy, using 40 Gy or 45 Gy delivered in 16 fractions and in 25 fractions, respectively, with a conformal three field technique. The target volume (GTV) was outlined using MRI slices coregistered with the CT data obtained on radiotherapy CT simulator. The CTV included the GTV as well as the perirectal and any macroscopically enlarged pelvic nodes with a 3–5 cm margin, depending on the proximity of critical organs such as bowel or anal sphincter.

A 2-week break was given after external beam therapy, followed by repeat pelvic MRI, which was repeated every 2 weeks until maximum tumor thickness of 1 cm or less was observed. At that time, the BT boost treatment was initiated.

Three boost treatments of 10 Gy each were delivered on a weekly schedule to the entire tumor bed using a combination of endoscopically placed radio-opaque clips (above and below the tumor bed) and the initial pelvic MRI for determination of treatment length. The treatment planning was carried out in a similar fashion as described for preoperative HDREBT.

The median patient age was 83.5 (77–90) years. Pretreatment staging revealed 12 T3 and six T2 tumors. Acute toxicity consisted of grade 2 proctitis in 61% and grade 1 proctitis in 39% of patients. The incidence of grade ≥2 dermatitis was 16.6%. Three patients received only two out of the three planned boost treatments (one patient refused and the other two patients had a circumferential tumor). During a median follow-up time of 23 months (range 4–40 months), five patients (26.3%) had persistent local tumor, and 13 patients (72.2%) had no evidence of disease (NED) when examined by both biopsy and CT scan/MRI imaging. Rectal stenosis was observed in three patients (16.6%). Two patients without evidence of disease experienced long-term proctitis with intermittent rectal bleeding.

HDREBT as a boost to external beam radiation therapy alone appears to be a tolerable treatment, and our preliminary results suggest a benefit in local control for patients with inoperable rectal cancer or for those refusing surgery. In circumferential tumors, rectal stenosis remains a serious toxicity. Further follow-up has been initiated in this group of patients.

HDREBT as a Neoadjuvant Modality to Promote SPS for Patients with Low-Lying Rectal Cancer

Contemporary data do not consistently support the benefit of neoadjuvant chemotherapy and external radiation therapy in facilitating sphincter preservation in patients with low-lying rectal cancer. We conducted a phase II study to test the feasibility of SPS for patients with low-lying rectal cancer following neoadjuvant HDREBT for patients with curable rectal cancer.

Patients with newly diagnosed adenocarcinoma of the rectum located at 6 cm or less from the anal verge, during every rigid rectoscopy measurement, are eligible for the study as long as their referring surgeon is a colorectal surgeon trained in technical skills for SPS.

Fifty patients were enrolled. Forty-four had T3, and the remaining six had T2 tumors. All patients received their planned treatment. Grade 1–2 proctitis was observed in all patients. There were no perforations. One patient died of a cardiac arrest after surgery. The sphincter preservation rate was 77%. The anastomotic leak rate was 8%, and in those patients who underwent abdominoperineal resection, the incidence of wound healing problems was 8%. During a median-follow up of 27 months (3–45 months), one patient developed local recurrence at the site of the initial tumor bed, and 12% of the patients developed systemic metastases. Based on this data, it appears that neoadjuvant HDREBT for patients with low-lying rectal cancer leads to a high SPS rate without increasing the postoperative complication rate.

HDREBT as a Neoadjuvant Treatment for Patients with Previous Pelvic Radiation Therapy for Other Malignancies (Prostate, Gynecological, Testicular Cancers)

Presently, this patient population has limited options with regard to further radiation treatments in efforts to prevent local recurrence, despite the risk associated with the newly diagnosed rectal cancer. However, given the fact that HDREBT represents a highly conformal radiation treatment modality targeting the tumor bed and with dose contained within the mesorectum, it is postulated that these heavily irradiated tissues will be removed by TME.

We treated 17 patients diagnosed with T3–4 rectal tumors who were previously irradiated for prostate (9), gynecological (4), and bladder cancers (2) and non Hodgkin's lymphoma (2) with 26 Gy in four fractions using HDREBT. All patients had negative circumferential resection margins at resection, and during a median follow-up time of 25 months, local recurrence was reported in only one patient.

CONCLUSION

HDREBT is a highly conformal, 3D image-guided BT technique. This highly targeted radiation modality allows treatment of most rectal cancers either as a neoadjuvant or a boost modality. It is considered useful for patients and as a physician-friendly technology. Although the potential clinical applications are numerous, they should be formally tested within clinical protocols.

REFERENCES

1. Papillon J. Endocavitary irradiation in the curative treatment of early rectal cancers. *Dis Colon Rectum.* 1974;17(2):172–180.
2. Gerard JP, Romestaing P, Ardiet JM, Mornex F. Sphincter preservation in rectal cancer. Endocavitary radiation therapy. *Semin Radiat Oncol.* 1998;8(1):13–23.
3. Ishikawa H, Fujii H, Koyama F, et al. Long-term results of high-dose extracorporeal and endocavitary radiation therapy followed by abdominoperineal resection for distal rectal cancer. *Surg Today.* 2004;34(6):510–517.
4. Evans MDC, Pla C, Podgorsak EB. Rectal and oesophageal treatment by the selectron high dose rate afterloader. *Med Dosimetry.* 1988;13:79–81.
5. Kaufman N, Nori D, Shank B, et al. Remote afterloading intraluminal brachytherapy in the treatment of rectal, rectosigmoid, and anal cancer: a feasibility study. *Int J Radiat Oncol Biol Phys.* 1989;17: 663–668.
6. Vuong T, Belliveau P, Michel R, et al. Conformal preoperative endorectal brachytherapy treatment for locally advanced rectal cancer. *Dis Colon Rectum.* 2002;45:1486–1495.
7. Vuong T, Devic S, Moftah B, Evans M, Podgorsak EB. High dose rate endorectal brachytherapy in the treatment of locally advanced rectal carcinoma: technical aspects. *Brachytherapy.* 2005;4:230–235.
8. Devic S, Vuong T, Moftah B, et al. Image guided high dose rate endorectal brachytherapy. *Med Phys.* 2007;34:4451–4458.
9. Devic S, Vuong T, Evans M, Podgorsak E. Endorectal high dose rate brachytherapy quality assurance. *Nowotwory J Oncol.* 2008;58:53e-54e.

10. Ryan R, Gibbons D, Hyland JMP, et al. Pathological response following long-course neoadjuvant chemoradiotherapy for locally advanced rectal cancer. *Histopathology*. 2005;47:141–146.
11. NIH Consensus Conference. Adjuvant therapy for patients with colon and rectal cancer. *JAMA*. 1990;264:1444–1450.
12. Glimelius B, Isacsson U, Jung B, Pahlman L. Radiotherapy in addition to radical surgery in rectal cancer: evidence for a dose response effect favouring preoperative treatment. *Int J Radiat Oncol Biol Phys*. 1997;37:281–287.

18 Radiation Therapy: Technical Innovations

Brian G. Czito and Christopher G. Willett

INTRODUCTION

Although surgery is the backbone of rectal cancer therapy, clinical trials have established the roles of radiation therapy and chemotherapy as critical elements in the care of these patients by improving rates of sphincter preservation, local control and survival *(1–4)*. Studies have shown that these treatments further enhance local control even in the setting of the optimized surgical technique of total mesorectal excision (TME) *(5)*. Additionally, phase III trials have demonstrated improved outcomes with neoadjuvant vs. adjuvant radiation therapy *(6,7)*.

Innovations in radiation therapy techniques for treatment of rectal cancer patients have also progressed. Initially, radiation therapy plans were based on two-dimensional (2D) planning, where treatment fields were defined using orthogonal X-ray images and known anatomical landmarks. With improvements in imaging and computer capabilities, three-dimensional (3D) treatment planning became available in the late 1980s. An advanced form of 3D planning, intensity-modulated radiation therapy (IMRT), was implemented in clinical practice in the late 1990s *(8,9)*.

By virtue of the strict dose conformality afforded by IMRT, further reduction in normal tissue irradiation and target radiation dose escalation may be achieved. Normal tissue toxicity is the primary dose-limiting factor in radiation therapy planning. In the treatment of rectal cancer, critical normal tissues include small bowel, bladder, femoral heads, genitalia, skin, and the pelvic bone marrow. IMRT allows the radiation oncologist and radiation physicist to limit dose to these normal structures (discussed below). By sparing these normal tissues, IMRT may also permit dose escalation to the target tissues. However, to justify the use of IMRT for a given tumor site, its ability to limit normal tissue radiation dose must be demonstrated and, where appropriate, demonstration of dose escalation to be beneficial.

From: *Current Clinical Oncology: Rectal Cancer*,
Edited by: B.G. Czito and C.G. Willett, DOI: 10.1007/978-1-60761-567-5_18,

RADIATION THERAPY PLANNING AND IMRT

The radiation oncologist has two aims in radiation planning: (1) to achieve appropriate coverage of the tumor (target) volume and (2) minimization of the dose to the normal tissues adjacent to the target (avoidance structures). Conventional 2D and 3D radiotherapy planning makes use of multiple static fields. With these techniques, it is difficult to conform radiation dose coverage to target tissues (including the primary tumor and at-risk lymphatic basins) that may be irregularly shaped. IMRT makes use of multiple "fields-within-fields" that more accurately conform radiation dose to the target while sparing avoidance (normal) structures *(10)*. The success of IMRT-based treatment is strongly dependent on accurate target delineation. To accomplish this, the treating physician uses physical (digital, nodal) examination, endoscopy/endoscopic ultrasound, CT, PET-CT, and/or MRI findings to define the primary/gross disease [the gross target volume (GTV)], tissues at risk for subclinical tumor involvement (based on established patterns of spread and recurrence), including draining nodal basins [the clinical target volume (CTV)], as well as a third volume encompassing the GTV and CTV, allowing additional "margin" to account for organ motion and daily positional differences [the planning target volume (PTV)]. Digital examination facilitates definition of the extent of the primary disease (i.e., distance proximal to the anal verge) which can be correlated to the planning CT scan, particularly if anal verge marker is used. Similarly, inguinal lymph node examination may signal adenopathy, which if proven to harbor disease on biopsy, influences radiation dose to this region (i.e., is included in the GTV). Similarly, endoscopy and endoscopic ultrasound aid in defining extent of primary disease as well as suspicious perianal/perirectal lymph nodes, which would also mandate delivery of higher radiation doses (GTV) relative to subclinical sites of disease (CTV). CT and MRI may identify anatomically abnormal sites of disease including the primary tumor as well as enlarged lymph nodes. CT and MRI also aid the radiation oncologist in delineating pertinent locoregional lymph node basins (including inguino-femoral, external, internal and perirectal/perianal nodes) which potentially harbor subclinical sites of disease that are included in the CTV.

PET and combined PET/CT represent a further advancement in the staging and treatment of anorectal cancer. Several series have demonstrated that PET detected nodal metastases occur in 17–24% of patients deemed to be clinically lymph node negative by CT *(11,12)*. In the absence of PET, these sites would generally receive "subclinical" doses of radiation therapy to the CTV, as compared to higher doses used to treat gross disease (GTV). Anderson et al described 23 patients with anorectal cancer receiving chemoradiotherapy. All patients underwent PET/CT fusion to facilitate radiation planning. In 25% of patients, PET detected distant metastases and changed overall patient management. Importantly, PET/CT also altered the PTV and radiation treatment plan in approximately one-fourth of patients (*13*).

Modern radiation treatment planning is performed using computer-based planning programs. In addition to the previously described target volumes, adjacent normal structures at risk are defined. With IMRT, dose constraints are then assigned to these organs along with a desired (prescription) dose to the GTV, CTV and PTV. IMRT planning software can then be used to perform "inverse planning," whereby computer search algorithms establish multiple (and sometimes unconventional) beam/field designs, with the ultimate goal of meeting the prescribed target dose and normal tissue dose constraints. Individual fields are treated with multiple, small beams rather than one uniform beam, and each beam delivers a different dose (intensity) to the different parts of the target. This allows close conformation of radiation dose to the shape of the target and preferential sparing of normal surrounding organs from the high-dose areas.

Radiation oncologists and physicists critically evaluate numerous plans until dose constraints are satisfactorily met. The result should be a series of radiation doses that closely conform to the target volumes while minimizing normal tissue dose (Figs. 1 and 2). In certain situations, these techniques allow for safe tumor dose escalation with improved avoidance of normal tissues, theoretically leading to an improved therapeutic ratio.

The use of IMRT for rectal cancer patients requires delineation of the target volumes described above as well as critical normal structures such as bladder, small bowel, large bowel, genitalia and femoral heads. However, the greater the number of avoidance structures, the more difficult it is to meet all dose constraints. Radiation oncologists must determine which structures are most critical and weight them appropriately during the treatment planning process.

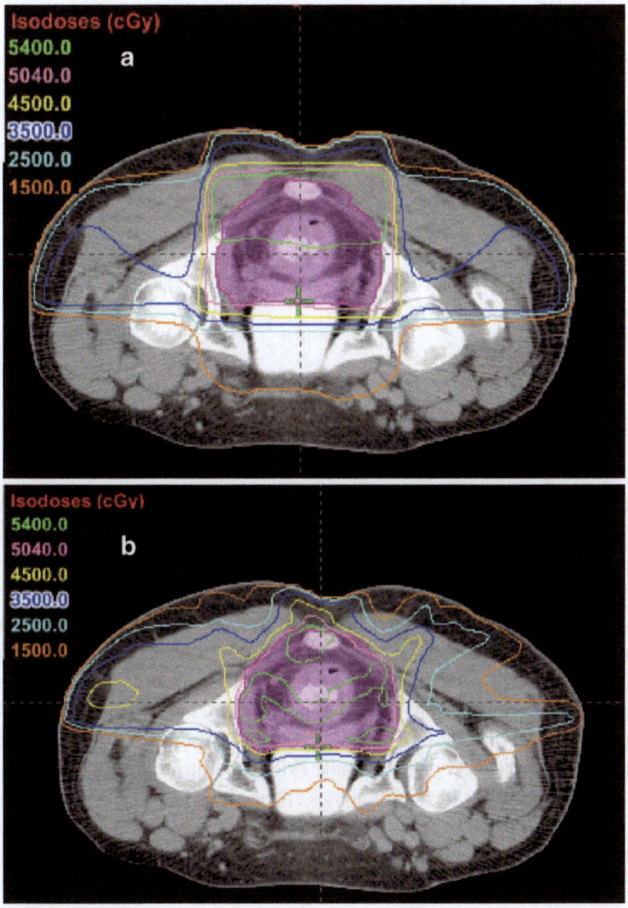

Fig. 1. Dosimetric comparison of conventional 3D and IMRT plans for the treatment of a 38-year-old man with T3N1 rectal cancer receiving preoperative radiotherapy. In the case of the 3D plan, the block edge is approximately 1 cm beyond the target volume in all beam projections. The (final) planning target volume is shaded in *pink*. Prescribed dose to the target volume was 5,040 cGy. (**a**) Axial slice of the conventional 3D plan. (**b**) Axial slice of the IMRT plan. (**c**) Dose–volume histogram (DVH) analysis of the 3D and IMRT plans. For essentially equivalent PTV coverage, IMRT spares the normal structures better than the 3D plan. *PTV* planning target volume.

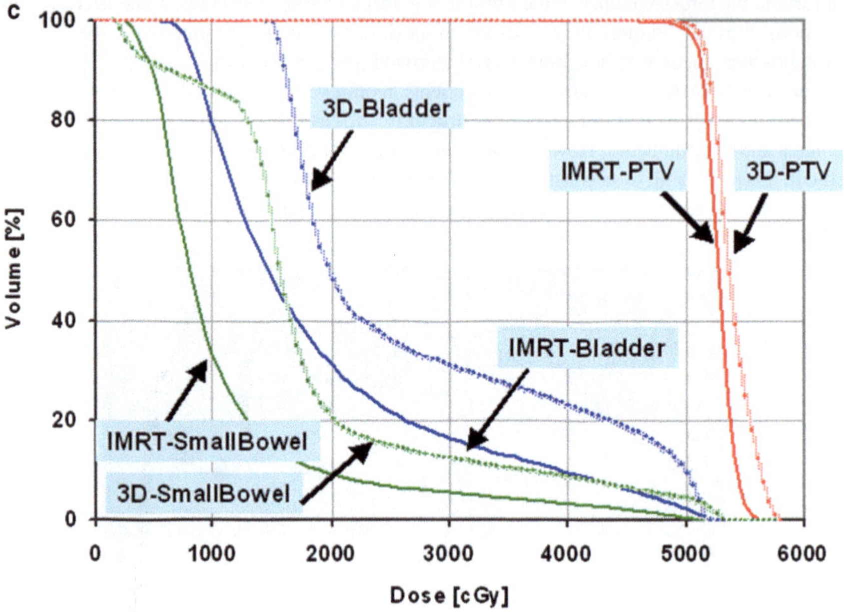

Fig. 1. (continued)

Proper margins are added to accommodate deviations related to patient set-up/positioning and physiological processes (accounted for in the PTV). Typically, patients are set up in either the prone or supine position. At each daily set-up, target volumes are in close proximity to critical normal structures. Clinical data from 3D real-time imaging in the treatment room have shown that pelvic structures vary in size, shape, and location between radiation fractions *(14–16)*. These include organ variation with respiration, changes in the size and shape of the rectum with gas filling/emptying as well as changes in the position of the rectum/anus associated with bladder filling/emptying. Unless organ motion is taken into account, tightly conformal IMRT fields could potentially result in underdosing of disease sites. As an example, deCrevoisier et al performed CT scans before and immediately after a single IMRT treatment in prostate cancer patients. Scan comparison showed rectal and bladder volumes changed a mean of 6 and 125 cm^3, respectively, resulting in displacement of the target (prostate and seminal vesicles) volumes by as much as 1.5 cm^3 in some instances *(17)*. Similarly, Nuyttens et al evaluated adjuvantly treated rectal cancer patients with weekly treatment planning CT. These authors found that the CTV varied by greater than 1 cm in some patients *(18)*. These and other data demonstrate the importance of careful delineation of target volumes in IMRT planning and the challenge of accurate localization of treatment target volumes prior to irradiation for both rectal and anal cancers. Compared to conventional film imaging, 2D "real-time" digital imaging, with or without implanted fiducial markers, has advantages in minimizing both random and systematic set-up deviations. Furthermore, advances in 3D tomographic imaging (CT on-rails, cone-beam CT, megavoltage CT, digital tomosynthesis, etc.) in the radiation treatment suite have made it possible to accurately target and measure target/normal organ deviations in real-time *(14–16,19)*. Therefore, adequacy of margins added to the treatment targets and critical organs should be judged and determined based on the methods of immobilization and localization techniques *(20,21)*.

DOSE ESCALATION

Dose–Response Relationship in Rectal Cancer

Most contemporary radiation therapy regimens for rectal cancer use doses of 45–54 Gy to treat gross disease and 45 Gy for subclinical disease sites. When radiation is delivered preoperatively with chemotherapy (usually fluoropyrimidine-based) to patients with locally advanced rectal cancer, pathologic complete response rates ranging from 4 to 67% have been

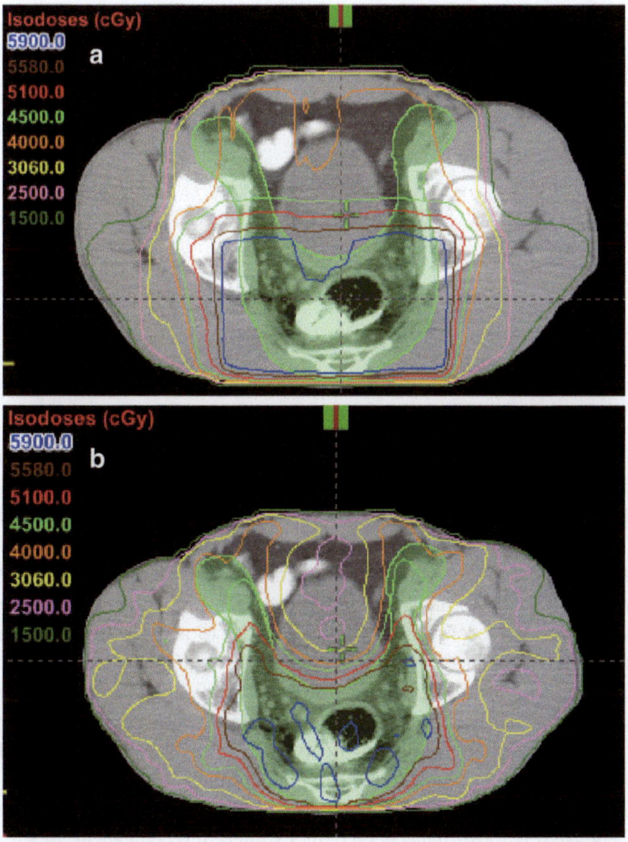

Fig. 2. Dosimetric comparison of conventional 3D and IMRT plans for the treatment of a 61-year-old HIV positive man with T3N0 anal canal cancer. For appropriate comparison between the two treatment modalities (3D and IMRT), the same target volumes were used to create appropriate plans. In the case of the 3D plan, the block edge is approximately 1 cm beyond the target volume in all beam projections. The planning target volume (PTV3060) is shaded in *green*. Prescribed dose to the final target volume was 5,580 cGy. (**a**) Axial slice of the conventional 3D plan. (**b**) Axial slice of the IMRT plan. (**c**) DVH analysis of the 3D and IMRT plans. IMRT spares the femurs and bladder more than the 3D plan. However, results for small bowl sparing are mixed; IMRT tends to deliver less dose in the high-dose region and more in the low-dose region. This case exemplifies the difficulties of matching all dose constraints during IMRT planning. *RFH* right femoral head, *LFH* left femoral head, *PTV* planning target volume.

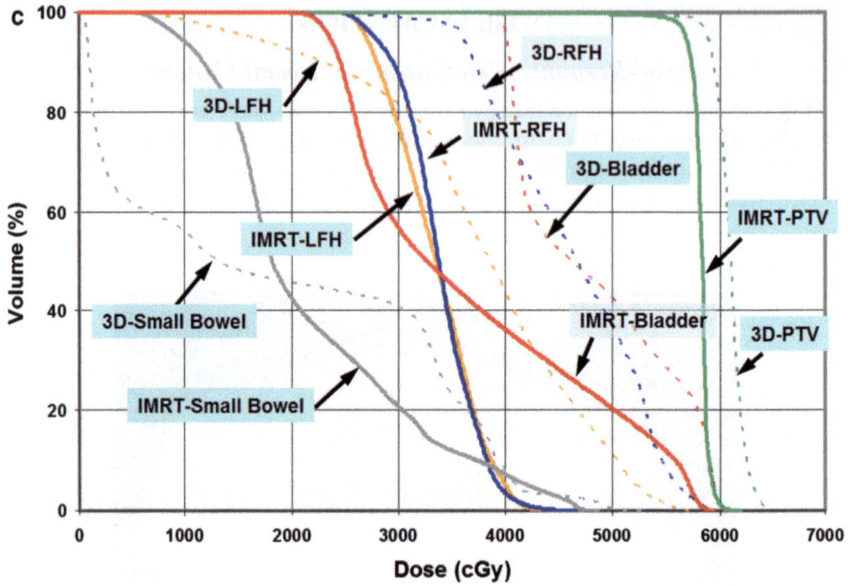

Fig. 2. (continued)

achieved *(22)*. In combination with TME, such regimens have produced 5-year actuarial local control rates of 94% *(7)*.

With such high rates of local control, it is appropriate to question whether radiation dose escalation is necessary and/or beneficial in the treatment of this disease. One potential reason for dose escalation is the finding that patients achieving pathologic complete responses have improved outcomes relative to patients with uninvolved surgical margins but residual tumor *(23–26)*. Another reason to consider dose escalation is to achieve improved rates of tumor regression and thereby enhance rates of sphincter-preserving surgery. This concept is supported by a recent randomized German trial where a significant number of patients with low-lying rectal tumors initially deemed to require abdominoperineal resection underwent sphincter-preserving resection following preoperative radiation therapy and chemotherapy *(7)*. Finally, there is a subset of patients with complete tumor response following preoperative chemoradiotherapy who will be long-term disease-free survivors without resection *(27)*.

A dose–response relationship has been demonstrated in rectal cancer. In a review of three phase II studies at Princess Margaret Hospital, a statistical trend toward increased pathologic complete response rates in patients receiving 50 Gy (vs. 46 and 40 Gy) was seen *(28)*. Additionally, Mohiuddin et al found a significantly higher rate of pathologic complete response in patients receiving 55–60 Gy vs. patients receiving 50 Gy or less (44 vs. 13%), with no significant increase in normal tissue toxicity *(29)*.

Overgaard and colleagues described 113 patients with recurrent, residual or inoperable colorectal cancer treated with varying doses up to 73 Gy. Patients receiving ≥56 Gy showed improved subjective response. Additionally, the frequency and duration of complete responses showed a marked dose–response relationship, with patients receiving ≥56 Gy showing a 2-year complete response rate of 40% vs. 7%, 4%, and 0% at doses of 46–55,

36–46 and ≤35 Gy, respectively. This dose–response relationship to local control was also shown to influence survival rate *(30)*.

Radiation dose escalation for nonsurgical patients has also been achieved through the use of brachytherapy (the temporary or permanent insertion of radioactive sources into a tumor and/or peritumoral tissues) and contact therapy (focal low-energy X-ray therapy). The goal of these techniques is to avoid high dose circumferential irradiation of the rectum. For example, Papillon described 90 patients with "limited" T1-2 rectal cancers treated with combined contact X-ray therapy and iridium brachytherapy, without planned surgery. Five-year disease-free survival and anal preservation rates were 78 and 74%, respectively. Among cured patients, the anal preservation rate was 96%. Similar reports from Europe and North America have also shown high rates of local control and disease response with these techniques *(31)*. These and other data suggest dose escalation may be beneficial in rectal cancer patients

Ultimately, it is unclear if dose escalation beyond 60 Gy in combination with 5-FU will provide clinically meaningful advances in surgically treated rectal cancer. However, improvements in radiosensitizing chemotherapy or targeted agents in combination with high-dose radiation therapy may allow for improvement in sphincter preservation in patients with distal cancers, higher rates of pathologic complete response and, potentially, the possibility for chemoradiation therapy alone to become primary therapy in highly selected patients. Preliminary studies have suggested this latter approach may be feasible and result in long-term disease-free survival in patients achieving clinical complete response following chemoradiotherapy *(27)*. Such dose escalation will likely mandate the use of radiation technologies that can more closely conform radiation to the tumor volume than is capable with 2D or conventional 3D radiotherapy.

NORMAL TISSUE TOXICITY

Rectal cancer exemplifies a malignancy where normal tissue toxicity induced by chemoradiotherapy frequently prevents the timely delivery and intensity of therapy. Additionally, local failure remains a predominant failure pattern in this disease. The use of IMRT to avoid normal tissues at risk (small bowel, femoral heads, bladder, and skin/genitalia) may allow for increased tolerance of combined modality treatment, timely treatment delivery, and potential radiation dose intensification. The following section reviews available dose–response relationships for normal tissues at risk in the treatment of rectal and anal canal cancer. Data from preliminary studies using IMRT to spare these tissues are highlighted.

Femur

The head and neck of the femur are exposed to radiation in classical radiation portals for rectal cancer. Bony vascular damage may result in avascular necrosis, leading to hip fracture with attendant morbidity, particularly in elderly populations *(32,33)*. Although there is no thoroughly established tolerance dose for the head and neck of the femur, most radiation oncologists limit the dose to 45–50 Gy *(34)*. A recent review of the Surveillance, Epidemiology, and End Results (SEER) database showed that elderly women undergoing pelvic radiation therapy for anal, cervical, and rectal cancer were at significantly higher risk for pelvic (notably hip) fractures *(35)*. Although information regarding field sizes and radiation dose was not given, this study suggests a significant correlation between pelvic irradiation and subsequent hip fracture.

Experience with IMRT

Chen and colleagues published a dosimetric comparison of conventional radiation therapy and IMRT plans for treating anal cancer *(36)*. These authors evaluated the commonly used radiation portals of a narrow posterior–anterior field with wide anterior–posterior field, using superficial electron radiation therapy to the groins, allowing for adequate inguino-femoral nodal dosing. For the IMRT plan, the investigators stipulated dose constraints for the femoral head and neck. Compared to the conventional plans, mean and maximum doses to the femurs were significantly lower in the IMRT plan, without significant decrease in target volume dose coverage. However, data describing long-term clinical outcomes with respect to pelvic bony injury in patients treated with IMRT are lacking.

Small Bowel

Small bowel is frequently the dose-limiting structure in pelvic radiotherapy administration. Acute and late sequelae of small bowel treatment include diarrhea, malabsorption, bowel obstruction, and perforation *(37)*. The established radiation tolerance of small bowel is approximately 45–50 Gy. Additionally, factors including concomitant use of chemotherapy and prior pelvic surgery may lower this tolerance *(38–40)* Studies by Baglan et al and Tho et al have analyzed dose–volume parameters associated with acute small bowel toxicity in patients undergoing treatment with 5-FU-based chemoradiation therapy for rectal cancer. Both studies found strong correlations between acute toxicity and the amount of small bowel irradiated at each dose level analyzed *(41,42)*. Another analysis by Gunnlaugsson et al evaluating rectal cancer patients treated preoperatively with chemoradiotherapy showed a strong correlation between the occurrence of severe diarrhea and irradiated small bowel volume, surmising that limiting the volume of small bowel receiving greater than 15 Gy may significantly improve treatment tolerance *(43)*.

As described previously, neoadjuvant chemoradiation therapy followed by TME is currently used in the treatment of locally advanced rectal cancer, as established in the German Rectal Cancer trial *(7)*. In this large trial, 12% of patients receiving preoperative therapy experienced grade 3/4 acute GI toxicity (diarrhea), whereas 9% of patients developed grade 3/4 late GI toxicity. Presently, there is active investigation of combination novel chemotherapeutic and "targeted" agents with radiation therapy in the neoadjuvant therapy of rectal cancer. Data from phase I and phase II trials integrating novel agents such as oxaliplatin, irinotecan and EGFR inhibitors suggest that the addition of these agents may significantly increase grade 3/4 gastrointestinal toxicity rates relative to conventional neoadjuvant chemoradiotherapy regimens, further emphasizing the importance of careful radiation planning with respect to normal tissue sparing in these patients *(44–46)*.

Experience with IMRT

IMRT-based reduction in small bowel irradiation has been primarily studied in patients with prostate and gynecologic cancers receiving whole pelvic radiotherapy. Investigators from Memorial Sloan-Kettering found dosimetric superiority of IMRT to conventional 3D planning for small bowel sparing in the treatment of prostate cancer, particularly in the high-dose (>45 Gy) range *(47)*. Clinically, acute GI toxicities were reduced in the group treated with IMRT-based therapy vs. non-IMRT 3D planning. Comparing patients with gynecologic malignancies who underwent pelvic radiotherapy using conventional radiation planning and more recently IMRT-based treatment, University of Chicago investigators found significantly lower chronic GI toxicity in the latter group, with 11% of women treated with IMRT experiencing grade 1–3 toxicity (0% grade 3) vs. 50% in the non-IMRT group *(48)*.

Guerrero Urbano and colleagues studied the impact of IMRT on bowel dosimetry in five patients with rectal cancer *(49)*. The volume of small bowel in the high-dose range (45–50 Gy) was reduced with the use of IMRT without compromise in coverage of the target volume. Comparing IMRT with conventional 3D planning in patients with rectal cancer, Duthoy et al found significant reduction in the mean small bowel dose (17.0 vs. 12.4 Gy) *(50)*. The volume of small bowel receiving radiation doses in the high-dose range (>90% of the prescribed dose) was also reduced in the IMRT group. Other investigators have also reported on the ability of IMRT (and inverse planning) to spare small bowel *(42,51)*. Kim et al found even further reduction of small bowel irradiation using IMRT in conjunction with a "belly board" (false-tabletop), facilitating displacement of bowel out of the radiation field *(52)*. In a large series, Salama and colleagues described 53 patients with anal carcinoma treated with IMRT-based chemoradiotherapy. Median radiation dose to the pelvis and primary disease was 45 and 52 Gy, respectively. Fifteen percent of patients experienced acute grade 3 gastrointestinal toxicity with no grade 4 toxicity observed, comparing favorably to observed rates of severe gastrointestinal toxicity in contemporary randomized trials using conventional radiation planning *(53)*. This is especially notable given the significantly higher pelvic doses delivered in patients receiving IMRT in this series. This data suggests that intentional small bowel sparing significantly decreases acute gastrointestinal toxicity despite higher doses delivered.

Skin and External Genitalia

One of the main advantages of megavoltage photon radiotherapy is its skin-sparing properties. However, dermatologic toxicity may be a significant dose-limiting side effect during chemoradiotherapy for rectal cancer patients, secondary to skin folds and fluctuating skin contours in the inguinal, gluteal, and perineal region. For example, in an EORTC randomized trial, 29% of patients with anal cancer experienced ≥grade 3 acute skin toxicity in the group treated with radiation, 5-FU, and mitomycin-C *(54)*. Similar high rates of dermatologic toxicity have been observed in other large series *(55–57)*.

Experience with IMRT

Milano et al demonstrated the ability of IMRT to spare the perineum and external genitalia in patients with anal cancer.*(58)* In their study, these structures were limited to a dose of 50 Gy or less, with no more than 50–60% of their volumes receiving >40 Gy. The mean dose to these organs was significantly lower compared to conventional anterior–posterior/posterior–anterior planning. Clinically, no patients experienced >grade 2 dermatologic toxicity, or required treatment break secondary to skin toxicity. In a study by Chen et al, mean external genitalia doses were lower in the IMRT group as compared to the conventional groups *(36)*. In the previously described multi-institutional experience of 53 anal cancer patients treated with IMRT-based chemoradiotherapy, grade 3 skin toxicity was seen in 38% of patients with no grade 4 toxicity observed. This compares favorably to higher grade 3+ dermatologic toxicity rates seen in similar patients treated with non-IMRT techniques *(53,59,60)*. It should also be remembered that these toxicities may necessitate a treatment break during the treatment course, potentially decreasing treatment efficacy.

Bladder

In contrast to other pelvic organs, the bladder is more "radiotolerant," particularly when small volumes are treated. Patients with cervical cancer routinely receive doses ≥70 Gy to small volumes of the bladder (through combination of external beam radiation and brachytherapy), as do patients with prostate cancer. Tolerance dose for whole bladder irradiation is approximately 65 Gy *(61)*.

As a result of this tolerance, late high-grade bladder toxicity is relatively uncommon. As reported in German Rectal Cancer trial, only 2% of patients undergoing preoperative radiation therapy and chemotherapy experienced grade 3–4 bladder toxicity *(7)*.

Experience with IMRT

IMRT treatment of prostate cancer has led to improvements in bladder dosimetry, with lower bladder volumes irradiated to high doses (65–75 Gy) vs. conventional planning *(62)*. In the largest series of patients with prostate cancer treated to high doses (>80 Gy) with IMRT, Zelefsky et al reported that <1% of patients experienced grade 3 acute or late genitourinary toxicity *(63)*. Radiation doses employed in rectal cancer treatment are lower than those used in prostate treatment. Therefore, the incidence of chronic bladder toxicity would be expected to be less in rectal patients compared to patients receiving high-dose therapy in prostate cancer. Given this, the magnitude of benefit of IMRT with regard to chronic genitourinary toxicity may be modest. However, rates of acute toxicity (frequency, urgency, dysuria, etc.) may be significantly reduced. Results from previously described multi-institutional study of Salama and colleagues evaluating 53 anal cancer patients treated with IMRT-based chemoradiotherapy showed a grade 3+ genitourinary urinary toxicity rate of 0%, with only 11% experiencing grade 2 toxicity *(53)*. If dose escalation is pursued in the treatment of rectal cancer, the benefit of IMRT-based radiation therapy for bladder sparing may become more apparent.

Bone Marrow

Approximately 40% of the body's active bone marrow is located in the pelvis, and acute and chronic hematologic toxicity is a well-described phenomenon in large-field pelvic radiotherapy *(64)*. The plasma half-lives of erythrocytes, leucocytes, and platelets are short, and combined chemotherapy and radiotherapy place the bone marrow at high risk for suppression with resultant anemia, infection, and hemorrhage *(65,66)*. Such toxicity may also mandate treatment delays, reducing treatment efficacy.

In contrast to anal cancer, hematologic toxicity has been less prominent in the treatment of rectal cancer, likely because the chemotherapy agents employed are less myelosuppressive, are often delivered in a continuous (vs. bolus) fashion, and irradiated bony volumes are less. The German Rectal Cancer Trial exemplifies this, where grade 3+ hematologic toxicity was observed in only 6% of patients *(7)*.

Experience with IMRT

There is a growing experience evaluating bone marrow as an avoidance structure in IMRT planning. In an analysis of patients with gynecologic malignancies treated with whole pelvic radiotherapy and cisplatin, Mell et al found the volume of marrow receiving low-dose irradiation (≥10 Gy, the V(10) value) correlated with increased risk of leucopenia and neutropenia *(67)*. This finding is consistent with the known radiosensitivity of the hematopoietic stem cells.

Clinical reports assessing the ability of IMRT to spare pelvic marrow in patients with receiving radiation therapy are few. Brixey et al found patients who underwent pelvic radiation therapy and cisplatin had lower rates of acute hematologic toxicity when IMRT was employed (even when bone marrow was not specified as an avoidance structure) *(68)*. Conversely, Milano et al were unable to significantly limit marrow dose in the treatment of 17 patients with anal cancer, and grade 4 hematologic toxicity rates remained high (38%). Of note, patients in this series received 45 Gy to subclinical nodal basins, potentially making marrow sparing more difficult *(58)*. In the series of anal cancer patients from Salama and colleagues, the rate of grade 3–4 acute hematologic toxicity was 59%, which is comparable to the 60% rate seen with 5-FU/mitomycin in randomized trials *(53)*. A recent analysis of 48 anal cancer patients treated with IMRT-based chemoradiotherapy showed that 56, 50, 8, and 27% of patients experienced acute grade 3/4 leucopenia, neutropenia, anemia, and thrombocytopenia, respectively. In this study, the volume of pelvic bone marrow receiving 5, 10, 15, and 20 Gy was significantly associated with increasing leucopenia and neutrophil nadirs. The authors concluded that increasing doses of low-dose radiation to pelvic bone marrow is associated with increasing acute hematologic toxicity and that the volume of treated pelvic and lumbosacral bone marrow is associated with acute leucopenia and neutropenia *(69)*.

Further clinical studies are underway evaluating the role of IMRT in sparing of bone marrow. Establishing dose–response relationships for radiation-induced marrow suppression in combination with various chemotherapy agents will remain an important aspect of these studies.

Disease-Related Outcomes and Future

Because the use of IMRT in the treatment of rectal malignancies was only recently introduced, data evaluating long-term clinical outcomes are lacking. A small prospective phase II trial recently reported the results of preoperative capecitabine and accelerated synchronous integrated boost (SIB) IMRT in eight patients with locally advanced rectal cancer. Patients with clinical stage II or III adenocarcinoma of the rectum received capecitabine (825 mg/m^2 PO BID, 5 days/week × 5 weeks) and SIB-IMRT delivering 55 Gy (2.2 Gy/fraction) to the gross tumor while simultaneously delivering 45 Gy (1.8 Gy/fraction) to the regional lymph nodes and areas at risk for harboring microscopic disease. TME followed 6 weeks later. A single pathologist analyzed the resected tumor's TNM stage and Mandard regression/response scores. The primary end point was pathologic complete response (pCR) rate. Ten subjects were enrolled, two of which were ineligible (one screening failure and one unrelated cerebrovascular accident occurring early in treatment). The remaining eight patients were evaluable. All eight completed chemoradiation with strict compliance to the protocol schedule and then went on to surgical resection. At a median follow-up of 26 months (range, 15–40), all patients were alive without evidence of recurrent disease. The crude pCR rate was 38% with 50% achieving downstaging. Of three patients who had tumors within 5 cm of the anal verge, two underwent sphincter-sparing procedures. Grade 4 diarrhea occurred in 1 of 8 (13%) patients. The remaining toxicities were grade 1 or 2. Preoperative chemoradiation with capecitabine and SIB-IMRT appeared to be well tolerated and resulted in an encouraging pCR rate for patients with locally advanced rectal cancer in this series *(70)*. Currently, the Radiation Therapy Oncology Group (RTOG 0822) is enrolling patients onto a phase II study combining capecitabine, oxaliplatin with IMRT-based radiotherapy in rectal cancer patients. Primary trial endpoints are to determine if the combined rates of grade 2+ gastrointestinal toxicity can be significantly reduced relative to contemporaneously, "conventionally" treated patients. Other endpoints include analysis of rates of other grade 2–3 toxicities, determination of the feasibility of this approach in a cooperative group setting, pathological response rates, rates of abdominoperineal resection as well as determination of preliminary disease-related outcomes in these patients.

PARTICLE RADIOTHERAPY

Traditional radiotherapy utilizes photons to deliver dose to target tissues. Photons deposit their maximal energy in tissues at relatively superficial depths, with gradual "fall-off" with increasing depth in tissue. However, charged particles such as protons and heavier ions (such

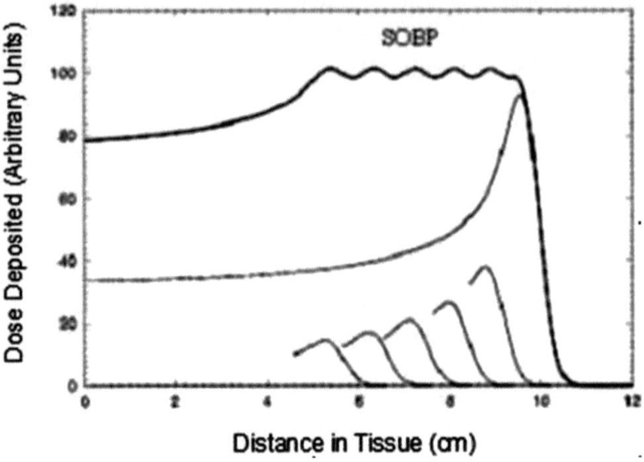

Fig. 3. Proton depth–dose curve. Protons of a given energy have a discrete range in tissue, with maximum dose occurring over a narrow range called the Bragg peak. In order to treat large tumors, beam degraders are used to yield protons of varying energies, and thus ranges, that sum together during a treatment to yield a spread-out Bragg peak (SOBP) (Figure courtesy of Judith Adams, Francis H. Burr Proton Therapy Center, Massachusetts, MA).

as helium, carbon, silicon, and neon) deposit low doses of energy initially followed by a sharp rise in energy transfer (and dose), known as the Bragg peak, toward the end of their course. Protons of a given energy have a discrete range in tissue; soon after the proton Bragg peak there is no further delivered dose in "downstream" tissues (i.e., no exit dose). Clinically, since the Bragg peak is over a narrow distance, protons of varying energies (and thus ranges) are summed together during a treatment to yield a "spread-out Bragg peak" (Fig. 3) *(71)*. As a result, proton beams can yield a lower integral dose to patients as compared to photons. In rectal cancer, there is thus the potential to deliver less dose to nontarget organs such as non-target large and small bowel, femoral heads and bladder. This may allow for tumor dose escalation without significant increases in complication rates and may reduce toxicity-related treatment breaks. The use of chemotherapy or targeted agents concurrent with radiation therapy may also be better tolerated relative to photon therapy. The risk of late effects (e.g., bowel stricture, liver or kidney damage, etc.) can also be minimized. Reduced integral doses may also lower the risk for radiation-induced malignancies *(72)*. As in photon therapy, intensity modulation methods can also be applied to charged particle radiotherapy *(73)*. The relative biological effectiveness of protons is quite similar to photons, with a generic value for tumor eradication of about 1.1 *(74)*. Therefore, proton dose is sometimes expressed as Gray equivalent (GyE) (with 1 Gy from protons equal to 1.1 GyE).

Use of proton and ion beam radiotherapy for more common malignancies has been less frequently reported (with the notable exception of prostate and lung tumors), in part because there are few oncology centers with the technology required to perform this type of treatment *(75,76)*. Particle accelerators (cyclotrons) are expensive to purchase and maintain. However, this will likely change in the upcoming years with the advent of new and less costly technology for production of particle beams, *(77,78)* providing opportunities for well-designed clinical studies to define the true role of proton and ion beam radiotherapy in the treatment of rectal cancer.

There is evidence that dose escalation is beneficial in patients with rectal cancer, yielding higher response rates (see prior dose escalation discussion). Preclinical studies have shown that, for a fixed normal tissue complication probability, protons can allow for higher doses delivered to the tumor in comparison to standard photon therapy in the adjuvant, locally recurrent, and locally advanced settings of rectal cancer *(79–81)*. In the latter situations, dose escalation may allow for downstaging, facilitating potentially curative resection. However, presently, there is limited clinical data regarding the efficacy of proton irradiation in rectal cancer. Investigators from the Harvard cyclotron reported on a series of 17 patients with rectal and anal cancer, some of whom were treated to high doses (>70 Gy) of radiation therapy *(82)*. Long-term follow-up results describing disease control and treatment-related toxicities have not, to our knowledge, been published.

As with photon therapy, one potential advantage of proton use in the treatment of rectal cancer is the opportunity to safely escalate the radiation dose concurrent with novel radiosensitizing agents. In rectal cancer, pathologic complete responses to standard doses (about 50 Gy) with photons and chemotherapy are a relatively uncommon but certainly recognized event. The introduction of newer systemic and targeted radiosensitizing agents could result in higher pathologic response rates. With elevated radiation doses and new, potentially more potent radiosensitizers, there is the possibility that selected patients may be able to undergo definitive therapy with chemoradiation alone.

In summary, it appears likely that there will be a significant increase in the number of oncology facilities offering charged particle radiotherapy in upcoming years. As detailed above, this interest lies in the unique characteristics of energy deposition in tissue seen with protons and heavier ions. The underlying goal is to yield improvements in the ratio of tumor control to normal tissue toxicity. Truly widespread adoption of proton and ion beam technology will be indicated if this improvement is convincingly demonstrated.

CONCLUSION

Radiation therapy remains an integral component in the multidisciplinary management of patients with rectal cancer. Normal tissue toxicity remains a significant obstacle in the radiotherapeutic management of rectal cancer, resulting in patient morbidity and impeding tumor control by limiting the timely delivery and intensity of radiation dose. Avoiding normal tissues while delivering therapeutic target doses are fundamental goals of the radiation oncologist. IMRT is an advanced radiation technique allowing improved dose conformation to target structures while limiting radiation dose to surrounding normal tissues and represents a potentially significant advance in achieving these goals. The application of this technology in the treatment of rectal cancer is attractive given the significant toxicities encountered with traditional chemoradiotherapy approaches. Potential advantages of IMRT include reduced normal organ irradiation and target radiation dose escalation. This would theoretically result in improvement in ultimate tumor control, cancer-related outcomes and rates of acute and chronic treatment-related toxicity rates. IMRT requires careful target delineation using available clinical, endoscopic, and radiographic data, as well as knowledge of surrounding normal tissue tolerances. IMRT-based radiation therapy will likely be increasingly utilized in the treatment of rectal malignancies.

There are potential limitations to these therapies. In IMRT planning, increasing the number of avoidance structures and thus constraints can lead to difficulty in delivery of a homogenous dose to the target volume. With the close proximity of normal pelvic tissues, it may be necessary to prioritize sparing of one or two structures and relax constraints for others so as to allow adequate target coverage. IMRT also requires a high capital cost commitment.

Collectively, early clinical results in anorectal cancer using IMRT-based chemoradiotherapy have shown significant decreases in treatment-related toxicities with disease-related outcomes similar to conventional radiotherapy approaches. The role of IMRT in rectal cancer patients is presently being evaluated in the cooperative group setting. Future strategies in the treatment of rectal malignancies would include combining IMRT-based radiation therapy with novel chemotherapeutic and "targeted" systemic therapies. These techniques will require further demonstration of meaningful clinical benefit in patient outcomes to further solidify their routine use in clinical practice.

Proton and heavy ion therapy offer potential advantages over photon therapy in terms of further reducing dose to normal tissues, potentially facilitating reductions in treatment-related toxicities/improving tolerance, as well as allowing dose escalation in the context of novel radiosensitizers. The role of protons and heavy ions in rectal cancer therapy will likely become increasingly clear as their use increases.

Acknowledgments: The authors acknowledge Leigh O'Neill and Kim Light for generating the 3D plans, as well as Sua Yoo for her assistance in generating the IMRT plans.

REFERENCES

1. Randomised trial of surgery alone versus radiotherapy followed by surgery for potentially operable locally advanced rectal cancer. Medical Research Council Rectal Cancer Working Party. *Lancet.* 1996;348:1605–1610.
2. Fisher B, Wolmark N, Rockette H, et al. Postoperative adjuvant chemotherapy or radiation therapy for rectal cancer: results from NSABP protocol R-01. *J Natl Cancer Inst.* 1988;80:21–29.
3. Prolongation of the disease-free interval in surgically treated rectal carcinoma. Gastrointestinal Tumor Study Group. *N Engl J Med.* 1985;312:1465–1472.
4. Krook JE, Moertel CG, Gunderson LL, et al. Effective surgical adjuvant therapy for high-risk rectal carcinoma. *N Engl J Med.* 1991;324:709–715.
5. Kapiteijn E, Marijnen CA, Nagtegaal ID, et al. Preoperative radiotherapy combined with total mesorectal excision for resectable rectal cancer. *N Engl J Med.* 2001;345:638–646.
6. Frykholm GJ, Glimelius B, Pahlman L. Preoperative or postoperative irradiation in adenocarcinoma of the rectum: final treatment results of a randomized trial and an evaluation of late secondary effects. *Dis Colon Rectum.* 1993;36:564–572.
7. Sauer R, Becker H, Hohenberger W, et al. Preoperative versus postoperative chemoradiotherapy for rectal cancer. *N Engl J Med.* 2004;351:1731–1740.
8. Bortfeld T, Boyer AL, Schlegel W, et al. Realization and verification of three-dimensional conformal radiotherapy with modulated fields. *Int J Radiat Oncol Biol Phys.* 1994;30:899–908.
9. Burman C, Chui CS, Kutcher G, et al. Planning, delivery, and quality assurance of intensity-modulated radiotherapy using dynamic multileaf collimator: a strategy for large-scale implementation for the treatment of carcinoma of the prostate. *Int J Radiat Oncol Biol Phys.* 1997;39:863–873.
10. Stein J, Bortfeld T, Dorschel B, et al. Dynamic X-ray compensation for conformal radiotherapy by means of multi-leaf collimation. *Radiother Oncol.* 1994;32:163–173.
11. Trautmann TG, Zuger JH. Positron Emission Tomography for pretreatment staging and posttreatment evaluation in cancer of the anal canal. *Mol Imaging Biol.* 2005;7:309–313.
12. Cotter SE, Grigsby PW, Siegel BA, et al. FDG-PET/CT in the evaluation of anal carcinoma. *Int J Radiat Oncol Biol Phys.* 2006;65:720–725.
13. Anderson C, Koshy M, Staley C, et al. PET-CT fusion in radiation management of patients with anorectal tumors. *Int J Radiat Oncol Biol Phys.* 2007;69:155–162.
14. Letourneau D, Martinez AA, Lockman D, et al. Assessment of residual error for online cone-beam CT-guided treatment of prostate cancer patients. *Int J Radiat Oncol Biol Phys.* 2005;62:1239–1246.
15. Godfrey DJ, Yin FF, Oldham M, et al. Digital tomosynthesis with an on-board kilovoltage imaging device. *Int J Radiat Oncol Biol Phys.* 2006;65:8–15.

16. Gao S, Zhang L, Wang H, et al. A deformable image registration method to handle distended rectums in prostate cancer radiotherapy. *Med Phys*. 2006;33:3304–3312.
17. de Crevoisier R, Melancon AD, Kuban DA, et al. Changes in the pelvic anatomy after an IMRT treatment fraction of prostate cancer. *Int J Radiat Oncol Biol Phys*. 2007;68:1529–1536.
18. Nuyttens JJ, Robertson JM, Yan D, et al. The variability of the clinical target volume for rectal cancer due to internal organ motion during adjuvant treatment. *Int J Radiat Oncol Biol Phys*. 2002;53:497–503.
19. Kupelian PA, Langen KM, Zeidan OA, et al. Daily variations in delivered doses in patients treated with radiotherapy for localized prostate cancer. *Int J Radiat Oncol Biol Phys*. 2006;66:876–882.
20. Yin FF, Das S, Kirkpatrick J, et al. Physics and imaging for targeting of oligometastases. *Semin Radiat Oncol*. 2006;16:85–101.
21. Yan D, Lockman D, Martinez A, et al. Computed tomography guided management of interfractional patient variation. *Semin Radiat Oncol*. 2005;15:168–179.
22. Hartley A, Ho KF, McConkey C, et al. Pathological complete response following pre-operative chemoradiotherapy in rectal cancer: analysis of phase II/III trials. *Br J Radiol*. 2005;78:934–938.
23. Valentini V, Coco C, Picciocchi A, et al. Does downstaging predict improved outcome after preoperative chemoradiation for extraperitoneal locally advanced rectal cancer? A long-term analysis of 165 patients. *Int J Radiat Oncol Biol Phys*. 2002;53:664–674.
24. Kaminsky-Forrett MC, Conroy T, Luporsi E, et al. Prognostic implications of downstaging following preoperative radiation therapy for operable T3-T4 rectal cancer. *Int J Radiat Oncol Biol Phys*. 1998;42:935–941.
25. Berger C, de Muret A, Garaud P, et al. Preoperative radiotherapy (RT) for rectal cancer: predictive factors of tumor downstaging and residual tumor cell density (RTCD): prognostic implications. *Int J Radiat Oncol Biol Phys*. 1997;37:619–627.
26. Theodoropoulos G, Wise WE, Padmanabhan A, et al. T-level downstaging and complete pathologic response after preoperative chemoradiation for advanced rectal cancer result in decreased recurrence and improved disease-free survival. *Dis Colon Rectum*. 2002;45:895–903.
27. Habr-Gama A, Perez RO, Proscurshim I, et al. Patterns of failure and survival for nonoperative treatment of stage c0 distal rectal cancer following neoadjuvant chemoradiation therapy. *J Gastrointest Surg*. 2006;10:1319–1328. discussion 1328–1329.
28. Wiltshire KL, Ward IG, Swallow C, et al. Preoperative radiation with concurrent chemotherapy for resectable rectal cancer: effect of dose escalation on pathologic complete response, local recurrence-free survival, disease-free survival, and overall survival. *Int J Radiat Oncol Biol Phys*. 2006;64:709–716.
29. Mohiuddin M, Regine WF, John WJ, et al. Preoperative chemoradiation in fixed distal rectal cancer: dose time factors for pathological complete response. *Int J Radiat Oncol Biol Phys*. 2000;46: 883–888.
30. Overgaard M, Overgaard J, Sell A. Dose-response relationship for radiation therapy of recurrent, residual, and primarily inoperable colorectal cancer. *Radiother Oncol*. 1984;1:217–225.
31. Papillon J, Montbarbon JF, Gerard JP, et al. Interstitial curietherapy in the conservative treatment of anal and rectal cancers. *Int J Radiat Oncol Biol Phys*. 1989;17:1161–1169.
32. Miller CW. Survival and ambulation following hip fracture. *J Bone Joint Surg Am*. 1978;60:930–934.
33. Cummings SR, Melton LJ. Epidemiology and outcomes of osteoporotic fractures. *Lancet*. 2002;359:1761–1767.
34. Martenson JA Jr, Gunderson LL. External radiation therapy without chemotherapy in the management of anal cancer. *Cancer*. 1993;71:1736–1740.
35. Baxter NN, Habermann EB, Tepper JE, et al. Risk of pelvic fractures in older women following pelvic irradiation. *JAMA*. 2005;294:2587–2593.
36. Chen YJ, Liu A, Tsai PT, et al. Organ sparing by conformal avoidance intensity-modulated radiation therapy for anal cancer: dosimetric evaluation of coverage of pelvis and inguinal/femoral nodes. *Int J Radiat Oncol Biol Phys*. 2005;63:274–281.
37. Nguyen NP, Antoine JE, Dutta S, et al. Current concepts in radiation enteritis and implications for future clinical trials. *Cancer*. 2002;95:1151–1163.
38. Eifel PJ, Levenback C, Wharton JT, et al. Time course and incidence of late complications in patients treated with radiation therapy for FIGO stage IB carcinoma of the uterine cervix. *Int J Radiat Oncol Biol Phys*. 1995;32:1289–1300.

39. Potish RA, Jones TK Jr, Levitt SH. Factors predisposing to radiation-related small-bowel damage. *Radiology*. 1979;132:479–482.
40. Rotman M, Moon S, John M, et al. Extended field para-aortic radiation in cervical carcinoma: the case for prophylactic treatment. *Int J Radiat Oncol Biol Phys*. 1978;4:795–799.
41. Baglan KL, Frazier RC, Yan D, et al. The dose-volume relationship of acute small bowel toxicity from concurrent 5-FU-based chemotherapy and radiation therapy for rectal cancer. *Int J Radiat Oncol Biol Phys*. 2002;52:176–183.
42. Tho LM, Glegg M, Paterson J, et al. Acute small bowel toxicity and preoperative chemoradiotherapy for rectal cancer: investigating dose-volume relationships and role for inverse planning. *Int J Radiat Oncol Biol Phys*. 2006;66:505–513.
43. Gunnlaugsson A, Kjellen E, Nilsson P, et al. Dose-volume relationships between enteritis and irradiated bowel volumes during 5-fluorouracil and oxaliplatin based chemoradiotherapy in locally advanced rectal cancer. *Acta Oncol*. 2007;46:937–944.
44. Ryan DP, Niedzwiecki D, Hollis D, et al. Phase I/II study of preoperative oxaliplatin, fluorouracil, and external-beam radiation therapy in patients with locally advanced rectal cancer: Cancer and Leukemia Group B 89901. *J Clin Oncol*. 2006;24:2557–2562.
45. Mohiuddin M, Winter K, Mitchell E, et al. Randomized phase II study of neoadjuvant combined-modality chemoradiation for distal rectal cancer: Radiation Therapy Oncology Group Trial 0012. *J Clin Oncol*. 2006;24:650–655.
46. Czito BG, Willett CG, Bendell JC, et al. Increased toxicity with gefitinib, capecitabine, and radiation therapy in pancreatic and rectal cancer: phase I trial results. *J Clin Oncol*. 2006;24:656–662.
47. Ashman JB, Zelefsky MJ, Hunt MS, et al. Whole pelvic radiotherapy for prostate cancer using 3D conformal and intensity-modulated radiotherapy. *Int J Radiat Oncol Biol Phys*. 2005;63:765–771.
48. Mundt AJ, Mell LK, Roeske JC. Preliminary analysis of chronic gastrointestinal toxicity in gynecology patients treated with intensity-modulated whole pelvic radiation therapy. *Int J Radiat Oncol Biol Phys*. 2003;56:1354–1360.
49. Guerrero Urbano MT, Henrys AJ, Adams EJ, et al. Intensity-modulated radiotherapy in patients with locally advanced rectal cancer reduces volume of bowel treated to high dose levels. *Int J Radiat Oncol Biol Phys*. 2006;65:907–916.
50. Duthoy W, De Gersem W, Vergote K, et al. Clinical implementation of intensity-modulated arc therapy (IMAT) for rectal cancer. *Int J Radiat Oncol Biol Phys*. 2004;60:794–806.
51. Nuyttens JJ, Robertson JM, Yan D, et al. The influence of small bowel motion on both a conventional three-field and intensity modulated radiation therapy (IMRT) for rectal cancer. *Cancer Radiother*. 2004;8:297–304.
52. Kim JY, Kim DY, Kim TH, et al. Intensity-modulated radiotherapy with a belly board for rectal cancer. *Int J Colorectal Dis*. 2007;22:373–379.
53. Salama JK, Mell LK, Schomas DA, et al. Concurrent chemotherapy and intensity-modulated radiation therapy for anal canal cancer patients: a multicenter experience. *J Clin Oncol*. 2007;25:4581–4586.
54. Bartelink H, Roelofsen F, Eschwege F, et al. Concomitant radiotherapy and chemotherapy is superior to radiotherapy alone in the treatment of locally advanced anal cancer: results of a phase III randomized trial of the European Organization for Research and Treatment of Cancer Radiotherapy and Gastrointestinal Cooperative Groups. *J Clin Oncol*. 1997;15:2040–2049.
55. Flam M, John M, Pajak TF, et al. Role of mitomycin in combination with fluorouracil and radiotherapy, and of salvage chemoradiation in the definitive nonsurgical treatment of epidermoid carcinoma of the anal canal: results of a phase III randomized intergroup study. *J Clin Oncol*. 1996;14:2527–2539.
56. Epidermoid anal cancer: results from the UKCCCR randomised trial of radiotherapy alone versus radiotherapy, 5-fluorouracil, and mitomycin. *Lancet*. 1996;14:2527–2539.
57. Ajani J, Winter K, Gunderson L, et al. Intergroup RTOG 98–11: A phase III randomized study of 5-fluorouracil (5-FU), mitomycin, and radiotherapy versus 5-fluorouracil, cisplatin, and radiotherapy in carcinoma of the anal canal. *Proc Am Soc Clin Oncol*. 2006;24:18S.
58. Milano MT, Jani AB, Farrey KJ, et al. Intensity-modulated radiation therapy (IMRT) in the treatment of anal cancer: toxicity and clinical outcome. *Int J Radiat Oncol Biol Phys*. 2005;63:354–361.
59. John M, Pajak T, Flam M, et al. Dose escalation in chemoradiation for anal cancer: preliminary results of RTOG 92–08. *Cancer J Sci Am*. 1996;2:205–211.

60. Gunderson L, Winter K, Ajani J, et al. In intergroup RTOG 98–11 phase III comparison of chemoradiation with 5-FU and Mitomycin versus 5-FU and cisplatin for anal canal carcinoma: impact on disease-free survival, overall and colostomy-free survival. *Annual meeting of the American Society of Therapeutic Radiology and Oncology*. Philadelphia, PA; 2006.
61. Emami B, Lyman J, Brown A, et al. Tolerance of normal tissue to therapeutic irradiation. *Int J Radiat Oncol Biol Phys*. 1991;21:109–122.
62. Luxton G, Hancock SL, Boyer AL. Dosimetry and radiobiologic model comparison of IMRT and 3D conformal radiotherapy in treatment of carcinoma of the prostate. *Int J Radiat Oncol Biol Phys*. 2004;59:267–284.
63. Zelefsky MJ, Fuks Z, Hunt M, et al. High-dose intensity modulated radiation therapy for prostate cancer: early toxicity and biochemical outcome in 772 patients. *Int J Radiat Oncol Biol Phys*. 2002;53:1111–1116.
64. Ellis RE. The distribution of active bone marrow in the adult. *Phys Med Biol*. 1961;5:255–258.
65. Sacks EL, Goris ML, Glatstein E, et al. Bone marrow regeneration following large field radiation: influence of volume, age, dose, and time. *Cancer*. 1978;42:1057–1065.
66. Mauch P, Constine L, Greenberger J, et al. Hematopoietic stem cell compartment: acute and late effects of radiation therapy and chemotherapy. *Int J Radiat Oncol Biol Phys*. 1995;31:1319–1339.
67. Mell LK, Kochanski JD, Roeske JC, et al. Dosimetric predictors of acute hematologic toxicity in cervical cancer patients treated with concurrent cisplatin and intensity-modulated pelvic radiotherapy. *Int J Radiat Oncol Biol Phys*. 2006;66:1356–1365.
68. Brixey CJ, Roeske JC, Lujan AE, et al. Impact of intensity-modulated radiotherapy on acute hematologic toxicity in women with gynecologic malignancies. *Int J Radiat Oncol Biol Phys*. 2002;54: 1388–1396.
69. Mell LK, Schomas DA, Salama JK, et al. Associated between bone marrow dosimetric parameters and acute hematologic toxicity in anal cancer patients treated with concurrent chemotherapy and intensity-modulated radiotherapy. *Int J Radiat Oncol Biol Phys*. 2008;70:1431–1437.
70. Ballonoff A, Kavanagh B, McCarter M, et al. Preoperative capecitabine and accelerated intensity-modulated radiotherapy in locally advanced rectal cancer: a phase II trial. *Am J Clin Oncol*. 2008;31:264–270.
71. Khan F. *The physics of radiation therapy*. 3rd ed. Philadelphia: Lippincott Williams & Wilkins; 2003:75–77.
72. Hall EJ. Intensity-modulated radiation therapy, protons, and the risk of second cancers. *Int J Radiat Oncol Biol Phys*. 2006;65:1–7.
73. Lomax AJ, Boehringer T, Coray A, et al. Intensity modulated proton therapy: a clinical example. *Med Phys*. 2001;28:317–324.
74. Paganetti H, Niemierko A, Ancukiewicz M, et al. Relative biological effectiveness (RBE) values for proton beam therapy. *Int J Radiat Oncol Biol Phys*. 2002;53:407–421.
75. Slater JD, Rossi CJ Jr, Yonemoto LT, et al. Proton therapy for prostate cancer: the initial Loma Linda University experience. *Int J Radiat Oncol Biol Phys*. 2004;59:348–352.
76. Bush DA, Slater JD, Shin BB, et al. Hypofractionated proton beam radiotherapy for stage I lung cancer. *Chest*. 2004;126:1198–1203.
77. Fourkal E, Shahine B, Ding M, et al. Particle in cell simulation of laser-accelerated proton beams for radiation therapy. *Med Phys*. 2002;29:2788–2798.
78. Hede K. Research groups promoting proton therapy "lite". *J Natl Cancer Inst*. 2006;98:1682–1684.
79. Tatsuzaki H, Urie MM, Willett CG. 3-D comparative study of proton vs. x-ray radiation therapy for rectal cancer. *Int J Radiat Oncol Biol Phys*. 1992;22:369–374.
80. Isacsson U, Montelius A, Jung B, et al. Comparative treatment planning between proton and X-ray therapy in locally advanced rectal cancer. *Radiother Oncol*. 1996;41:263–272.
81. Santoni R, Scoccianti S, Galardi A, et al. Comparison of different external beam treatment techniques to deliver high-dose irradiation to local recurrent rectal carcinoma. *Tumori*. 2004;90:310–316.
82. Munzenrider JE, Austin-Seymour M, Blitzer PJ, et al. Proton therapy at Harvard. *Strahlentherapie*. 1985;161:756–763.

[illegible] New York, 2007.

[illegible] (Ann Arbor) 2008;[illegible]

[illegible]

[illegible]

[illegible] Stereotact Funct Neurosurg [illegible]

Index

MIX
Papier aus verantwortungsvollen Quellen
Paper from responsible sources
FSC® C105338
FSC
www.fsc.org

If you have any concerns about our products,
you can contact us on
ProductSafety@springernature.com

In case Publisher is established outside the EU,
the EU authorized representative is:
Springer Nature Customer Service Center GmbH
Europaplatz 3, 69115 Heidelberg, Germany

Printed by Libri Plureos GmbH
in Hamburg, Germany